Machine Learning Techniques for Medical Imaging

Machine Learning Techniques for Medical Imaging

Edited by Hubert Henson

hayle medical

New York

Hayle Medical,
750 Third Avenue, 9th Floor,
New York, NY 10017, USA

Visit us on the World Wide Web at:
www.haylemedical.com

ISBN: 978-1-64647-533-9

Cataloging-in-Publication Data

Machine learning techniques for medical imaging / edited by Hubert Henson.
p. cm.
Includes bibliographical references and index.
ISBN 978-1-64647-533-9
1. Diagnostic imaging. 2. Imaging systems in medicine. 3. Radiography, Medical.
4. Diagnosis, Radioscopic. I. Henson, Hubert.
RC78.7.D53 H36 2023
616.075 4--dc23

Table of Contents

Preface

Medical imaging or radiology is the field of medical science that involves the recreation of images of human body parts for the purpose of diagnosing and treating different medical conditions. There are various types of medical imaging procedures such as X-ray, magnetic resonance imaging (MRI), ultrasound, etc. The area of study within artificial intelligence which focuses on providing the computers with the capability to learn without being explicitly programmed is known as machine learning. Some radiological applications of machine learning include identification, portrayal and observation of infections, image classification, object detection, image segmentation and registration, image generation, and image transformation. Machine learning and artificial intelligence tools are used extensively for identifying cardiovascular abnormalities, neurological diseases, and detecting fractures and other musculoskeletal injuries. This book outlines the applications of machine learning in the field of medical imaging. It will prove to be immensely beneficial to medical students and researchers involved in this field.

All of the data presented henceforth, was collaborated in the wake of recent advancements in the field. The aim of this book is to present the diversified developments from across the globe in a comprehensible manner. The opinions expressed in each chapter belong solely to the contributing authors. Their interpretations of the topics are the integral part of this book, which I have carefully compiled for a better understanding of the readers.

At the end, I would like to thank all those who dedicated their time and efforts for the successful completion of this book. I also wish to convey my gratitude towards my friends and family who supported me at every step.

Editor

1

Coronary Artery Disease Detection by Machine Learning with Coronary Bifurcation Features

Xueping Chen [1,†], Yi Fu [2,†], Jiangguo Lin [1,†], Yanru Ji [1], Ying Fang [1,*] and Jianhua Wu [1,*]

1 Institute of Biomechanics, School of Bioscience and Bioengineering, South China University of Technology, Guangzhou 510006, China; bichenxueping@mail.scut.edu.cn (X.C.); linjiangguo@gdph.org.cn (J.L.); 201530781142@mail.scut.edu.cn (Y.J.)

2 Collaborative Innovation Center for Biomedicines & School of Medical Instruments, Shanghai University of Medicine & Health Sciences, Shanghai 200237, China; fuy_18@sumhs.edu.cn

* Correspondence: yfang@scut.edu.cn (Y.F.); wujianhua@scut.edu.cn (J.W.)

† X. Chen, Y. Fu and J. Lin contributed equally to this work.

Abstract: *Background:* Early accurate detection of coronary artery disease (CAD) is one of the most important medical research areas. Researchers are motivated to utilize machine learning techniques for quick and accurate detection of CAD. *Methods:* To obtain the high quality of features used for machine learning, we here extracted the coronary bifurcation features from the coronary computed tomography angiography (CCTA) images by using the morphometric method. The machine learning classifier algorithms, such as logistic regression (LR), decision tree (DT), linear discriminant analysis (LDA), k-nearest neighbors (k-NN), artificial neural network (ANN), and support vector machine (SVM) were applied for estimating the performance by using the measured features. *Results:* The results showed that in comparison with other machine learning methods, the polynomial-SVM with the use of the grid search optimization method had the best performance for the detection of CAD and had yielded the classification accuracy of 100.00%. Among six examined coronary bifurcation features, the exponent of vessel diameter (n) and the area expansion ratio (AER) were two key features in the detection of CAD. *Conclusions:* This study could aid the clinicians to detect CAD accurately, which may probably provide an alternative method for the non-invasive diagnosis in clinical.

Keywords: coronary artery disease; coronary bifurcations; machine learning; morphological features; classification performance

1. Introduction

Coronary artery disease (CAD) is one of the leading causes of death in the world [1,2]. Early detection of CAD could save patients' lives and reduce the cost of healthcare, which is of great clinical significance. Many tools have been developed for CAD diagnosis [3–5], among which the cardiac catheterization is the most direct and reliable approach [3]. However, cardiac catheterization is costly and time-consuming, and it is also an invasive and risky surgical operation. Hence, few CAD patients prefer to choose cardiac catheterization as their diagnostic method. Therefore, finding a reliable and non-invasive method for early detection of CAD is very desirable. Although some non-invasive diagnostic approaches like coronary computed tomography angiography (coronary CTA, CCTA), echocardiography, and nuclear magnetic resonance imaging (MRI) could accurately detecting CAD, they lack the ability to detect CAD at early stage. On the other hand, these methods usually require assistance from medical experts. Thus, they have not been effectively used for the early detection of CAD. Our previous study found that the changes in the morphological features of coronary arterial trees were highly correlated to the degrees of CAD lesion (unpublished yet). Moreover, these morphological changes had probably occurred before the CAD lesion developed [6]. Machine learning methods are widely used for pattern recognition and binary classification problems which can be used to classify common diseases with positive or negative attributes [7]. Therefore, it is of great potential to build a machine learning classifier by using the coronary morphological features for the non-invasive detection of CAD at its early stages.

In recent decades, various machine learning algorithms were used for quick and non-invasive CAD detection, such as k-nearest neighbors (k-NN), decision tree (DT), artificial neural network (ANN) and support vector machine (SVM) [8–11]. The comparison of performances of CAD detection by current machine learning methods with the use of different algorithms and medical features is shown in Table A1 (see Appendix A). Machine learning comprised of various steps: collecting the original features data, preprocessing of the data, choosing a machine learning model, training the selected model and parameter tuning, evaluating the selected model, and finally making predictions. The features selection is the first step and plays a crucial role in machine learning, which can impact the detection accuracy of the machine learning classifier [12]. Studies suggested that many features were clinically associated with CAD and varied with the degrees of diseases, including physiological-based features such as blood pressure, blood glucose, blood lipids, age, obesity degree, and overweight [1], signal-based features such as electrocardiogram (ECG) and phonocardiogram (PCG) signals [13], computer imaging-based features such as "gray value" [14], and morphological features such as diameter stenosis [15]. Although all these features were potentially used in machine learning for the detection of CAD, the performance of the machine learning classifier depended on the quality of features used. Selecting the most important features could significantly improve the accuracy of the medical diagnosis. Previous studies had proposed numerous feature selection algorithms to analyze the most important features among CAD datasets. For example, Li et al. developed a signal feature selection method and obtained the accuracy, sensitivity, specificity, and G-mean of 95.62%, 98.48%, 89.17%, and 93.69%, respectively with the use of the dual-input neural network [13]. Wosiak et al. proposed an unsupervised features selection method from the medical datasets and obtained relatively good diagnosis results [16]. Nasarian et al. proposed a heterogeneous hybrid feature selection algorithm and had yielded the classification accuracy of 81.23% with SMOTE and XGBoost classifier [12]. However, the medical significance behind these selected features data is not well known. Previous studies suggested different features were associated with CAD in different correlation degrees [12]. In addition, morphological features were the most direct features for characterizing CAD in clinical [4]. In other words, the coronary arteries with CAD lesion has special morphological features that are different from the normal arteries. Therefore, morphological features of the coronary arterial trees may be of great potential to build a machine learning classifier for the detection of CAD.

The aim of this paper is to propose a new methodology (a combination of using machine learning algorithms and imaging-based morphological measurement methods) for the detection of CAD, which may help to detect CAD at the early stage in a non-invasive way and provide a tool to save more lives. To collect morphological features dataset, we reconstructed three-dimensional (3D) coronary arteries from CCTA images of CAD patients and healthy individuals and measured the morphological features from the reconstructed 3D coronary arterial trees. To evaluate the quality of the morphological features, machine learning algorithms such as logistic regression (LR), DT, linear discriminant analysis (LDA), k-NN, ANN, and support vector machines (SVMs) were then applied to build classifiers for the detection of CAD. The accuracy of these machine learning algorithms was used to evaluate the prediction capability of classification algorithms. Moreover, the algorithm with best performance was further used to find the most important features in detecting CAD. In addition, the effects of the kernel function selection, data sampling, training dataset amount, and the dimension of input features on the classification performances of the machine learning model were also studied. The main contributions of this work were: (1) combined utilization of machine learning and morphological measurement method for CAD detection, (2) achieved superior classification performance compared with existing studies, (3) found the most two important morphological features for CAD detection.

2. Materials and Methods

We here proposed a morphometric methodology to collect the morphological features dataset for the detection of CAD. Then, we evaluated these features by different commonly used machine learning algorithms to find the best-fitted classifier for the detection of CAD. Finally, we applied the best algorithm to evaluate all the morphological features to seek the most important features for the detection of CAD.

2.1. Morphometric Features Data Collection and Selection

With the development of hardware and software of angiographic techniques, the CCTA imaging has been successfully applied to the visualization of coronary arteries in recent decades [17,18]. We can obtain many features from the CCTA images, such as geometric features, size of calcified plaque, and diameter stenosis rate, etc. Selecting the most important features has a significant impact on the medical diagnostic process. It helps to get an accurate and quick diagnosis. In this study, we selected the morphometric features data for building the machine learning classifiers. These features were measured from the CCTA images of the Southern Chinese populations. In this study, we totally collected morphometric features datasets with 1163 variables (features data), among which 571 variables were from patients with CAD lesion (CAD subjects) and 592 variables were from individuals without CAD lesion (non-CAD subjects). This study was approved by the Ethics Committee of the College of Basic Medicine, Southern Medical University and the Ethics Committee of the Guangdong General Hospital, Guangdong Academy of Medical Sciences, and was performed per the Declaration of Helsinki.

The morphological features were obtained from the coronary bifurcations and the method of data collection was shown in Figure 1. Morphometric data of coronary arterial trees were extracted from CCTA images with MIMICS software (Materialize). In the MIMICS software, centerlines were formed by a series of center points that located at the center of the cross-sectional plane of the 3D coronary artery. Subsequently, the best fit diameter was calculated as twice of the average radius from the points of the centerlines to the contour of the 3D coronary artery. The original morphometric data of mother vessel diameters (D_m), larger daughter vessel diameters (D_l), smaller daughter vessel diameters (D_s), and bifurcation angles (α), were determined at all bifurcations of arterial trees. Table 1 showed the definitions of six morphological features (α, n, $\frac{D_s^3}{D_m^3}$, $\frac{D_l^3}{D_m^3}$, $\frac{D_s^3}{D_l^3}$, and AER). The morphological features of n and AER represented the exponent of vessel diameter and area expansion ratio of the coronary bifurcations, respectively. They were calculated from mother vessel diameters and two daughter vessel diameters. These six morphological features were selected since they were highly correlated with atherosclerotic lesion in previous researches [19,20] or were of potential clinical importance as indicated by medical experts.

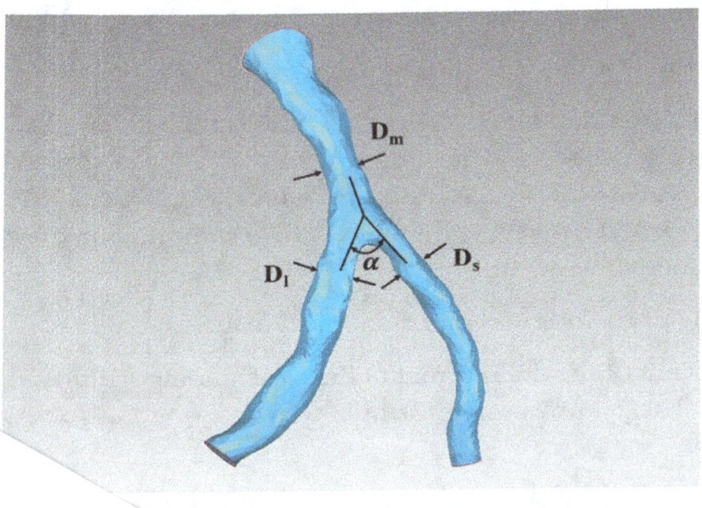

…ion of the coronary bifurcation geometry and the method for

Table 1. The definitions of the coronary morphological features.

Features	Definitions
D_m	Diameter of mother vessel.
D_l	Diameter of larger daughter vessel.
D_s	Diameter of smaller daughter vessel.
α	Bifurcation angle between larger and smaller vessel axes.
n	The exponent of vessel diameter: $D_m^n = D_l^n + D_s^n$.
$\frac{D_s^3}{D_m^3}$	Ratio of diameters between smaller daughter and mother vessels.
$\frac{D_l^3}{D_m^3}$	Ratio of diameters between larger daughter and mother vessels.
$\frac{D_s^3}{D_l^3}$	Ratio of diameters between smaller and larger daughter vessels.
AER	Area expansion ratio: $AER = \frac{D_l^2+D_s^2}{D_m^2}$.

2.2. Machine Learning Modeling Processes and Algorithms Evaluation

The aim of this study was to obtain the best machine learning classifier and to find the most important morphological features for the detection of CAD. Moreover, to evaluate the quality of the selected morphological features for the detection of CAD, several commonly used classifier algorithms were applied for classification, namely LR, DT, LDA, k-NN, ANN, and SVM, respectively. In this study, the classification performances of the SVM model for three different kernel functions (namely linear, polynomial, and radial basis function (RBF)) were first studied to find the best kernel function for the detection of CAD. We named these three sub-algorithms as linear-SVM, polynomial-SVM, and RBF-SVM, respectively. Moreover, the accuracies among the best sub-algorithm of SVM and the other machine learning algorithms were further compared to assess the capability of all algorithms we used. This aim was to select the best machine learning algorithm for the following up researches. To find the most important features for the detection of CAD, we then applied the selected best algorithm to evaluate the classification performance of the specific feature(s) or their combinations.

The process flow diagram of our proposed machine learning approach was shown in Figure 2. The main steps of the proposed approach were summarized below.

Step 1. Collecting the original morphological features;

In this study, we totally collected six original morphological features (α, n, $\frac{D_s^3}{D_m^3}$, $\frac{D_l^3}{D_m^3}$, $\frac{D_s^3}{D_l^3}$, and AER). These morphological features were selected since they had been shown highly correlating with CAD.

Step 2. Dividing all the features into four equal groups;

The morphological feature datasets for both CAD subjects and non-CAD subjects were randomly divided into four equal-sized subsets. The subsets of the non-CAD subjects were designated as $A1$, $A2$, $A3$, and $A4$; while the subsets of the CAD subjects were designated as $B1$, $B2$, $B3$, and $B4$ (Figure 2). This part was aimed to prepare for studying the effect of data sampling on the classification performance of the machine learning model.

Step 3. Preprocessing of the original morphological features;

To meet the requirement of the data format of the classifier algorithms, the original morphometric data were preprocessed. The preprocessing formula was described as follows:

where x_{max} and x_{min} were the maximum and minimum values of each morphological feature, respectively. After data preprocessing, the values of original morphometric data were normalized to values ranging from −1 to 1.

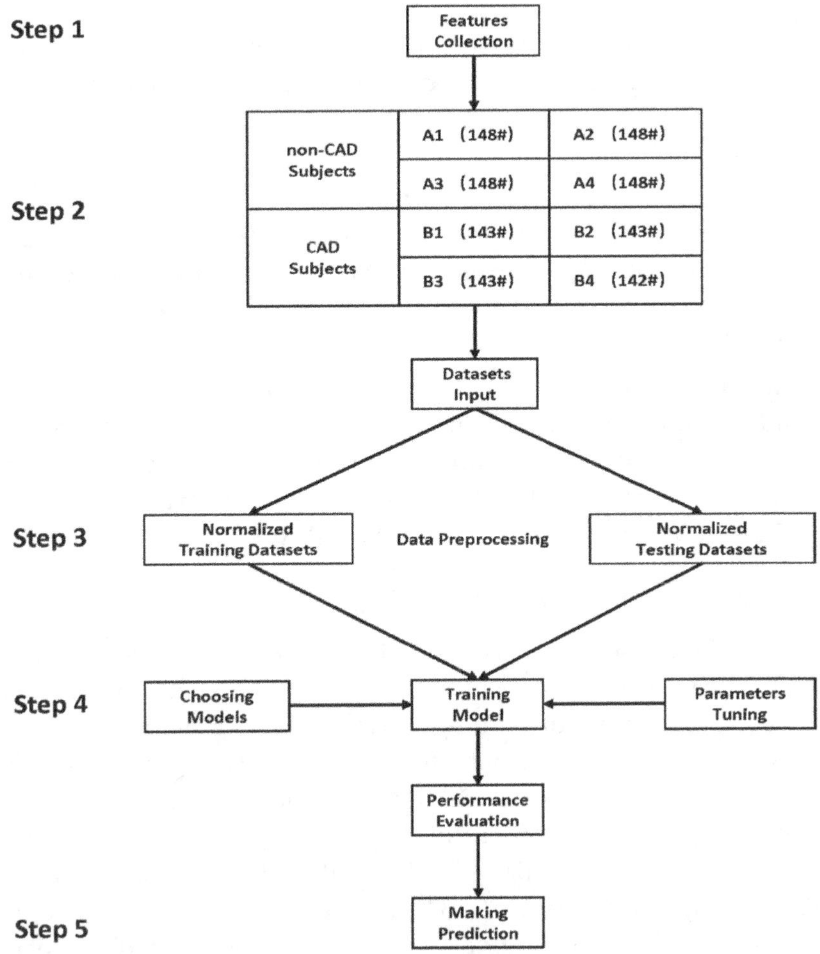

Figure 2. The flow diagram of the machine learning modeling. The morphological data for both non-coronary heart disease (CAD) subjects and CAD subjects were divided into four equal-sized subsets. The subsets of the non-CAD subjects were designated as *A*1, *A*2, *A*3 and *A*4; and the subsets of the CAD subjects were designated as *B*1, *B*2, *B*3 and *B*4. non-CAD: non-coronary artery disease; CAD: coronary artery disease; PSO: particle swarm optimization; SVM: support vector machine.

Step 4. Choosing a machine learning model, training the selected model, and parameter tuning;

Different classification algorithms (LR, DT, LDA, k-NN, ANN, linear-SVM, polynomial-SVM, and RBF-SVM) were applied for training under the use of same morphological features (75% of data for training, the remaining for testing). The cross-validation was set as 10-fold (in subsets with proportional data quantities for both classes). For the SVM classifiers, two key parameters, C and g, were needed to be pre-optimized to establish the best SVM model. There were two common algorithms for parameter optimization, namely grid search and particle swarm optimization (PSO) [21]. In this study, the given range of grid search algorithm was set from 2^{-8} to 2^{8}, and the maximum iteration number of PSO algorithm was set to 200 to find the near-optimal parameters.

Step 5. Evaluating the models and making the predictions;

The calculations of the statistical metrics on the results of models were defined as follows [22]:

$$Accuarcy = \frac{TP + TN}{TP + FN + TN + FP} \quad (2)$$

$$Sensitivity = \frac{TP}{TP + FN} \tag{3}$$

$$Specificity = \frac{TN}{TN + FP} \tag{4}$$

Accuracy showed the ratio of correctly classified samples to the total number of tested samples. *TP*, *FN*, *TN*, and *FP* represented true positives, false negatives, true negatives, and false positives, respectively.

2.3. Features Evaluation

In this study, the effects of the data sampling, the volume of the training dataset, and the dimension of input features, on the classification performances of machine learning were further analyzed.

2.3.1. Effects of Data Sampling

To examine the impact of data sampling on the classification performances, we randomly selected one subset from CAD subjects and one subset from non-CAD subjects as the testing datasets, respectively. All the remaining subsets were used as the training datasets. This process was repeated 16 times for each algorithm. In this part, we only studied the classification performances of the polynomial-SVM algorithm as it showed good performances (see Results below).

2.3.2. Effects of the Volume of Training Dataset

There were three cases in this section. *Case 0* was that 75% of data (444 from non-CAD subjects and 429 from CAD subjects) were used for training, *Case 1* was that 50% of data (296 from non-CAD subjects and 286 from CAD subjects) were used for training, and *Case 2* was that 25% of data (148 from non-CAD subjects and 143 from CAD subjects) were used for training. Given that the different data sampling did not affect the classification performances (See Results below), in order to simplify the subsequent description, we further defined the subsets of non-CAD subjects as $C1 = A1 + A2$, $C2 = A3 + A4$; and the subsets of CAD subjects as $D1 = B1 + B2$, $D2 = B3 + B4$. *Case 0*: we randomly selected three subsets from ($A1$, $A2$, $A3$, $A4$) and ($B1$, $B2$, $B3$, $B4$) as training data sets, respectively, the remaining morphometric data were used as the testing data sets; *Case 1*: we randomly selected one subset from ($C1$, $C2$) and ($D1$, $D2$) as training data sets, respectively, the remaining subsets were used as the testing data sets; *Case 2*: similarly, we randomly selected one subset from ($A1$, $A2$) and ($B1$, $B2$) as training data sets, respectively, the remaining morphometric data (including ($A3$, $A4$) and ($B3$, $B4$)) were used as the testing data sets. This part performed by using the best classification algorithm among the algorithms given above.

2.3.3. Effects of the Dimension of Input Features

Six different morphological features were available to generate the classifier. There were C_6^k ($k \in [1, 6]$) possible combinations for the specific input features, where k was the number of morphological features selected from six morphological features. This part performed by using the best classification algorithm with 75% of morphometric data used for training.

The best classification algorithm was further applied to train each morphological feature to find the most important features for the detection of CAD.

2.4. Models Running Approaches

The proposed machine learning methods were performed on a PC with 2.60 GHz Intel Core i7 CPU, 16 GB RAM, and a windows 7 operating system. All the machine learning models were run in the MATLAB software (Math Works, Natick, MA, USA) with the use of the classification learner codes and the computational time of each model can be completed within ~30 min. Moreover, libSVM [23], an open-source library, was applied to build the SVM models. The results of the machine learning classification were analyzed in the following subsections.

3. Results

3.1. Polynomial-SVM Model with Grid Search Optimization Showed the Best Performance in the Detection of CAD

In this study, the classification performances of linear-SVM, polynomial-SVM, and RBF-SVM were first studied to choose the best SVM algorithm for the following investigation. Previous studies suggested that the SVM model could not achieve best classification outcomes if the kernel functions and parameters were not selected properly [21]. To find the best SVM algorithm for the detection of CAD, we compared the classification performances of linear-SVM, polynomial-SVM, and RBF-SVM algorithm with the use of three different parameter setting methods of default method, grid search and PSO (Table 2). The results showed that although all SVM algorithms worked well with the default parameters, the classification performances of the SVM models were improved remarkably through parameter optimizations with both grid search and PSO. Moreover, for all the SVM models, the performances optimized by grid search were better than those by PSO (Table 2). On the other hand, the classification performances of polynomial-SVM were much better than those of linear-SVM and RBF-SVM (Table 2). This suggested that polynomial-SVM with the parameter optimization method of grid search achieved the best performance among three given SVM models.

To compare the performances among the best SVM algorithm (polynomial-SVM) and the other machine learning algorithms, the accuracies of the polynomial-SVM algorithm and other machine learning algorithms (LR, DT, LDA, k-NN, and ANN) were further studied (Table 3). The aim of this part was to assess the classification capability of all used algorithms. The results indicated that the polynomial-SVM model achieved the best performance in the detection of CAD, followed by ANN. The classification accuracy of LR, DT, LDA, k-NN, ANN, and polynomial-SVM were 96.30%, 97.00%, 92.30%, 95.70%, 98.40% and 100.00%, respectively. This suggested that polynomial-SVM was the best algorithm for the detection of CAD among all these algorithms. Hence, the following studies will be mainly based on the polynomial-SVM model (with the parameter optimization of grid search) for further research.

Table 2. The comparison of the classification performances of three different SVM models (linear-SVM, polynomial-SVM, and radial basis function (RBF)-SVM) with the use of different parameter setting methods.

Results	Parameter Setting Methods / SVM Kernel Functions	Default	Grid Search	PSO
Training Accuracy (%)	Linear	90.86	96.56	95.24
	Polynomial	95.19	100	98.99
	RBF	88.81	99.77	97.99
Testing Accuracy (%)	Linear	90.29	96.92	94.88
	Polynomial	95.23	100	99.86
	RBF	88.05	99.66	97.65
Testing Sensitivity (%)	Linear	90.39	98.65	97.94
	Polynomial	91.64	100	99.80
	RBF	88.42	99.32	97.55
Testing Specificity (%)	Linear	87.25	95.10	91.86
	Polynomial	94.09	100	99.83
	RBF	90.09	100	97.51

RBF: radial basis function.

Table 3. The comparison of the classification accuracy among the polynomial-SVM model and other machine learning methods with the use of the same training datasets (75% of morphometric datasets for training).

Methods	LR	DT	LDA	k-NN	ANN	Polynomial-SVM
Accuracy (%)	96.30	97.00	92.30	95.70	98.40	100.00

Here, LR, DT, LDA, k-NN, and ANN represented logistic regression, decision tree, linear discriminant analysis, k-nearest neighbors and artificial neural network classifiers, respectively. The parameter optimization method of the polynomial-SVM applied the grid search.

3.2. The Performance of the SVM Models Was Not Affected by Data Sampling

To examine whether the classification performances of the polynomial-SVM model were dependent on data sampling, 75% morphometric data from both non-CAD and CAD subjects were randomly selected as the training datasets, and the other morphometric data were selected as the testing datasets. The results in Table 4 indicated that the values of the classification performances (including training accuracy, testing accuracy, testing sensitivity, and testing specificity) for the polynomial-SVM model were similar in all sampling cases. Moreover, the fluctuation of the classification performances of the polynomial-SVM model was less than 1‰. This suggested that the classification performances were not affected by the data sampling. Furthermore, the results also showed that all classification performances (accuracy, sensitivity, and specificity) of the polynomial-SVM model were close to 100%. This suggested that polynomial-SVM model was very effective and stable to detect CAD by combining the measured morphological features. Table A2 also showed the comparison of the classification performances among linear-SVM, polynomial-SVM, and RBF-SVM under using different sampling methods. The fluctuations of the classification performances of all the SVM models were within 5%. This further suggested that the classification performances of all SVM algorithms were not affected by the data sampling, especially for the polynomial-SVM algorithm (see Appendix A).

Table 4. The classification performances of the polynomial-SVM model with 75% of morphometric datasets for training.

Results	CAD \ non-CAD	A(1,2,3)	A(1,2,4)	A(1,3,4)	A(2,3,4)	Mean
Training Accuracy (%)	B(1,2,3)	100	100	100	100	100
	B(1,2,4)	100	100	100	100	100
	B(1,3,4)	100	100	100	100	100
	B(2,3,4)	100	100	100	100	100
	Mean	100	100	100	100	100
Testing Accuracy (%)	B(1,2,3)	100	100	100	100	100
	B(1,2,4)	100	100	99.66	100	99.92
	B(1,3,4)	100	100	100	100	100
	B(2,3,4)	100	100	100	100	100
	Mean	100	100	99.92	100	99.98
Testing Sensitivity (%)	B(1,2,3)	100	100	100	100	100
	B(1,2,4)	100	100	100	100	100
	B(1,3,4)	100	100	100	100	100
	B(2,3,4)	100	100	100	100	100
	Mean	100	100	100	100	100
Testing Specificity (%)	B(1,2,3)	100	100	100	100	100
	B(1,2,4)	100	100	99.31	100	99.83
	B(1,3,4)	100	100	100	100	100
	B(2,3,4)	100	100	100	100	100
	Mean	100	100	99.83	100	99.96

Note: $A(i_1, i_2, i_3)$ (where $i_1, i_2, i_3 \in [1,4]$ *and* $i_1 < i_2 < i_3$) represented the features data from the non-CAD subjects; while $B(j_1, j_2, j_3)$ (where $j_1, j_2, j_3 \in [1,4]$ *and* $j_1 < j_2 < j_3$) represented the features data from the CAD subjects. The data combinations of $A(i_1, i_2, i_3)$ and $B(j_1, j_2, j_3)$ represented the training datasets.

3.3. *Adequate Training Data Volume Was Necessary and Sufficient to Obtain High Detecting Performance*

Although polynomial-SVM algorithm had exhibited high performances in classification events, this model had speed limitation for training larger datasets [24]. However, excessively reducing the volume of training data might affect the classification performance of the polynomial-SVM model. A reasonable training data volume should not only guarantee the running efficiency but also retain the high classification performance. To study the effect of the training data volume on the classification performances, 75% (*Case 0*), 50% (*Case 1*) and 25% (*Case 2*) of morphometric data were selected as training datasets (see "Methods" section; please note that the results of *Case 0* were presented in Table 4). As shown in Table 5, although the performance of the training accuracy was not affected by the training datasets volume, the performances of testing accuracy, testing sensitivity, and testing specificity were sensitive to the volume of training datasets. In addition, when the volume of training data was sufficient (≥50%), all the performances of the polynomial-SVM model reached the best (close to 100%) and were not affected by the training datasets volume and the sampling method (Tables 4 and 5 (*Case 1*)). These results suggested that adequate training datasets volume (≥50%) was necessary and sufficient to obtain high detecting performance.

Table 5. The classification performances of the polynomial-SVM model with the use of different training data volumes.

Case 1	Results	CAD \ non-CAD	C1	C2	Mean
50% Datasets for Training	Training Accuracy (%)	D1	100	100	100
		D2	100	100	100
		Mean	100	100	100
	Testing Accuracy (%)	D1	99.83	100	99.92
		D2	100	100	100
		Mean	99.92	100	99.96
	Testing Sensitivity (%)	D1	99.66	100	99.83
		D2	100	100	100
		Mean	99.83	100	99.92
	Testing Specificity (%)	D1	100	100	100
		D2	100	100	100
		Mean	100	100	100

Case 2	Results	CAD \ non-CAD	A1	A2	Mean
25% Datasets for Training	Training Accuracy (%)	B1	100	100	100
		B2	100	100	100
		Mean	100	100	100
	Testing Accuracy (%)	B1	84.88	97.59	91.24
		B2	87.29	92.78	90.04
		Mean	86.09	95.19	90.64
	Testing Sensitivity (%)	B1	73.65	96.62	85.14
		B2	81.08	92.57	86.83
		Mean	77.37	94.60	85.98
	Testing Specificity (%)	B1	96.50	98.60	97.55
		B2	93.71	93.01	93.36
		Mean	95.11	95.81	95.46

Note: *Case 1* and *Case 2* indicated the 50% and 25% volume of morphometric data for training, respectively.

3.4. *The Effect of the Dimension and Combination of Morphological Features on the Classification Performances*

To examine the effect of the input features dimension (features number of a combination) on the classification performances, all the combinations of the six morphological features were examined with the polynomial-SVM model. When the dimension was k, there were C_6^k possible combinations that can be used to build model (see "Methods" section). Each scatted point in Figure 3a–d represented a detection result for the specific combination. The results showed that the performances of training accuracy, testing accuracy, testing sensitivity, and testing specificity exhibited a similar trend. The classification performances of the model were improved as the dimension of input features increased (Figure 3). When the dimension ≥4, all the classification performances achieved a high level (over 95%) and were not susceptible to the combination approach. However, when the dimension <4, the classification performances increased rapidly as the number of the dimension increased, and the classification performances exhibited large dispersion among different feature combinations for a specific dimension. This suggested that the feature combination approach was also a factor affecting the classification performances of the machine learning model when the dimension <4.

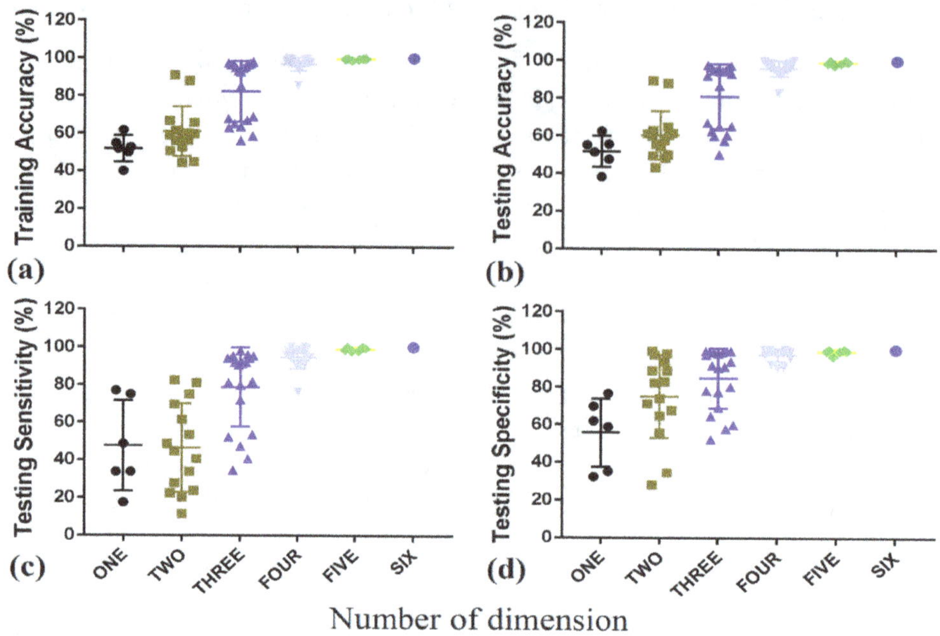

Figure 3. (**a**–**d**) The classification performances of polynomial-SVM model with various feature dimensions. (**a**) Training accuracy, (**b**) testing accuracy, (**c**) testing sensitivity, and (**d**) testing specificity.

3.5. Bifurcation Diameter Exponent (n) and Area Expansion Ratio (AER) Were Two Key Features for the CAD Detection

To find out which morphological feature(s) was the most important feature for the detection of CAD, we compared the classification performances of the polynomial-SVM model among each single morphological feature (Table 6). The results showed that the morphological feature n exhibited the best performance among the six morphological features, followed by AER, while the $\frac{D_s^3}{D_m^3}$ had the worst performance. Moreover, it was worth noting that, in the cases of combinations of two input features, there were two points of the classification performances that were significantly higher than the other points (see Figure 3). This suggested that those two detection results of the polynomial-SVM model achieved pretty good performances than the other results under the two-dimensional combination. Hence, in order to find out which features were selected of these two detections, we further compared the classification performances of the polynomial-SVM model for the combinations with two features (Table 7). The results showed that the combinations of (n & AER) and (n & $\frac{D_l^3}{D_m^3}$) achieved the testing accuracy of 89.31% and 87.93%, which were significantly higher than the third-ranked combination of n & $\frac{D_s^3}{D_m^3}$ (with the testing accuracy of 64.83%) (Table 7). These results suggested that the polynomial-SVM model with the use of feature n and AER may have great clinical application prospects in the early detection of CAD.

Table 6. The comparison of the classification performances of the polynomial-SVM model for each morphological feature. The morphological feature n exhibited the best performance among the six morphological features, followed by AER, while the $\frac{D_s^3}{D_m^3}$ had the worst.

Variables	Training Accuracy (%)	Testing Accuracy (%)	Testing Sensitivity (%)	Testing Specificity (%)
n	61.63	62.41	48.65	76.76
AER	54.75	55.52	75.00	35.21
a	52.69	55.17	77.03	32.39
$\frac{D_l^3}{D_m^3}$	51.89	51.38	33.78	69.72
$\frac{D_s^3}{D_l^3}$	49.94	47.59	33.78	69.73
$\frac{D_s^3}{D_m^3}$	40.09	38.28	17.57	58.86

Table 7. The comparison of the classification performances of the plynomial-SVM model for each combination with two features. The combinations of (n & AER) and (n & $\frac{D_l^3}{D_m^3}$) performed better than the other combinations.

Combinations	Training Accuracy (%)	Testing Accuracy (%)	Testing Sensitivity (%)	Testing Specificity (%)
n, AER	90.95	89.31	81.08	97.89
$n, \frac{D_l^3}{D_m^3}$	87.97	87.93	82.43	93.66
$n, \frac{D_s^3}{D_m^3}$	66.78	64.83	33.78	97.18
a, AER	61.40	62.76	69.59	55.63
$\frac{D_s^3}{D_m^3}, \frac{D_l^3}{D_m^3}$	59.91	61.38	40.54	83.10
n, a	65.75	61.03	48.65	73.94
$n, \frac{D_s^3}{D_l^3}$	59.91	60.34	53.38	67.61
$\frac{D_l^3}{D_m^3}, \frac{D_s^3}{D_l^3}$	59.68	59.97	20.27	99.30
$\frac{D_l^3}{D_m^3}, AER$	58.88	57.59	44.59	71.13
$a, \frac{D_s^3}{D_m^3}$	56.01	55.51	23.65	88.73
$a, \frac{D_s^3}{D_l^3}$	52.69	54.48	27.70	82.39
$\frac{D_s^3}{D_l^3}, AER$	56.24	50.07	75.00	28.17
$\frac{D_s^3}{D_m^3}, AER$	50.63	49.31	11.49	88.73
$a, \frac{D_l^3}{D_m^3}$	44.33	48.28	61.49	34.51
$\frac{D_s^3}{D_m^3}, \frac{D_s^3}{D_l^3}$	44.79	43.10	22.30	64.79

4. Discussion

Diversity is one of the properties of medical features dataset and greatly increased the difficulty of medical data mining. In this study, we utilized the commonly used machine learning models (such as LR, DT, LDA, k-NN, ANN, linear-SVM, polynomial-SVM, and RBF-SVM) for the detection of CAD by using the image-based morphometric features. Six measured morphological features were applied to generate the machine learning models. These morphological features were representative of the detailed quantitative topological information of the coronary bifurcations. The results showed that the polynomial-SVM algorithm with the use of the grid search optimization method showed the best performance for the detection of CAD and yielded the classification accuracy of 100.00%. It was worth noting that adequate training data volume and input feature dimensions were necessary for obtaining high classification performances of machine learning. Moreover, when the volume of training dataset was large enough, the classification performances were not susceptible to the data sampling method. In addition, we further found that the exponent of vessel diameter (n) and the area expansion ratio (AER) were the most two important features for the detection of CAD, especially for their combination.

Remarkable progress have been made in applying different machine learning algorithms with medical features for detecting different diseases such as various types of cancer and cardiovascular diseases [12–14,25–27]. Abdar et al. proposed a nested ensemble nu-support vector classification (NE-nu-SVC) model for the diagnosis of CAD [26]. The proposed model provided accuracies of 94.66% and 98.60% for two different datasets (Z-Alizadeh Sani and Cleveland CAD datasets), respectively. Singh et al. [27] applied extreme learning machine (ELM) to detect CAD with 100% accuracy when constructing the classifier with 31 input features. However, the detection accuracy of ELM was drastically decreased to 68.48% when the number of input features was reduced to 24. Nasarian et al.'s summarized the existing machine learning methods for the detection of CAD with the use of various medical databases [12]. It showed that the detection accuracy of different algorithms varied with the medical databases. This suggested that both machine learning algorithms and features selection method would play significant roles in the medical diagnostic process. Table A1 (see Appendix A) summarized the comparisons of machine learning performances for the detection of CAD with different classifier algorithms and medical features, which also supported Nasarian et al.'s study that both features and machine learning algorithms could significantly affect the performances of machine learning. In this study, we hence comprehensively compared the prediction performance of existing commonly used algorithms to select the best algorithm for the evaluation of the features.

The SVM model is one of the most well-known supervised machine learning techniques that have been widely used in pattern recognition and binary classification problems [28]. Since the SVM algorithm was invented, a large number of studies have been done by previous researchers on its optimization [21,29,30]. Syarif et al. showed that SVM parameter optimization using grid search was powerful to improve classification accuracy [21]. Our findings showed that although SVM worked well with the default parameters, and the performances of SVM could be significantly improved by using parameter optimizations with both grid search and PSO. Liu et al. found that the RBF-SVM achieved the best accuracy in the classification of fasting plasma glucose level ≥ 126 mg/dL vs. fasting plasma glucose level < 126 mg/dL, and the linear-SVM performed the best in the classification of fasting plasma glucose level ≥ 100 mg/dL vs. fasting plasma glucose level < 100 mg/dL by applying support vector machine modeling to predict diabetes disease [29]. The study by Patle et al. revealed that the RBF-SVM was better than the polynomial-SVM for the classification task when the data set was very large [30]. In this paper, we found that the polynomial-SVM with grid search optimization method performed the best in the detection of CAD by using six measured morphological features to build the SVM classifiers (Table 2).

Previous studies showed that features used for building the machine learning classifier can be extracted from the diagnostic images (such as MRI, CTA and ultrasound) by automatic algorithms [31]. However, the clinical significance of these features was unknown and difficult to be interpreted. Moreover, for a given image, automatic algorithms can generate a large number of features. It was suggested that reducing the number of features in machine learning to speed up the training was of great importance especially when dealing with large datasets [32]. However, this process may degrade the classification results. A reasonable method for feature selection was of great significance for building a high-performance classification model. There are various automatic algorithms for the feature extraction or selection, such as F-score and SVM-RFE [33,34]. These methods were helpful to efficiently select the features for the machine learning. However, the F-score algorithm did not provide any mutual information among the features [33], while the SVM-RFE algorithm can only be used to linear kernel SVM [34]. In the present study, the six morphometric features were selected because they had exhibited great clinical significance in terms of atherosclerosis [20] or indicated by medical experts. The results showed that our features achieved high classification performances with using only six morphological features for building the machine learning models, especially for polynomial-SVM (close to 100.00%) (Tables 2–4 and Figure 3 and Table A2). This suggested that reasonable and targeted selection of features for building machine learning models could greatly improve the classification performances. To the best of our knowledge, this study was the first report that the machine learning models successfully detected CAD by using the measured morphological features from the reconstructed 3D coronary bifurcations.

Trivedi et al. found that the SVM model achieved an accuracy of 98.5% with 1358 dimensions of feature while the accuracy below 85.2% with 158 dimensions of feature, by studying the effect of feature dimension on the ability to detect email spams [35]. Our present modeling strategy showed a similar phenomenon that the average testing accuracy with the lowest (one) and highest (six) dimensions of the feature were 51.83% and 99.98%, respectively (Figure 3). Moreover, we found that the morphological feature n achieves the best classification performances among the six morphological features, followed by AER, while the $\frac{D_s^3}{D_m^3}$ achieves the worst (Table 6). The results also indicated that two combinations in the two-dimensional section achieved the testing accuracy as high as 90% (Figure 3). This classification accuracy was remarkably higher than that of the other combinations with two input features. Further studies suggested that these two combinations were (n & $\frac{D_l^3}{D_m^3}$) and (n & AER) (Table 7). These results were consistent with our recent study which predicts that the $\left|\frac{n-3}{3}\right|$ and AER were the best two indicators for CAD prediction (data not shown). Our results further indicated that the volume of training data was another factor that can impact the classification performance (Table 5). A study by Rudd et al. indicated that the whole data were split into 80% (1652# of 2066#) for training and the remaining 20% for testing achieved high accuracy of 97.5% [31]. Our present strategy showed similar high performances when no less than 50% of the morphometric data were used for training. In addition, the performance did not improve significantly as the volume of training datasets further increases from 50% to 75% (Tables 4 and 5 (*Case 1*)). Specifically, 50% and 75% of morphometric data were selected for training resulting in a mean testing accuracy of 99.96% and 99.98%, respectively. These results were obtained by the polynomial-SVM model. These suggest that the polynomial-SVM model was a stable and powerful approach for the detection of coronary artery disease.

Although the polynomial-SVM model performed the best in this study, this algorithm could also have its inherent pros and cons. Compared to other models used in this study, the most pros of the polynomial-SVM model is that it has the best performances when combined with measured morphological features. However, it also has its cons side. For instance, to have the best classification performances, parameters tuning is necessary for the polynomial-SVM model. In addition, when dealing with large amounts of datasets, the polynomial-SVM model will be time-consuming [24]. A survey study by Leo et al. indicated that different types of features data could suit for different machine learning models [36]. Our present study demonstrated that, compared to other considered models, the polynomial-SVM model is the best for detecting the changes of the morphological features, however, whether it is also the best for detecting other types of features needs further exploration.

5. Conclusions

In this work, the detection of CAD based on machine learning models with the measured morphological features were proposed. The experimental results demonstrated that among all the considered machine learning models, the polynomial-SVM model performed the best; and, moreover, the exponent of vessel diameter (n) and the area expansion ratio (AER) were the two most important features for the detection of CAD; in addition, the combinations of (n & $\frac{D_l^3}{D_m^3}$) and (n & AER) can significantly decrease the dimension of input features without losing much detection accuracy. This study was proposed a new methodology that combined using machine learning techniques and imaging-based morphological measurement methods for the detection of CAD and obtained the high detection accuracy, which could aid the clinicians to detect CAD accurately in a non-invasive way at the early stages. The proposed methodology may also be applied to earlier detection of other diseases related to morphology change, such as carotid artery disease. Moreover, as the change of the morphological features of nervous tissue usually occurred before the disease happened [37], then it also could be potentially used for the early detection of neurological diseases, such as Parkinson's disease. For future work, we will be committed to developing an automatic method for the measurements of morphological features to speed up the original data acquisition process. Moreover, the proposed method will be applied for more different vascular disease detection to verify the feasibility of our given strategy.

Author Contributions: Conceptualization, X.C., Y.F. (Ying Fang) and J.W.; methodology, X.C., Y.F. (Yi Fu) and J.L.; validation, X.C., Y.F. (Yi Fu), J.L., Y.J., Y.F. (Ying Fang) and J.W.; data curation, X.C., Y.F. (Yi Fu) and J.L.; writing—original draft preparation, X.C.; writing—review and editing, Y.F. (Yi Fu), J.L. and Y.J.; funding acquisition, Y.F. (Ying Fang), J.W. and J.L. All authors have read and agreed to the published version of the manuscript.

Acknowledgments: We here thank Jingxing Dai (Southern Medical University) and Yueheng Wu (Guangdong General Hospital) provided the original CTA imaging data for this study.

Appendix A

Table A2 listed classification performances of linear-SVM, polynomial-SVM, and RBF-SVM, by using the parameter optimization method of grid search. The results indicated that the values of the classification performances (training accuracy, testing accuracy, testing sensitivity, and testing specificity) for the specific SVM model were similar in all sampling cases. Moreover, the fluctuations of the classification performances of all the SVM models were within 5%. The fluctuation of these classification performances was even less than 1‰ of the polynomial-SVM model. This suggested that the classification performances were not significantly affected by the data sampling, no matter what SVM algorithm was used. Moreover, the results showed that classification performances of accuracy, sensitivity, and specificity of all the SVM models were over 95%, and the values of polynomial-SVM were the best (almost all were 100%). This suggested that SVM models were very effective and stable to detect CAD by combining the measured morphological features, especially for polynomial-SVM.

Table A1. The comparison of existing machine learning performances in the detection of CAD with the use of different algorithms and medical features. The comparison results in the table showed that selection of appropriate algorithms and medical features for machine learning had a significant impact on the accuracy of CAD detection.

Study	Year	Machine Learning Algorithms	Medical Features Datasets	Accuracy (%)
Nasarian et al. [12]	2020	Decision tree (DT)	Long beach dataset selected by ADASYN	77.53
		Gaussian Naive Bayes (GNB)		79.44
		Random Forest (RF)		80.45
		Extreme Gradient Boosting (XGBoost)		80.41
		DT	Z-Alizadeh Sani dataset selected by ADASYN	88.12
		GNB		88.72
		RF		91.56
		XGBoost		92.35
Chen et al. [14]	2020	Deep learning (DL)	Coronary computed tomography angiography (CCTA)	87.10
Aouabed et al. [26]	2019	Nested ensemble nu-Support Vector Classification (NE-nu-SVC)	Cleveland	98.60
Subramaniyam et al. [38]	2019	Taylorgradient descent (TGD)-based actor critic neural network (ACNN)	Hungarian	82.55
Zomorodi-moghadam et al. [39]	2019	Hybrid particle swarm optimization (PSO)	Z-Alizadeh Sani	84.2
Li et al. [13]	2019	Dual-input neural network	Electrocardiogram (ECG) and phonocardiogram (PCG) signals	95.62
Betancur et al. [40]	2019	DL	Myocardial perfusion imaging (MPI)	84.8
Abdar et al. [25]	2019	N2Genetic-nuSVM	Z-Alizadeh Sani	93.08
	2019	NE-nu-SVC	Z-Alizadeh Sani and Cleveland	94.66 and 98.60
Qin et al. [41]	2017	Ensemble algorithm based on multiple feature selection (EA-MFS)	Z-Alizadeh Sani	93.70
Raghavendra et al. [42]	2017	Double Density-Dual Tree DWT (DD-DTDWT)	Ultrasound images	96.05
Alizadehsani et al. [43,44]	2016	Support Vector Machine (SVM)	Z-Alizadeh Sani	86.14
	2013	Sequential Minimal Optimization (SMO)		94.08
Acharya et al. [45]	2013	Gaussian Mixture Model (GMM)	Echocardiography images	100.00
		DT		88.90
		Fuzzy sugeno (FS)		90.70
		KNN		86.30
		Naive Bayes classifier (NBC)		94.4
		Radial basis probabilistic neural network (RBPNN)		82.4

Table A2. The classification performances of all SVM models (linear-SVM, polynomial-SVM, and RBF-SVM) with the parameter optimization method of grid search (75% of morphometric datasets for training).

Results	SVM Kernel Functions	CAD \ non-CAD	A(1,2,3)	A(1,2,4)	A(1,3,4)	A(2,3,4)	Mean
Training Accuracy (%)	Linear	B(1,2,3)	96.33	96.56	96.22	96.33	96.36
		B(1,2,4)	96.90	96.67	96.67	95.56	96.45
		B(1,3,4)	96.45	96.56	96.33	96.22	96.39
		B(2,3,4)	96.56	96.33	96.11	96.79	96.45
		Mean	96.56	96.53	96.33	96.25	96.41
	Polynomial	B(1,2,3)	100	100	100	100	100
		B(1,2,4)	100	100	100	100	100
		B(1,3,4)	100	100	100	100	100
		B(2,3,4)	100	100	100	100	100
		Mean	100	100	100	100	100
	RBF	B(1,2,3)	100	99.78	99.89	99.89	99.89
		B(1,2,4)	99.31	99.77	99.89	99.89	99.47
		B(1,3,4)	100	99.77	99.66	99.31	99.69
		B(2,3,4)	99.89	99.77	100	99.89	99.89
		Mean	99.80	99.77	99.61	99.75	99.73
Testing Sensitivity (%)	Linear	B(1,2,3)	98.65	98.65	99.32	100	99.16
		B(1,2,4)	98.65	98.65	99.32	100	99.16
		B(1,3,4)	98.65	98.65	100	100	99.32
		B(2,3,4)	97.97	98.65	99.32	100	98.99
		Mean	98.48	98.65	99.49	100	99.16
	Polynomial	B(1,2,3)	100	100	100	100	100
		B(1,2,4)	100	100	100	100	100
		B(1,3,4)	100	100	100	100	100
		B(2,3,4)	100	100	100	100	100
		Mean	100	100	100	100	100
	RBF	B(1,2,3)	98.65	99.32	99.32	91.61	97.22
		B(1,2,4)	98.65	98.65	98.65	99.32	98.82
		B(1,3,4)	98.65	99.32	99.32	99.32	99.15
		B(2,3,4)	98.65	99.32	98.65	100	99.16
		Mean	98.65	95.15	98.99	97.56	98.59

Results	SVM Kernel Functions	CAD \ non-CAD	A(1,2,3)	A(1,2,4)	A(1,3,4)	A(2,3,4)	Mean
Testing Accuracy (%)	Linear	B(1,2,3)	96.22	96.22	96.22	95.88	96.14
		B(1,2,4)	95.53	95.88	95.88	96.22	95.88
		B(1,3,4)	96.91	96.92	97.25	97.25	97.08
		B(2,3,4)	94.83	95.17	95.17	95.86	95.26
		Mean	95.87	96.05	96.13	96.30	96.09
	Polynomial	B(1,2,3)	100	100	100	100	100
		B(1,2,4)	100	100	99.66	100	99.92
		B(1,3,4)	100	100	100	100	100
		B(2,3,4)	100	100	100	100	100
		Mean	100	100	99.92	100	99.98
	RBF	B(1,2,3)	98.97	99.31	99.31	99.66	99.31
		B(1,2,4)	97.59	98.26	98.97	98.97	98.45
		B(1,3,4)	99.31	99.66	99.66	99.66	99.57
		B(2,3,4)	98.97	99.66	98.97	100	99.40
		Mean	98.71	99.23	99.23	99.58	99.18
Testing Specificity (%)	Linear	B(1,2,3)	93.71	93.71	93.01	91.61	93.01
		B(1,2,4)	92.31	93.01	92.31	92.31	92.49
		B(1,3,4)	95.10	95.10	94.41	94.41	94.76
		B(2,3,4)	91.55	91.55	90.85	91.55	91.38
		Mean	93.17	93.34	92.65	92.47	92.91
	Polynomial	B(1,2,3)	100	100	100	100	100
		B(1,2,4)	100	100	99.31	100	99.83
		B(1,3,4)	100	100	100	100	100
		B(2,3,4)	100	100	100	100	100
		Mean	100	100	99.83	100	99.96
	RBF	B(1,2,3)	99.31	99.30	99.30	99.30	99.30
		B(1,2,4)	96.50	98.60	99.30	98.60	98.25
		B(1,3,4)	100	100	100	100	100
		B(2,3,4)	99.30	100	99.30	100	99.65
		Mean	98.78	99.48	99.48	99.48	99.30

References

1. Benjamin, E.J.; Muntner, P.; Alonso, A.; Bittencourt, M.S.; Callaway, C.W.; Carson, A.P.; Chamberlain, A.M.; Chang, A.R.; Cheng, S.; Das, S.R.; et al. Heart Disease and Stroke Statistics-2019 Update: A Report From the American Heart Association. *Circulation* **2019**, *139*, e1–e473. [CrossRef]
2. Benjamin, E.J.; Blaha, M.J.; Chiuve, S.E.; Cushman, M.; Das, S.R.; Deo, R.; de Ferranti, S.D.; Floyd, J.; Fornage, M.; Gillespie, C.; et al. Heart Disease and Stroke Statistics-2017 Update: A Report From the American Heart Association. *Circulation* **2017**, *135*, e146–e603. [CrossRef]
3. Tavakol, M.; Ashraf, S.; Brener, S.J. Risks and complications of coronary angiography: A comprehensive review. *Glob. J. Health Sci.* **2012**, *4*, 65–93. [CrossRef] [PubMed]
4. Nie, K.; Chen, J.H.; Yu, H.J.; Chu, Y.; Nalcioglu, O.; Su, M.Y. Quantitative analysis of lesion morphology and texture features for diagnostic prediction in breast MRI. *Acad. Radiol.* **2008**, *15*, 1513–1525. [CrossRef]
5. De Filippo, M.; Capasso, R. Coronary computed tomography angiography (CCTA) and cardiac magnetic resonance (CMR) imaging in the assessment of patients presenting with chest pain suspected for acute coronary syndrome. *Ann. Transl. Med.* **2016**, *4*, 255. [CrossRef] [PubMed]
6. Carita, P.; Guaricci, A.I.; Muscogiuri, G.; Carrabba, N.; Pontone, G. Prognostic Value and Therapeutic Perspectives of Coronary CT Angiography: A Literature Review. *Biomed. Res. Int.* **2018**, *2018*, 6528238. [CrossRef] [PubMed]
7. Huang, S.; Cai, N.; Pacheco, P.P.; Narrandes, S.; Wang, Y.; Xu, W. Applications of Support Vector Machine (SVM) Learning in Cancer Genomics. *Cancer Genom. Proteom.* **2018**, *15*, 41–51. [CrossRef]
8. Poddar, M.G.; Kumar, V.; Sharma, Y.P. Automated diagnosis of coronary artery diseased patients by heart rate variability analysis using linear and non-linear methods. *J. Med. Eng. Technol.* **2015**, *39*, 331–341. [CrossRef]
9. Karimi, M.; Amirfattahi, R.; Sadri, S.; Marvasti, S.A. Noninvasive detection and classification of coronary artery occlusions using wavelet analysis of heart sounds with neural networks. In Proceedings of the 3rd IEE International Seminar on Medical Applications of Signal Processing (Ref. No. 2005-1119), London, UK, 3–4 November 2005; pp. 117–120.
10. Liu, N.; Lin, Z.; Koh, Z.; Huang, G.-B.; Ser, W.; Ong, M.E.H. Patient Outcome Prediction with Heart Rate Variability and Vital Signs. *J. Signal Process. Syst.* **2011**, *64*, 265–278. [CrossRef]
11. Asl, B.M.; Setarehdan, S.K.; Mohebbi, M. Support vector machine-based arrhythmia classification using reduced features of heart rate variability signal. *Artif. Intell. Med.* **2008**, *44*, 51–64. [CrossRef]
12. Nasarian, E.; Abdar, M.; Fahami, M.A.; Alizadehsani, R.; Hussain, S.; Basiri, M.E.; Zomorodi-Moghadam, M.; Zhou, X.; Pławiak, P.; Acharya, U.R.; et al. Association between work-related features and coronary artery disease: A heterogeneous hybrid feature selection integrated with balancing approach. *Pattern Recognit. Lett.* **2020**, *133*, 33–40. [CrossRef]
13. Li, H.; Wang, X.; Liu, C.; Wang, Y.; Li, P.; Tang, H.; Yao, L.; Zhang, H. Dual-Input Neural Network Integrating Feature Extraction and Deep Learning for Coronary Artery Disease Detection Using Electrocardiogram and Phonocardiogram. *IEEE Access* **2019**, *7*, 146457–146469. [CrossRef]
14. Chen, M.; Wang, X.; Hao, G.; Cheng, X.; Ma, C.; Guo, N.; Hu, S.; Tao, Q.; Yao, F.; Hu, C. Diagnostic performance of deep learning-based vascular extraction and stenosis detection technique for coronary artery disease. *Br. J. Radiol.* **2020**, *93*, 20191028. [CrossRef] [PubMed]
15. Fan, T.; Zhou, Z.; Fang, W.; Wang, W.; Xu, L.; Huo, Y. Morphometry and hemodynamics of coronary artery aneurysms caused by atherosclerosis. *Atherosclerosis* **2019**, *284*, 187–193. [CrossRef] [PubMed]
16. Wosiak, A.; Zakrzewska, D. Integrating Correlation-Based Feature Selection and Clustering for Improved Cardiovascular Disease Diagnosis. *Complexity* **2018**, *2018*, 2520706. [CrossRef]
17. Kigka, V.I.; Rigas, G.; Sakellarios, A.; Siogkas, P.; Andrikos, I.O.; Exarchos, T.P.; Loggitsi, D.; Anagnostopoulos, C.D.; Michalis, L.K.; Neglia, D.; et al. 3D reconstruction of coronary arteries and atherosclerotic plaques based on computed tomography angiography images. *Biomed. Signal Process. Control* **2018**, *40*, 286–294. [CrossRef]
18. Sharma, R.K.; Voelker, D.J.; Sharma, R.K.; Singh, V.N.; Bhatt, G.; Moazazi, M.; Nash, T.; Reddy, H.K. Coronary computed tomographic angiography (CCTA) in community hospitals: "Current and emerging role". *Vasc. Health Risk Manag.* **2010**, *6*, 307–316. [CrossRef]
19. Kaimovitz, B.; Huo, Y.; Lanir, Y.; Kassab, G.S. Diameter asymmetry of porcine coronary arterial trees: Structural and functional implications. *Am. J. Physiol. Heart Circ. Physiol.* **2008**, *294*, H714–H723. [CrossRef]

20. Huang, X.; Yin, X.; Xu, Y.; Jia, X.; Li, J.; Niu, P.; Shen, W.; Kassab, G.S.; Tan, W.; Huo, Y. Morphometric and hemodynamic analysis of atherosclerotic progression in human carotid artery bifurcations. mboxemphAm. J. Physiol. Heart Circ. Physiol. **2016**, *310*, H639–H647. [CrossRef]
21. Syarif, I.; Prugel-Bennett, A.; Wills, G. SVM Parameter Optimization using Grid Search and Genetic Algorithm to Improve Classification Performance. *Telkomnika* **2016**, *14*, 1502. [CrossRef]
22. Zhu, Y.; Wu, J.; Fang, Y. Study on application of SVM in prediction of coronary heart disease. *J. Biomed. Eng.* **2013**, *30*, 1180–1185.
23. Chang, C.C.; Lin, C.J. LIBSVM: A library for support vector machines. *ACM Trans. Intell. Syst. Technol.* **2011**, *2*, 27. [CrossRef]
24. Nalepa, J.; Kawulok, M. Selecting training sets for support vector machines: A review. *Artif. Intell. Rev.* **2018**, *52*, 857–900. [CrossRef]
25. Abdar, M.; Książek, W.; Acharya, U.R.; Tan, R.-S.; Makarenkov, V.; Pławiak, P. A new machine learning technique for an accurate diagnosis of coronary artery disease. *Comput. Methods Programs Biomed.* **2019**, *179*, 104992–105003. [CrossRef] [PubMed]
26. Abdar, M.; Acharya, U.R.; Sarrafzadegan, N.; Makarenkov, V. NE-nu-SVC: A New Nested Ensemble Clinical Decision Support System for Effective Diagnosis of Coronary Artery Disease. *IEEE Access* **2019**, *7*, 167605–167620. [CrossRef]
27. Singh, R.S.; Saini, B.S.; Sunkaria, R.K. Detection of coronary artery disease by reduced features and extreme learning machine. *Clujul Med.* **2018**, *91*, 166–175. [CrossRef]
28. Awad, M.; Khanna, R. Support Vector Machines for Classification. In *Efficient Learning Machines: Theories, Concepts, and Applications for Engineers and System Designers*; Awad, M., Khanna, R., Eds.; Apress: Berkeley, CA, USA, 2015; pp. 39–66. [CrossRef]
29. Yu, W.; Liu, T.; Valdez, R.; Gwinn, M.; Khoury, M.J. Application of support vector machine modeling for prediction of common diseases: The case of diabetes and pre-diabetes. *BMC Med. Inform. Decis. Mak.* **2010**, *10*, 16. [CrossRef]
30. Patle, A.; Chouhan, D.S. SVM kernel functions for classification. In Proceedings of the 2013 International Conference on Advances in Technology and Engineering (ICATE), Mumbai, India, 23–25 January 2013; pp. 1–9.
31. Rudd, J.M. Application of Support Vector Machine Modeling and Graph Theory Metrics for Disease Classification. *Model Assist. Stat. Appl.* **2017**, *13*, 341–349. [CrossRef]
32. Brank, J.; Grobelnik, M.; Milic-Frayling, N.; Mladenic, D. Feature selection using support vector machines. In *Data Mining III*; Zanasi, A., Ed.; WIT: Southampton, UK, 2002; pp. 261–273.
33. Chen, Y.-W.; Lin, C.-J. Combining SVMs with Various Feature Selection Strategies. *Feature Extr.* **2005**, *207*, 315–324. [CrossRef]
34. Cho, B.H.; Yu, H.; Kim, K.W.; Kim, T.H.; Kim, I.Y.; Kim, S.I. Application of irregular and unbalanced data to predict diabetic nephropathy using visualization and feature selection methods. *Artif. Intell. Med.* **2008**, *42*, 37–53. [CrossRef]
35. Trivedi, S.; Dey, S.; Shikhar, P. Effect of various kernels and feature selection methods on SVM performance for detecting email spams. *Int. J. Comput. Appl.* **2013**, *66*, 18–23.
36. Leo, M.; Carcagnì, P.; Mazzeo, P.L.; Spagnolo, P.; Cazzato, D.; Distante, C. Analysis of Facial Information for Healthcare Applications: A Survey on Computer Vision-Based Approaches. *Information* **2020**, *11*, 128. [CrossRef]
37. Pannese, E. Morphological changes in nerve cells during normal aging. *Brain Struct. Funct.* **2011**, *216*, 85–89. [CrossRef]
38. Subramaniyam, A.; Mahapatra, R.P.; Singh, P. Taylor and Gradient Descent-Based Actor Critic Neural Network for the Classification of Privacy Preserved Medical Data. *Big Data* **2019**, *7*, 176–191. [CrossRef]
39. Zomorodi-moghadam, M.; Abdar, M.; Davarzani, Z.; Zhou, X.; Pławiak, P.; Acharya, U.R. Hybrid particle swarm optimization for rule discovery in the diagnosis of coronary artery disease. *Expert Syst.* **2019**, *2019*, 1–17. [CrossRef]
40. Betancur, J.; Hu, L.H.; Commandeur, F.; Sharir, T.; Einstein, A.J.; Fish, M.B.; Ruddy, T.D.; Kaufmann, P.A.; Sinusas, A.J.; Miller, E.J.; et al. Deep Learning Analysis of Upright-Supine High-Efficiency SPECT Myocardial Perfusion Imaging for Prediction of Obstructive Coronary Artery Disease: A Multicenter Study. *J. Nucl. Med.* **2019**, *60*, 664–670. [CrossRef] [PubMed]

41. Qin, C.-J.; Guan, Q.; Wang, X.-P. Application of Ensemble Algorithm Integrating Multiple Criteria Feature Selection in Coronary Heart Disease Detection. *Biomed. Eng. Appl. Basis Commun.* **2017**, *29*. [CrossRef]
42. Raghavendra, U.; Fujita, H.; Gudigar, A.; Shetty, R.; Nayak, K.; Malpe, U.; Samanth, J.; Acharya, U.R. Automated technique for coronary artery disease characterization and classification using DD-DTDWT in ultrasound images. *Biomed. Signal Process. Control* **2017**, *40*, 324–334. [CrossRef]
43. Alizadehsani, R.; Habibi, J.; Hosseini, M.J.; Mashayekhi, H.; Boghrati, R.; Ghandeharioun, A.; Bahadorian, B.; Sani, Z.A. A data mining approach for diagnosis of coronary artery disease. *Comput. Methods Programs Biomed.* **2013**, *111*, 52–61. [CrossRef]
44. Alizadehsani, R.; Zangooei, M.H.; Hosseini, M.J.; Habibi, J.; Khosravi, A.; Roshanzamir, M.; Khozeimeh, F.; Sarrafzadegan, N.; Nahavandi, S. Coronary artery disease detection using computational intelligence methods. *Knowl. Based Syst.* **2016**, *109*, 187–197. [CrossRef]
45. Acharya, U.R.; Sree, S.V.; Muthu Rama Krishnan, M.; Krishnananda, N.; Ranjan, S.; Umesh, P.; Suri, J.S. Automated classification of patients with coronary artery disease using grayscale features from left ventricle echocardiographic images. *Comput. Methods Programs Biomed.* **2013**, *112*, 624–632. [CrossRef] [PubMed]

2

3D Deep Learning on Medical Images

Satya P. Singh [1,2], Lipo Wang [3], Sukrit Gupta [4], Haveesh Goli [4], Parasuraman Padmanabhan [1,2,*] and Balázs Gulyás [1,2,5]

1 Lee Kong Chian School of Medicine, Nanyang Technological University, Singapore 608232, Singapore; satya@ntu.edu.sg (S.P.S.); balazs.gulyas@ntu.edu.sg (B.G.)
2 Cognitive Neuroimaging Centre, Nanyang Technological University, Singapore 636921, Singapore
3 School of Electrical and Electronic Engineering, Nanyang Technological University, Singapore 639798, Singapore; elpwang@ntu.edu.sg
4 School of Computer Science and Engineering, Nanyang Technological University, Singapore 639798, Singapore; SUKRIT001@e.ntu.edu.sg (S.G.); HAVEESH001@e.ntu.edu.sg (H.G.)
5 Department of Clinical Neuroscience, Karolinska Institute, 17176 Stockholm, Sweden
* Correspondence: ppadmanabhan@ntu.edu.sg

Abstract: The rapid advancements in machine learning, graphics processing technologies and the availability of medical imaging data have led to a rapid increase in the use of deep learning models in the medical domain. This was exacerbated by the rapid advancements in convolutional neural network (CNN) based architectures, which were adopted by the medical imaging community to assist clinicians in disease diagnosis. Since the grand success of AlexNet in 2012, CNNs have been increasingly used in medical image analysis to improve the efficiency of human clinicians. In recent years, three-dimensional (3D) CNNs have been employed for the analysis of medical images. In this paper, we trace the history of how the 3D CNN was developed from its machine learning roots, we provide a brief mathematical description of 3D CNN and provide the preprocessing steps required for medical images before feeding them to 3D CNNs. We review the significant research in the field of 3D medical imaging analysis using 3D CNNs (and its variants) in different medical areas such as classification, segmentation, detection and localization. We conclude by discussing the challenges associated with the use of 3D CNNs in the medical imaging domain (and the use of deep learning models in general) and possible future trends in the field.

Keywords: 3D convolutional neural networks; 3D medical images; classification; segmentation; detection; localization

1. Introduction

Medical images have varied characteristics depending on the target organ and the suspected diagnosis. Common modalities used for medical imaging include X-ray, computed tomography (CT), diffusion tensor imaging (DTI), positron emission tomography (PET), magnetic resonance imaging (MRI), and functional MRI (fMRI) [1–4]. In the past thirty years, these radiological image acquisition technologies have enormously improved in terms of acquisition time, image quality, resolution [5–8] and have become more affordable. Despite improvements in hardware, all radiological images require subsequent image analysis and diagnosis by trained human radiologists [9]. Besides the significant time and economic costs involved in training radiologists, radiologists also suffer from limitations due to their lack of experience, time and fatigue. This becomes especially significant because of an increasing number of radiological images due to the aging population and more prevalent scanning technologies that put additional stress on radiologists [9–12]. This puts a focus on automated machine learning algorithms that can play a crucial role in assisting clinicians in alleviating their onerous workloads.

Deep learning refers to learning patterns in data samples using neural networks containing multiple interconnected layers of artificial neurons [11]. An artificial neuron by analogy to a biological neuron is something that takes multiple inputs, performs a simple computation and produces an output. This simple computation has the form of a linear function of the inputs followed by an activation function (usually non-linear). Examples of some commonly used non-linear activation functions are the hyperbolic tangent (tanh), sigmoid transformation and the rectified linear unit (ReLU) and their variants [13]. The development of deep learning can be traced back to Walter Pitts and Warren McCulloch (1943). Their work has been followed by significant advancements due to the development of the backpropagation model (1960), convolutional neural networks (CNN) (1979), long short-term memory (LSTM) (1997), ImageNet (2009) and AlexNet (2011) [14]. In 2014, Google presented GoogLeNet (Winner of ILSVRC 2014 challenge) [15], which introduced the concept of inception modules that drastically reduced the computational complexity of CNN. Deep learning is essentially a reincarnation of the artificial neural network where we stack layer upon layer of artificial neurons. Using the outputs of the terminal layers built on the outputs of previous layers, we can start to describe arbitrarily complex patterns. In the CNN [14], network features are generated by convolving kernels in a layer with outputs of the previous layers, such that the first hidden layer kernels perform convolutions on the input images. While the features captured by early hidden layers are generally shapes, curves or edges, deeper hidden layers capture more abstract and complex features.

Historical methods for automated classification of images involves extensive rule-based algorithms or manual feature handcrafting [16–21], which are time-consuming, have poor generalization capacity and require domain knowledge. All this changed with the advent and demonstrated the success of CNNs. CNNs are devoid of any manual feature handcrafting, require little preprocessing and are translation-invariant [22]. In CNNs, low-level image features are extracted by the initial layers of filters and progressively higher features are learnt by successive layers before classification. The commonly seen X-ray is an example of a two-dimensional (2D) medical image. The machine learning of these medical images is no different from CNNs applied to classify natural images in recent years, e.g., the ImageNet Large Scale Visual Recognition Competition [14]. With decreasing computational costs and powerful graphics processing (units (GPUs) available, it has become possible to analyze three-dimensional (3D) medical images, such as CT, DTI, fMRI, Ultrasound and MRI scans [14] using 3D deep learning. These scans give detailed three-dimensional images of human organs and can be used to detect infection, cancers, traumatic injuries and abnormalities in blood vessels and organs. The major drawback in the application of 3D deep learning on medical images is the limited availability of data and high computational cost. Further, there is a problem of the curse of dimensionality. However, with the recent advancements in neural network architectures, data augmentation techniques and high-end GPUs, it is becoming possible to analyze the volumetric medical data using 3D deep learning. Consequently, since 2012, we have seen exponential growth in the applications of 3D deep learning in different medical image modalities. Here, we present a systematic review of the applications of 3D deep learning in medical imaging with possible future directions. To the best of our knowledge, this is the first review paper of 3D deep learning on medical images.

2. Materials and Methods

In a very short time, deep learning techniques have become an alternative to many machine learning algorithms that were traditionally used in medical imaging. We explored various terms used in medical imaging literature to understand the trend in using deep learning in medical imaging applications. We searched for 'machine learning + medical' in the title and abstract in PubMed publication database (on 9 July 2020) and across a predictable trend of using more and more similar data in different approaches (Figure 1). We observed a similar trend for the query 'deep learning + medical', albeit with few publications before 2015. However, while searching for the query '3D deep learning + medical' in the title and abstract, we see a different scenario. An exponential increase can be seen for 'deep learning' and '3D deep learning' after 2015 and 2017 onwards, respectively. This signifies that, while there was not much work in the domain a few years ago, there has been an accelerated rise in the number of publications related to deep learning for both 2D and 3D images.

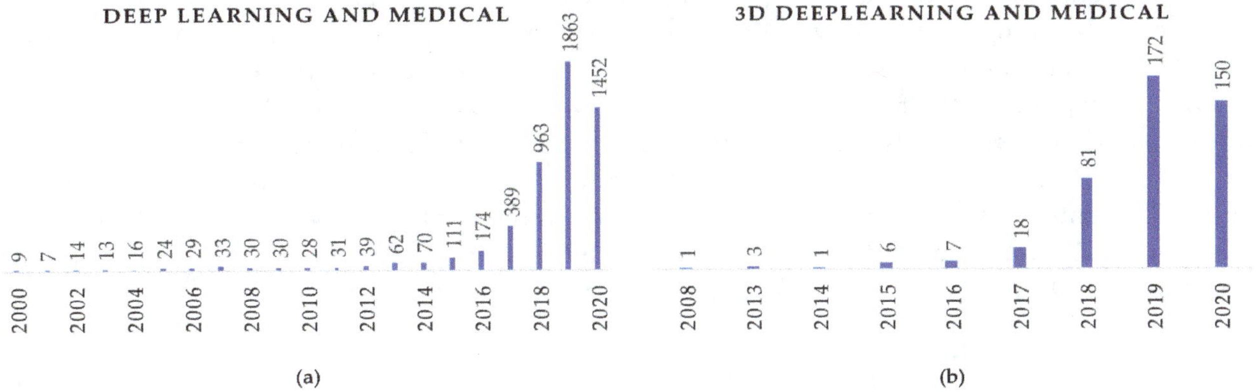

Figure 1. Year-wise number of publications in PubMed while searching for 'deep learning + medical' and '3D deep learning + medical' in the title and abstract in PubMed publication database (as at 1 July 2020).

In this systematic review, we searched for the applications of 3D deep learning in medical image segmentation, classification, detection and localization. For the literature search, we chose three database platforms, namely Google Scholar, PubMed and Scopus. The application of 3D CNN effectively came into the picture after the remarkable success of AlexNet in 2012, which was enabled by advanced parallel computing architecture. Between 2015 and 2016, we have seen exponential growth in the literature related to 3D deep learning in medical imaging, and therefore, we limited our search to after 1 January 2012. The first search was performed on 12 September 2019, and the second search on 1 January 2020, while the third search was performed on 1 July 2020. The literature search and selection for the study were done according to the preferred reporting items for systematic seviews and meta-analyses (PRISMA) statement [23]. We searched for title and abstract with different keyword combination of "3D CNN", "medical imaging", "classification", "segmentation", "detection" and "localization" and selected 31,576 records. 11,987 duplicate records were removed. After studying the title and abstract, we further removed 19,380 records. We further excluded 77 records. Finally, we collected 132 papers for our review purpose. The details about the inclusion and exclusion of papers according to the PRISMA statement is depicted in Figure 2.

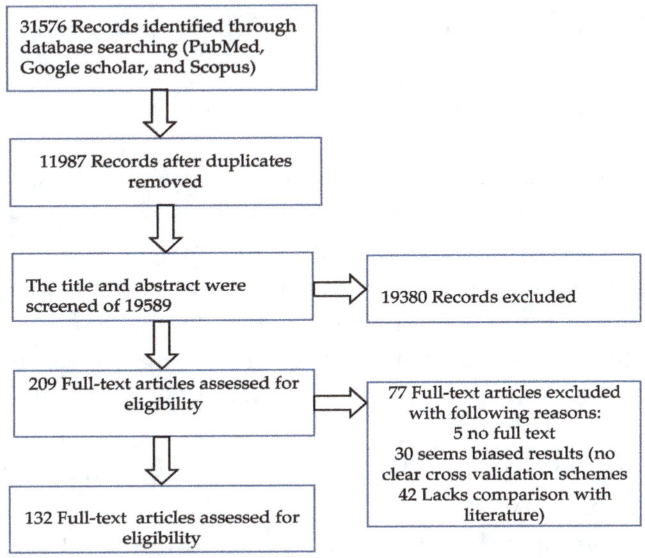

Figure 2. Criteria for literature selection for systematic review according to preferred reporting items for systematic seviews and meta-analyses (PRISMA) [23] guidelines.

2.1. A Typical Architecture of 3D CNN

A typical architecture of CNN may include four basic components: (1) local receptive field, (2) sharing weights, (3) pooling and (4) fully connected (fc) layers. Deep CNN architecture is constructed by stacking several convolutional layers and pooling layers and one or so fully connected layers at the end of the network [9,24]. While 1D CNN can extract spectral features from the data, 2D CNN can extract spatial features from the input data. However, 3D CNNs can take advantage of both 1D and 2D CNNs by extracting both spectral and spatial features simultaneously from the input volume. These 3D CNN features are very useful in analyzing the volumetric data in medical imaging. The mathematical formulation of 3D CNN is very similar to 2D CNN with an extra dimension added. The basic architecture of 3D CNN is shown in Figure 3. We briefly discuss the mathematical background of 3D CNN.

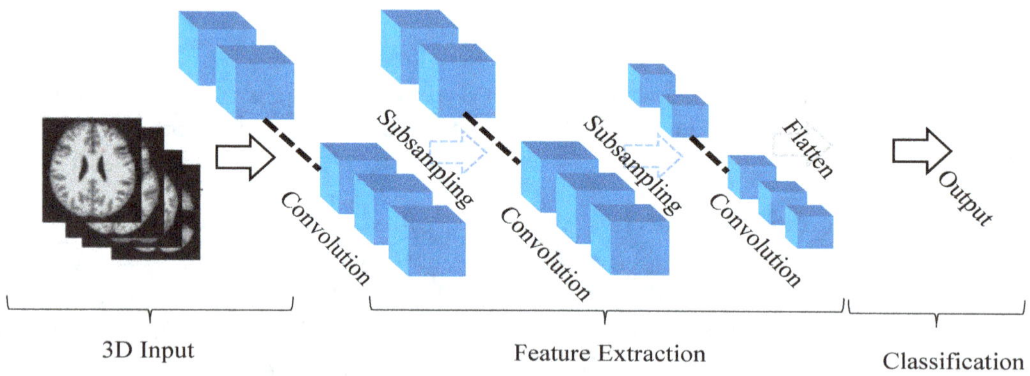

Figure 3. Typical architecture of 3D CNN.

Convolutional Layer: The basic definition, principle, and working equation of 3D CNN is quite similar to 2D CNN. We only add an extra dimension of depth to the working equation of 2D CNN. Suppose 3D CNN of input x has a dimension of $M \times N \times D$ with i, j, k as iterators. The kernel ω with dimensions $n1 \times n2 \times n3$ has iterator a, b, c. We denote ℓ is the ℓth, where $\ell = 1$ is the first layer and $\ell = L$ is the last layer. We denote y^{ℓ} and b^{ℓ} as the output and the bias unit the ℓth layer. To compute the nonlinear input $x^{\ell}_{i,j,k}$ to (i, j, k)th unit in layer ℓ, we add up the weight contribution from the previous layer as follows:

$$x^{\ell}_{i,j,k} = \sum_{a} \sum_{b} \sum_{c} \omega_{a,b,c} y^{\ell-1}_{(i+a)(j+b)(k+c)} + b^{\ell}. \tag{1}$$

The output of the (i, j)th unit in the 'ℓth' convolutional layer is given as follows:

$$y^{\ell}_{i,j,k} = f\left(x^{\ell}_{i,j,k}\right). \tag{2}$$

Pooling Layer: Each feature map in the convolutional layer of 3D CNN can be a pooling layer. There are two kinds of pooling. If the pooling layer averages across the group of input voxels, it is called average pooling, while if it obtains a maximum of the input voxels, it is called maximum pooling. The output of the pooling layer will be the input of the next layer. Since a small shift in the input image results in a shift in activation function, the pooling layer also introduces some translational invariance to the 3D CNN. To lower the sampling effect of pooling, we can remove the pooling layer by increasing the number of strides in the preceding CNN layer [25]. This will not result in any significant depreciation of the performance. However, by doing this, we significantly reduce the overlap in the CNN layer that precedes the pooling layer. This is simply equivalent to the pooling operation where only the top-left features are considered.

Dropout regularization: Deep neural networks with a large number of parameters are very dominant learning systems. Multiple deep nonlinear hidden layers allow them to learn complex relationships between input and outputs. However, with the limited training data, these complex relationships introduce sampling noise, which appears in training data sets but not in real test datasets even if both are drawn from the same distribution. This scenario leads to overfitting and there have been several strategies [26] to tackle the problem, such as early stopping of the training epochs and weight penalties (L1 and L2 regularizations, soft weight sharing, and pooling). Ensemble models of several CNNs with different configurations on the same dataset are known for their overfitting. However, this leads to extra computational and maintenance cost for training several models. Moreover, training a large network requires large datasets, but the availability of such datasets in the field of medical imaging is very rare. Even if one can train large networks with a versatile setting of parameters, testing these networks is not feasible in a real-time situation due to the nature of medical imaging systems. In the case of ensemble models, a CNN model can also simulate multiple configurations just by probabilistically dropping out edges and nodes. Dropout is a kind of regularization technique to reduce overfitting by temporarily dropping a unit out of the network [27]. This simple idea shows a significant improvement in CNN performance.

Batch normalization: The input of each hidden layer dynamically changes during training because the parameters in the previous layer update at each training epoch. If these changes are large, the search for an optimal hyperparameter becomes difficult for the network and may be computationally expensive to reach an optimal value. This problem can be solved by an algorithm called batch normalization, which was proposed by two researchers [28]. Batch normalization allows the use of a higher learning rate and thereby achieves the optimal value in less time. It facilitates the smooth training of deeper network architectures in less time. The normalization of data from a particular batch is about finding the mean and variance of the data points from mini-batch and normalizing them to have a zero mean and unit variance.

In backward pass, the CNN adjusts its weights and parameters according to the output by calculating the error through some loss functions, e (other names are cost function and error function) and backpropagating the error with some rules towards the input. The loss is calculated by taking the partial derivative of e w.r.t., which is the output of each neuron in that layer, such as $\partial e / y^{\ell}_{i,j,k}$ for the output, $y^{\ell}_{i,j,k}$ of $(i, j, k)^{th}$ unit in layer ℓ. The cFhain rule allows us to write and add up the contribution of each variable as follows:

$$\frac{\partial e}{\partial x^{\ell}_{i,j,k}} = \frac{\partial e}{\partial y^{\ell}_{i,j,k}} \frac{\partial f\left(y^{\ell}_{i,j,k}\right)}{\partial x^{\ell}_{i,j,k}} = \frac{\partial e}{\partial y^{\ell}_{i,j,k}} f'\left(x^{\ell}_{i,j,k}\right)\#. \tag{3}$$

Weights in the previous convolutional layer can be updated by backpropagating the error to the previous layer according to the following equation:

$$\frac{\partial e}{\partial y^{\ell-1}_{i,j,k}} = \sum_{a=0}^{n1-1} \sum_{b=0}^{n2-1} \sum_{c=0}^{n3-1} \frac{\partial e}{\partial x^{\ell}_{(i-a),(j-b),(k-c)}} \frac{\partial x^{\ell}_{(i-a),(j-b),(j-b)}}{\partial y^{\ell-1}_{i,j,k}}. \tag{4}$$

$$= \sum_{a=0}^{n1-1} \sum_{a=0}^{n2-1} \sum_{b=0}^{n3-1} \frac{\partial e}{\partial x^{\ell}_{(i-a),(j-b),(k-c)}} \omega_{a,b,c}. \tag{5}$$

Equation (5) allows us to calculate the error for the previous layer. Further, the above eq. makes sense for those points which are n times away from each side of the input data. This situation can be avoided by simply padding with zeros to the end of each side of the input volume.

2.2. *Breakthroughs in CNN Architectural Advances*

Several different versions of CNN have been proposed in the literature to improve model performance. In 2011, Krizhevsky et al. [14] presented a deep CNN architecture. A systematic architecture of AlexNet is shown in Figure 4. AlexNet has five convolutional layers and three fully connected layers (the last FC layer was the SoftMax layer). The network was trained on 1.2 million images with 60 million parameters. To tackle these large parameters, AlexNet was trained on a multi-GPU (2-GPUs, 3GB GTX-580) environment by systematically distributing the neurons on both the GPUs. Data augmentation and dropouts were used to avoid overfitting. Data augmentation was done in two ways: (1) image translations and horizontal reflections, and (2) changing the intensity of RGB channels. The AlexNet architecture has won ILSVRC-2012 (ImageNet Large Scale Visual Recognition Competition-2012) with a large margin. The difference between the top-five test errors of AlexNet (15.3%) and the second prize winner (26.2%) was around 10%.

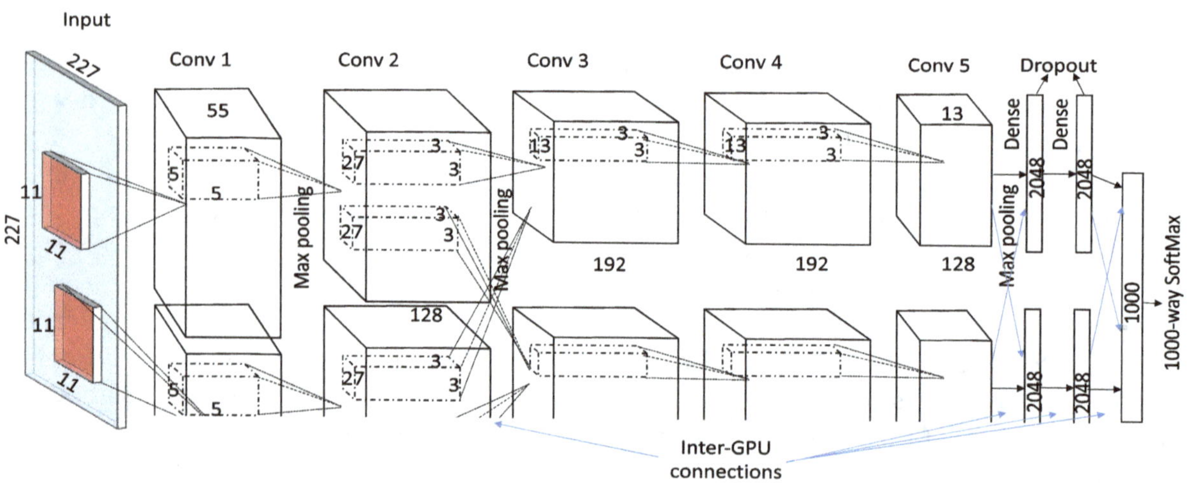

Figure 4. A typical architecture of AlexNet [14].

In 2014, Simonyan and Zisserman [29] presented a more profound deep network architecture called VGGNet (Visual Geometry Group Network) (16 layers and 19 layers) for the ImageNet Challenge 2014 and secured the first position for the localization task and the second position for the classification task. VGGNet uses 3 × 3 filters for convolutional layers and three consecutive fully connected layers 4096, 4096, and 1000 in size, respectively. The design of VGGNet is quite similar to AlexNet. Adding consecutive layers to the network increases the number of parameters that cause networks to suffer from errors and overfitting. In supervising learning, the deeper network requires large data for training and despite the use of data augmentation techniques, it may happen that the data is not sufficient. Further, annotating such a large amount of data can be quite expensive. Furthermore, because a linear increase in the filter emerges as a result of a quadratic increase in computational burden, deeper networks lead us to a computational explosion. In deeper layers, weights can be near zero and emerge as a waste of computational resources. Fast forwarding from 2012, in 2014, the designers at Google presented the concept of "Inception" based on the Hebbian principle and the intuition of multiple-scale processing, and the network was called GoogLeNet (also known as Inception-V1) [15]. The intuition behind the inception module (version V1) (Figure 5a) is that the optimal neural network topology can be built by clustering neurons to the correlation statistics in the input images. The authors analyzed the correlation statistics in the activations in the previous layer and clustered the neurons with highly correlated outputs for the next layer. In the images, the correlation tends to be local, and therefore, performing convolutions over the local patches can cluster the neurons. In lower layers, there exists a high correlation between local pixels in a surrounding patch. These pixels can be covered by a small 1 × 1 convolution. Besides, the correlation between a smaller number of spatially spread-out clusters can be quantified by 3 × 3 and 5 × 5 convolutions. In order take effect of 1 × 1, 3 × 3 and 5 × 5, the authors stacked them as a single output vector for the next layer (Figure 5a). In addition, to take the advantages of maximum (max)-pooling, they also concatenated a pooling layer in parallel (3 × 3 max pooling branch in Figure 5a). The model size of GoogLeNet was 12 times less than AlexNet's and required relatively net-lower memory and power than AlexNet. In addition,

GoogLeNet's computational cost was less than 2× that of AlexNet, while AlexNet was a network of eight layers and GoogLeNet was a network of 22 layers. Due to its high accuracy, fewer parameters and low power consumption, GoogLeNet was more suitable for mobile platforms. GoogLeNet has secured the first position in the ImageNet Large-Scale Visual Recognition Challenge 2014 (ILSVRC14). The concept of the inception module in GoogLeNet alleviates the problem of vanishing gradients and allows us to move deeper into the network. In the event of increasing computational complexity, the authors suggest reducing network dimensions by introducing Inception-V2 and Inception-V3. [30]. In inception-V2, inexpensive 1×1 convolution convolutions were inserted before the expensive 3×3 and 5×5 convolutions. In addition, in this module, the 1×1 convolution used ReLU activation. It was also suggested that the incorporation of inception layers would benefit if inserted in higher-order layers. Since the architecture of the GoogLeNet was rather deep, the designers were also concerned about the problem of gradient vanishing in the hidden layers during back-propagation. Since the intermediate layers in the network had a higher representation of the input image, they had more discriminative power. In Reference [31], the authors presented the concept of Inception-V4 by appending the auxiliary classifiers to the intermediate layers. Since the FC connected layers were generally prone to error, in order to avoid overfitting, the authors replaced the FC layers with average pooling layers.

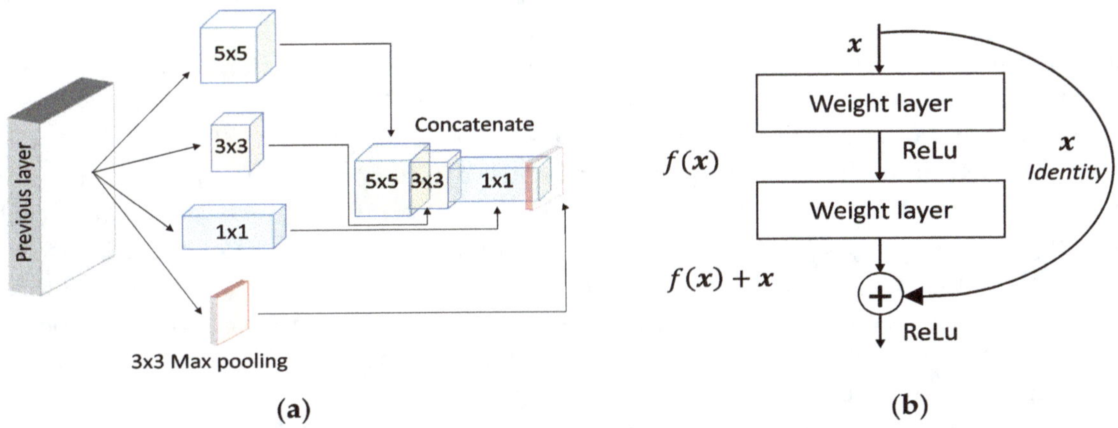

Figure 5. (**a**) The intuition behind the inception (V1) module in GoogLeNet. Screening local clusters with 1×1 convolutional operations, screening spread-out clusters with 3×3, screening even more spread-out clusters with 5×5 convolutional operations, and finally conceiving the inception module by concatenating (**b**) residual building block in ResNet.

Very deep architectural neural networks are often difficult to train due to the problem of vanishing and exploding gradients. Considering a shallow CNN and its deeper counterpart with more layers, a deeper model is theoretically just needed to copy the output from the shallow model with identity mappings. Therefore, the constructed solution suggests that the deeper model must not produce higher errors than the shallow model. However, the identity functions are not easy to learn, and therefore, in Reference [32], He et al. presented ResNet by reformulating the layers as residual learning functions. ResNet uses skip connections, which allows us to take the activation from one layer and suddenly feed it to another layer. Original ResNet uses batch normalization after each convolutional layer and before the activation. Using these skip connections, we can train very deep network architectures, ranging from 52 to 10,000 layers. ResNet is one of the most popular deep learning architectures in the literature. Figure 5b shows the basic concept of residual connection, which is the building block of ResNet. The authors trained 152 layers deep ResNet (11.3 billion FLOPs) on ImageNet against VGGNet-19 (15.3/19.3 billion FLOPs) and obtained state-of-the-art results. This was about eight times deeper than VGGNet, but in terms of the floating-point operation measurement, it has less computation. With a 3.57% test error on the ImageNet dataset, ResNet secured first place in ILSVRC-2015. Inspired by the power of the inception module from GoogLeNet and residual connections from ResNet [32], the research team from Google further presented Inception-ResNet [31]. They showed that the residual connections accelerate training in the inception network and thereby improved the performance of the Inception network. Continuous concatenation of convolutional layers on the top of activations will make the training worse. Ronneberger et al. [33] proposed U-Net, which was the winner of the ISBI cell tracking challenge 2015 for biomedical image segmentation tasks. U-Net can be trained with a relatively small number of samples and achieves high accuracy in a short time. U-Net involves the symmetrical expansion and contraction paths with skip connections. In 2016, Cicek et al. [34] presented a modified version of the original U-Net i.e., 3D U-Net for volumetric segmentation from sparse notation.

3. 3D Medical Imaging Pre-Processing

Preprocessing of the image dataset before feeding the CNN or other classifiers is important for all types of imaging modalities. Several preprocessing steps are recommended for the medical images before they are fed as input to the deep neural network model, such as (1) artifact removal, (2) normalization, (3) slice timing correction (STC), (4) image registration and (5) bias field correction. While all the steps, (1) to (5), help in getting reliable results, STC and image registration are very important in the case of 3D medical images (especially MR and CT images). Artifact removal and normalization are the most performed preprocessing steps across the modalities. We briefly discuss pre-processing steps above.

The first part of any preprocessing pipeline is the removal of artifacts. For example, we may be interested in removing skulls in brain CT scans before feeding to 3D CNN. Removal of extracerebral tissues is highly recommended before analyzing the T1 or T2 weighted MRI, and DTI modalities for brain images. fMRI data often contains transient spike artifacts or a slowed over drift time. Thus, the principal component analysis technique can be used to look at these spike related artifacts [3,35,36]. Before feeding the data for preprocessing to an automated pipeline, a manual check is also advisable. For example, if the input T1 anatomical data is large, the FSL's BET command will not perform proper brain region extraction, and if we use images with artifacts for the popular fMRI preprocessing tool fMRIprep [37], it fails as well. Therefore, to remove these extra neck tissues, we should perform other necessary preprocessing steps.

The brain and other body parts for the imaging of every person can vary in shape and size. Hence, it is advisable to normalize brain scans before further processing [4,38–41]. Due to the characteristics of imaging modalities, the same scanning device can essentially have different intensities even in the same patient's medical images. Since scanning of patients may be performed in different light conditions, intensity normalization also plays an important role in the performance of 3D CNN. Besides, for a typical CNN, each input channel (i.e., sequence) is normalized to have a zero mean and unit variance within the training set. Parameter normalization within the CNN also affects the CNN performance.

To create a volumetric representation of the brain, we often sample several slices in the brain for each repetition time (TR). However, each slice is typically sampled at slightly different time points as we acquire them sequentially [42,43]. Hence, even though the 3D brain volume should be scanned instantaneously, in practical terms, there is always some delay in sampling the first and the last slice. This is a key problem that needs to be considered and accounted before performing any further tasks like classification or segmentation. In this regard, STC is frequently employed for adjusting the temporal misalignment and is widely utilized by a range of software such as SPM and FSL [44]. Several types of techniques have been proposed based on data interpolation methods for STC, including cubic spline, linear and CNC interpolation [45]. In general, the STC methods based on interpolation techniques can be grouped as scene-based and object-based. In the scene-based approach, the interpolated pixel intensity is revealed by the pixel intensity of a slice. While the interpolation techniques are sub-standard, they are relatively simple and easy to implement. However, object-based methods have much better accuracy and are reliable, but they are computationally expensive. Subsequently, cubic spline and other polynomials were also found in medical image interpolation. Essentially, all these strategies perform strength averaging of the neighboring pixels without forming any feature deformation. Therefore, the resultant in-between pixels have negative blurring effects within the object boundary. Cubic interpolation is the standard technique selected in BrainVoyager [46] software.

Medical imaging is becoming increasingly multimodal, whereby images of the same patient from different modalities are acquired to provide information about different organ features. Additionally, situations also arise where multiple images of the same patient and location are acquired with different orientations. It was necessary to match the images by visual comparison in this case [47]. This alignment or registration of the images to a standard template can also be automated, which helps to locate repetitive locations of abnormalities. The image alignment not only makes it easier to manually analyze images and locate lesions or other abnormalities, but also makes it easier to train a 3D CNN on these images [48–50].

MRI images are corrupted by a low-frequency and smooth bias field signal produced by MRI scanners, thereby affecting pixel intensities to fluctuate [51,52]. The bias field usually appears due to improper image acquisition from the scanner, and influences machine learning algorithms that perform classification and segmentation using pixel intensities. It is, therefore, important to either remove the bias field artifacts from sample images or incorporate this artifact into the model before training on these images.

4. Applications in 3D Medical Imaging

4.1. Segmentation

For several years, machine learning and artificial intelligence algorithms have been facilitating radiologists in the segmentation of medical images, such as breast cancer mammograms, brain tumors, brain lesions, skull stripping, etc. Segmentation not only helps to focus on specific regions in the medical image, but also helps expert radiologists in quantitative assessment, and planning further treatment. Several researchers have contributed to the use of 3D CNN in medical image segmentation. Here, we focus on the important related works of medical image segmentation using 3D CNN.

Lesion segmentation is probably the most challenging task in medical imaging because lesions are rather small in most of the cases. Further, there are considerable variations in their sizes across different scans that can cause imbalances in training samples. In this regard, Deep Medic [53] is a popular work, which also won the ISLES 2015 competition. In DeepMedic, a 3D CNN architecture has been introduced for automatic brain lesion segmentation, which gives a state-of-the-art performance on 3D volumetric brain scans. The multiresolution approach has been utilized to include local as well as the spatial contextual information. The network gives a 3D map of where the network believes the lesions are located. DeepMedic was implemented on datasets where patients suffered from traumatic brain injuries due to accidents and were also shown to work well for classification and detection problems in head images to detect brain tumors. This work was carried forward by Kamnitsas et al. [54] during the brain tumor segmentation (BRATS) 2016 challenge where the authors took advantage of residual connections in 3D CNN (Figure 6). The results were impressive and were in the top 20 teams with median Dice scores of 0.898 (whole tumor, WT), 0.75 (tumor core, TC) and 0.72 (enhancing core, EC). Following DeepMedic, Casamitjana et al. [55] proposed a 3D CNN to process the entire 3D volume in a single pass to make predictions.

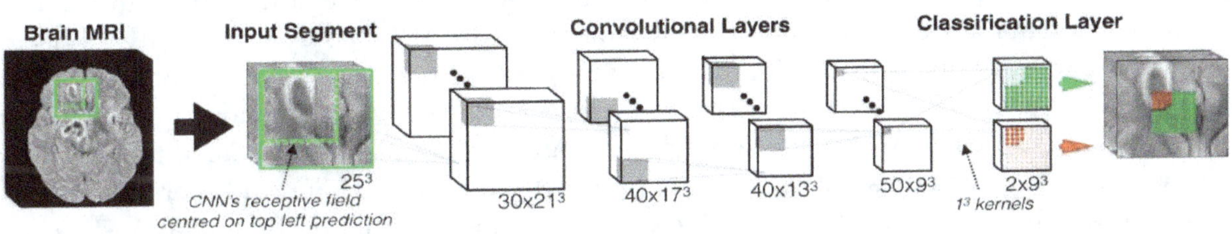

Figure 6. The baseline architecture of 3D convolution neural network (CNN) for lesion segmentation. The figure is slightly modified from [54].

Besides constraints in acquiring enough training samples, class imbalance also pervades in the medical imaging domain, whereby samples of the diseased patients are hard to come by. This issue is further exacerbated in problems related to the tumor or lesion segmentation because the sizes of tumors or lesions are usually small when compared to the whole scan volume. In this context, Zhou et al. [56] proposed 3D CNN (3D variant of FusionNet) for brain tumor segmentation on the BRATS 2018 challenge. The authors split the multiclass tumor segmentation problem into three separate segmentation tasks for the deep 3D CNN model, i.e., (i) coarse segmentation for whole tumor, (ii) refined segmentation for Wavelet transform (WT) and intraclass tumor, and (iii) precise segmentation for a brain tumor. Their model has ranked first for the BRATS 2015 dataset and third (among 64 teams) on the BRATS 2017 validation dataset. Ronneberger et al. proposed the U-Net architecture for the segmentation of 2D biomedical images [33] They made use of up-sampling layers, which in turn enabled the architecture for segmentation besides classification. However, the original U-Net was not too deep as there was a single pooling layer after the convolution layer. Further, this only analyzed 2D images and did not fully exploit the spatial and texture information that can be obtained from the 3D volumes. To solve these issues, Chen et al. [57] proposed a separable 3D U-Net for brain tumor segmentation. On BRATS 2018 challenge dataset, they achieved dice scores of 0.749 (EC), 0.893 (WT) and 0.830 (TC). Kayalibay et al. [58] presented a modified 3D U-Net architecture for brain tumor segmentation where they introduce some nonlinearity in the traditional U-Net architecture by inserting residual blocks during up-sampling, thus facilitating the gradients to flow easily. The proposed architecture also intrinsically handles the class imbalance problem that arises due to the use of the Jaccard loss function. However, the proposed architecture was computationally expensive owing to the large size of the receptive field used. Isensee et al. [59] proposed a 3D U-Net architecture, which consists of a perspective collection pathway for brain tumor segmentation. The strategy encodes progressively abstract interpretations of the input as we move deeper and adds a localization pathway that recombines these interpretations with features for lower layers. By hypothesizing that semantic features are easy to learn and process, Peng et al. [60] presented a multi-scale 3D U-Net for brain tumor segmentation. Their model consists of several 3D U-Net blocks for capturing long-distance spatial resolutions. The upsampling was done at different resolutions to capture meaningful features. On the BRATS 2015 challenge dataset, they achieved 0.893 (WT), 0.830 (TC) and 0.742 (EC). Some important developments in 3D CNN for brain tumor/lesion segmentation applications on BRATS challenges are summarized in Table 1.

While brain tumor or lesion segmentation is used to detect glioblastoma, brain stroke or traumatic brain injuries, multiple deep learning solutions are being proposed for the segmentation of brain lobes or deep brain structures. Milletari et al. [61] combined a Hough voting approach with 2D, 2.5D and 3D CNN to segment volumetric data of MRI scans. However, these networks still suffer from the class imbalance problem. In Reference [62], a 3D CNN was implemented for subcortical brain structure segmentation in MRI and this study was based on the effect of the size of the kernels in a network. In Reference [34], the authors applied 3D U-Net for dense volume segmentation. However, this network was not entirely in 3D because it used 2D annotated slices for training. Sato et al. [63] proposed 3D deep network for the segmentation of the head CT volume.

Liver cancer is one of the major causes of cancer deaths worldwide. Therefore, reliable and automated liver tumor segmentation techniques are needed to assist radiologists and doctors in hepatocellular carcinoma identification and management. Duo et al. [64] presented a fully connected 3D CNN for liver segmentation from 3D CT scans. The same network has also been tested on the whole heart and great vessel segmentation. Further, 3D U-Net has been applied in liver segmentation problems [65]. In Reference [66], 3D ResNet has been used for liver segmentation using the coarse-to-fine approach. Some other similar approaches for segmentation of the liver can be found in References [43,67–69]. In this sequence, another work, based on the 2D DenseUnet and hierarchical diagnosis approach (H-DensNet) for the segmentation of liver lesions, has been presented in Reference [70]. This network secured the first position in the LiTS 2017 leaderboard. The network has been tested on the 3D IRCADs database and achieved state-of-the-art outcomes, outperforming the other very well-established liver segmentation approaches. They have achieved dice scores of 0.982 and 0.93.7 for liver and tumor segmentation, respectively.

Table 1. 3D CNN for brain tumor/lesion segmentation on brain tumor segmentation (BRAST) challenges.

Ref.	Methods	Data	Task	Performance Evaluation
Zhou et al. [56]	A 3D variant of FusionNet (One-pass Multi-task Network (OM-Net))	BRATS 2018	brain tumor segmentation	0.916 (WT), 0.827 (TC), 0.807(EC)
Chen et al. [57]	Separable 3D U-Net	BRATS 2018	–do–	0.893(WT), 0.830(TC), 0.742(EC)
Peng et al. [60]	Multi-Scale 3D U-Nets	BRATS 2015	–do–	0.850(WT), 0.720(TC), 0.610(EC)
Kayalıbay et al. [58]	3D U-Nets	BRATS 2015	–do–	0.850 (WT), 0.872(TC), 0.610(EC)
Kamnitsas et al. [54]	11 layers deep 3D CNN	BRATS 2015 and ISLES 2015	–do–	0.898 (WT), 0.750 (TC), 0.720(EC)
Kamnitsas et al. 2016 [53]	3D CNN in which features extracted by 2D CNNs	BRATS 2017	–do–	0.918 (WT), 0.883(TC), 0.854 (EC)
Casamitjana et al. [55]	3D U-Net followed by fully connected 3D CRF	BRATS 2015	–do–	0.917(WT), 0.836(TC), 0.768(EC)
Isensee et al. [59]	3D U-Nets	BRATS 2017	–do–	0.850(WT), 0.740(TC), 0.640(EC)

3D CNNs are also being used in the segmentation of knee structures. In Reference [71], Ambellan et al. proposed a technique with 3D statistical shape models along with 2D to accomplish an effective and precise segmentation of knee structures. In Reference [72], the authors suggested a 3D CNN to segment cervical tumors on 3D PET images. Their architecture uses spatial information for segmentation purposes. The authors claimed highly precise results for segmenting cervical tumors on the 3D PET. In Reference [73], the authors proposed 3D convolution kernels for learning filter coefficients and spatial filter offsets simultaneously for 3D CT multi-organ segmentation work. The outcomes were compared to U-Net architectures and the authors claim that their architecture requires less trainable parameters and storage to obtain a high quality. In Reference [74], Chen et al. proposed 3D FC deep CNN (3D UNet) for the segmentation of six thoracic and abdominal organs (liver, spleen, and left/right kidneys and lungs) from dual-energy computed tomographic (DECT) images.

4.2. *Classification*

Classification of diseases using deep learning technologies on medical images has gained a lot of traction in the last few years. For neuroimaging, the major focus of 3D deep learning has been on detecting diseases from anatomical images. Several studies have focused on detecting dementia and its variants from different imaging modalities, including functional MRI and DTI. Alzheimer's Disease (AD) is the most common form of dementia, usually linked to the pathological amyloid depositions, structural-atrophy and metabolic variations in the chemistry of the brain. The timely diagnosis of AD plays an important role to intercept the progression of the disease.

Yang et al. [39] visualized the 3D CNN, trained to classify AD in terms of AD features, which can be a very good step in understanding the behavior of each layer of 3D CNN. They proposed three types of visual inspection approaches: (1) sensitivity analysis, (2) 3D class activation mapping and (3) 3D weighted gradient weighted mapping. The authors explained how visual inspection can improve accuracy and aid in deciding the 3D CNN architecture. In their work, some well-known baseline 2D deep architectures, such as VGGNet and ResNet, were converted to their 3D counterparts, and the classification of AD was performed using MRI data from the Alzheimer's Disease Neuroimaging Initiative (ADNI). In Reference [75], the authors trained an auto-encoder to derive an embedding from the input features of 3D patches. These features were extracted from the preprocessed MRI scans downloaded from the ADNI dataset. Their work demonstrated an improvement in results in comparison to the 2D approaches available in the literature. In Reference [76], the authors stacked recurrent neural network (long short-term memory) layers on 3D CNN layers for AD classification tasks using PET and MRI data. The 3D fully connected CNN layers obtained deep feature representations and the LSTM was applied on these features to improve the performance. In Reference [77], a deep 3D CNN was researched on a sizeable dataset for the classification of AD. Gao et al. [78] showed 87.7% accuracy in the classification of AD, lesion and normal aging by implementing a seven-layer deep 3D CNN on 285 volumetric CT head scans from Navy General hospital, China. In this study, the authors also compared their results from 3D CNN with hand-crafted features of 3D scale-invariant Fourier transform (SIFT) and showed that the proposed 3D CNN approach gives around four percent higher classification accuracy.

Besides detecting AD using head MRI (or other modalities), multiple studies have been performed to detect diseases from varied organs in the body. Nie et al. [79] took advantage of the 3D aspect of MRI by training a 3D CNN to evaluate the survival in patients going through high-grade gliomas. Zhou et al. [80] proposed a weakly-supervised 3D CNN for breast cancer detection. However, there are several limitations of the study: (1) the data was selective in nature, (2) the proposed architecture was only able to detect the tumor with high probability and (3) only structural features were used for the experiments. Jnawali et al. [41] demonstrated the performance of 3D CNN in the classification of CT brain hemorrhage scans. The authors constructed three versions of the 3D architectures based on CNNs. Two of these architectures are 3D versions of the VggNet and GoogLeNet. This unique research was done on a large private dataset and about 87.8% accuracy was demonstrated. In Reference [9], Ker et al. developed a three-layer shallow 3D CNN for brain hemorrhage classification. The proposed network was giving state-of-the-art results with small training time when compared to 3D VGGNet and 3D GoogLeNet. Ha et al. [81] modified 2D U-Net into 3D CNN to quantify the breast MRI fibro-glandular tissue (FGT) and background parenchymal enhancement (BPE). In Reference [58], Nie et al. proposed a multi-channel structure of 3D CNN for survival time prediction of Glioblastoma patients using multi-modal head images (T1 weighted MRI and diffusion tensor imaging, DTI). Recently, in Reference [82], the author presented a hybrid model for the classification and prediction of lymph node metastasis (LNM) in head and neck cancer. They combined the outputs of MaO-radiomics and 3D CNN architecture by using an evidential reasoning (ER) fusion strategy. In Reference [83], the authors presented a 3D CNN for predicting the maximum standardized uptake value of lymph nodes in patients suffering from cancer using CT images from a PET/CT examination. We summarized some important developments in 3D deep learning models for classification tasks in medical imaging in Table 2.

Table 2. 3D CNN for classification tasks in medical imaging.

Ref.	Task	Model	Data	Performance Measures
Yang et al. [39]	AD classification	3D VggNet, 3D Resnet	MRI scans from ADNI dataset (47 AD, 56 NC)	86.3% AUC using 3D VggNet and 85.4% AUC using 3D ResNet
Kruthika et al. [75]	–do–	3D capsule network, 3D CNN	MRI scans from ADNI dataset (345 AD, NC, 605, and 991MCI)	Acc. for AD/MCI/NC 89.1%
Feng et al. [76]	–do–	3D CNN + LSTM	PET + MRI scans from ADNI dataset (93 AD, 100 NC)	Acc. 65.5% (sMCI/NC), 86.4% (pMCI/NC), and 94.8 % (AD/NC)
Wegmayr et al. [77]	–do–	3D CNN	ADNI and AIBL data sets, 20000 T1 scans	Acc. 72% (MCI/AD), 86 % (AD/NC), and 67 % (MCI/NC)
Oh et al. [84]	–do–	3D CNN +transfer learning	MRI scans from the ADNI dataset (AD 198, NC 230, pMCI 166, and sMCI 101) at baseline.	74% (pMCI/sMCI), 86% (AD/NC), 77% (pMCI/NC)
Parmar et al. [10]	–do–	3D CNN	fMRI scans from ADNI dataset (30 AD, 30 NC)	Classification acc. 94.85 % (AD/NC)
Nie et al. [79]	Brain tumor	3D CNN with learning supervised features	Private, 69 patient (T1 MRI, fMRI, and DTI)	Classification acc. 89.85 %
Amidi et al. [85]	Protein shape	2-layer 3D CNN	63,558 enzymes from PDB datasets	Classification acc. 78%
Zhou et al. [80]	Breast cancer	Weakly supervised 3D CNN	Private, 1537 female patient	Classification acc. 78% 83.7%

4.3. *Detection and Localization*

Cerebral Microbleeds (CMBs) are small foci of chronic hemorrhages that can occur in the normal brains due to structural abnormalities of small blood vessels in the brain. Due to the differential properties of blood, MRI can detect CMBs. However, detecting cerebral micro-hemorrhages in brain tissue is a difficult and time-consuming task for radiologists, while recent studies employed 3D deep architectures to detect CMBs. Dou et al. [86] proposed a two-stage fully connected 3D CNN architecture to detect CMBs from the dataset of MRI susceptibility-weighted images (SWI). The network reduced many false-positive candidates. For training purposes, multiple 3D cubes were extracted from the preprocessed dataset. This study also examined the effect of the size of 3D patches on network performance. The study also focuses on the higher performance of 3D architectures in the detection of CMBs in comparison to their 2D architectures, such as Random Forest and 2D-CNN-SVM. Dou et al. further employed a fully 3D CNN to detect microscopic areas of a brain hemorrhage on MRI brain scans. This method had a sensitivity of 93% and outperformed prior methods of detection. Standvoss et al. [87] detected CMBs in traumatic brain injury. In their study, the authors prepared three types of 3D architectures with varying depths, i.e., three, five and eight layers. These models were quite simple and straight forward, with an overall best accuracy of 87%. The drawback of these studies was that they utilized a small dataset for training the network. In Reference [88], the author presented a

3D CNN to forecast the route and radius of an artery at any given point in a cardiac CT angiography image, which depends on the local image patch. This approach can precisely and effectively predict the path and the radius of coronary arteries through the details extracted from the image files.

Lung cancer is also the foremost cause of death worldwide. Nonetheless, the survival rate would be increased if we could detect lung cancer at an early stage. Subsequently, the past decade has seen considerable research into the detection, classification and localization of lung nodules using 3D deep learning approaches. In Reference [89], Anirudh et al. first proposed a 3D CNN for lung nodule detection using weakly labeled data. In 3D medical imaging, data labeling is quite complex and time-consuming when compared to 2D image modalities. The authors used a single-pixel point to unveil the data and used this single point information to grow the region using the thresholding and filtering of super-pixels. This process was performed on 2D slices and these slices were combined using 3D Gaussian filtering. Using the proposed 3D CNN, the authors showed an 0.80 sensitivity with 10 false positives per scan. However, the architecture of 3D CNN was not very deep in this work. Furthermore, the data were very small (70 scans), and therefore, the results may be biased. Dou et al. [90] exploited 3D CNN with multilevel contextual information for the false-positive reduction in pulmonary nodules in volumetric CT scans. The authors used 887 CT scans from a publicly available LIDC-IDRI dataset (LUNA16 challenge). Huang et al. [91] exploited 3D CNN to detect lung nodules in low-dose CT chest scans. The positive and negative cubes were extracted from CT data using a priori knowledge about the data and confounding the anatomical structure. The proposed design effectively reduced the complexity and showed a significant improvement in performance. Compared to the baseline approach, their approach showed 90% sensitivity, while a reduction in false positives from 35 to 5. Gruetzemacher et al. [12] used 3D UNet with residual blocks for detecting pulmonary nodules in CT scans from the LIDC-IDRI dataset. The authors used two 3D CNN models, one for each essential task, i.e., candidate generation and false-positive reduction. The model was experimented and evaluated with 888 CT scans. On the test data, an overall 89.3% detection and 1.79 false-positive rate was obtained. To tackle large variations in the size of the nodules, Gu et al. [92] proposed multi-scale prediction with a fusion scheme for 3D CNN (Figure 7). This work was also a part of the LUNA16 challenge and achieved 92.9% sensitivity with four false positives per scan.

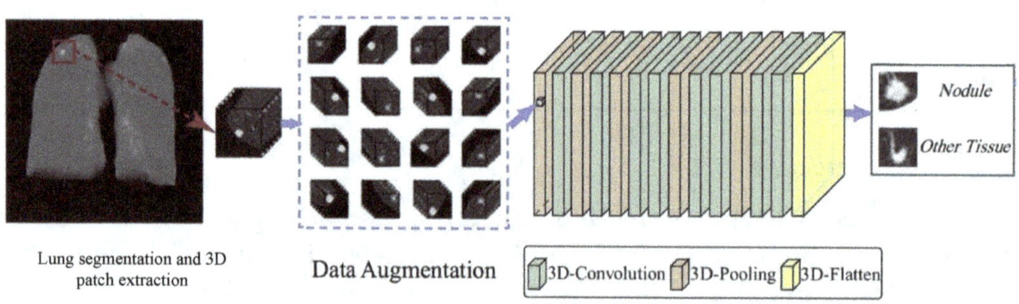

Figure 7. The basic procedure for lung nodule detection. The figure is modified from Reference [92].

To deal with the issue of limited data, Winkels and Cohen [93] proposed a 3D group convolutional neural network (3D-GCNNs). In this work, 3D rotations and reflections were used as input instead of translating a filter on the input (as in traditional 3D CNN). The authors showed that this approach needs only one-tenth of the data used in the conventional approach to obtain the same performance. In another work, Gong et al. [94] suggested a 3D CNN by exploiting the properties of ResNet and squeeze and excitation (SE) strategy. A 3D region proposal network using a UNet like structure was used for nodule detection, and then a 3D CNN was used for the reduction of false positives. The SE block increases the representation power of the network by focusing on channel-wise information. On the LIDC-IDRI dataset, 95.7% sensitivity was achieved with four false positives per scan. Pezeshk et al. [24] presented two-stage 3D CNN for automatic pulmonary nodule detection in CT scans. The first stage of

3D CNN was used for screening and candidate generation. The second stage was an ensemble of 3D CNNs trained with both positive and negative augmented patches.

The localization of biological architectures is a basic requirement for various initiatives in medical image investigation. Localization might be a hassle-free process for the radiologist, but it is usually a hard task for NNs that are vulnerable to variation in medical images induced by dissimilarities in the image acquisition process, structures and pathological differences among patients. Generally, a 3D volume is required for localization in medical images. Several techniques treat the 3D space as an arrangement of 2D orthogonal planes. Wolterink et al. [95] detected coronary artery calcium scoring in coronary CT angiography using a CNN based architecture. De Vos et al. [96] introduced the localization technique using a solitary CNN, and 2D CT image slices (chest CT, cardiac CT and abdomen CT) as inputs. While this work was related to a 3D localization approach, they did not use 3D CNN in a real sense. Further, the approach depended heavily on the accurate recognition of biological structures. Huo et al. [97] utilized the properties of a 3D fully connected CNN and presented a spatially localized atlas network tiles (SLANT) model for whole-brain segmentation on high-resolution multi-site images.

Intervertebral discs (IVDs) are modest joint parts that are located in between surrounding vertebrae and the localization of IVDs, which are usually important for spine disease analysis and measurement. In Reference [98], the authors presented a 3D detection for multiple brain structures in fetal neuro-sonography using fully connected CNNs and named it VP-Nets. They explained that the proposed strategy requires a comparatively less amount of data for training and can learn from coarsely annotated 3D data. Recently, a 3D CNN, based on regression, has been introduced in Reference [42] to assess the degree of enlarged perivascular spaces (EPVS) through 2000 basal ganglia scans from 3D head MRI. In Reference [99], the authors reported the human-level efficiency of 3D CNN in the landmark detection of clinical 3D CT data. In [100], Saleh et al. proposed a 3D CNN based regression models for 3D pose estimation of anatomy using T2 weighted imaging. They showed that the proposed network offers fine initialization for optimization-based techniques to increase the capture range of slice-to-volume registration. Xiaomeng et al. [101] presented fully connected, accurate and automatic 3D deep architecture for the localization and segmentation of IVDs using multimodal MR images. The work shows state-of-the-art performance in the MICCAI-2016 challenge for IVDs localization and segmentation section with a dice score of 0.912 for IVD segmentation. Cardiac magnetic resonance (CMR) imaging is popular in diagnosing various cardiovascular diseases. Vesel et al. [102] proposed a 3D DR-UNet (modified 3D UNet) for localization of cardiac structure in MRI volume. The model was evaluated on two datasets: the Automatic Cardiac Segmentation Challenge (ACDC) STACOM 2017, and Left Atrium Segmentation Challenge (LASC) STACOM 2018. Their model shows state-of-the-art results in terms of several performance indices.

4.4. Registration

Medical images of a single subject can be increasingly multi-modal in the same patient from CT, MRI T1 and MRI T2. Each imaging modality focuses on different features of the subject. Typically, a clinician is expected to view images of multiple modalities in different orientations to deduce a match between these images by visual comparison. The clinician is also expected to manually identify points in these images that have significant signal differences. Thus, two image analysis problems can be automated. First, the alignment or registration of datasets can be automated, and second, the automatic alignment of datasets can be made to modalities in which abnormalities are present. This allows us to identify prominent parts of an image for further review. In recent years, many efforts have been made in medical image registration using 3D deep learning. For example, Sokooti et al. successfully used 3D CNN for 3D nonrigid image registration in Reference [103]. For training the 3D CNN, 3D patches were extracted from 3D CT chest images. The network was trained on artificially generated displacement vector fields. The authors confirmed that their model outperformed a traditional B-spline registration method and performed on par with multi-resolution B-spline methods. However, for all the landmarks, multi-resolution B-spline methods outperformed their approach. Further, the capture range of their approach was limited to the size of the patches. A possible solution to increase the capture range of their method is to increase the size of the patches or to add more scales to the network. Torng et al. [104] showed the effectiveness of a shallow 3D CNN with three convolutional layers with filter sizes of 3x3, followed by 3D max-pooling layers and two fully connected layers with dropout for analyzing the interaction of amino acids to their neighboring microenvironment. The authors also proposed the CNN activation visualization technique called the atom importance map. For training and test data, 3D patches (local box) were extracted from the protein structure. Furthermore, the local structure was decomposed into five channels (inputs to 3D CNN), including oxygen, carbon, nitrogen and sulphur. The model shows a performance improvement of 20% when compared to the structure based on handcrafted biochemical features. To deal with the memory issue and computational cost, Blendowski and Heinrich [105] suggested a combination of MRF-based deformable registration and 3D CNN descriptors for lung motion estimation on non-rigidly deformed chest CT images.

There are several freely available medical image registration software and toolkits such as SimpleITK [106] and ANTs [107]. Typically, the registration process to these toolkits is done by iteratively updating the transformational parameters until a predefined similarity metric is optimized. These methods show a decent performance. However, their performance is limited by their slow registration process. To overcome this issue, several attempts have been made in the literature based on deep learning and 3D deep learning. Recently, Chee and Wu [108] used CNN as an affine image registration network (AIRNet) for MR brain image registration. AirNet, proposed by the authors, works in two parts, i.e., encoder and regressor. The architecture of the encoder part was drawn from DenseNet [109] with some modifications in filter structures (a mixture of 2D and 3D filters). The output of the encoder was then given to the regressor part. The proposed framework was compared to conventional registration algorithms used in the well-known software package SimpleITK [106]. The proposed framework shows significant improvements in J_{ac} and d_H. The authors claim that this method was 100 times faster than other traditional methods. Zhou et al. [110] proposed 3D CNN for serial electron microscopy images (experiments were performed on two databases, Cremi and FIB25) registration. Recently, Zhao et al. [111] presented a 3D Volume Tweening Network (VTN) for 3D medical image (liver CT and brain MRI dataset) registration in an unsupervised manner. Compared to the traditional optimization approaches (ANTs [107], Elastix [112] and VoxelMorph-2 [113]), their method was 880 times faster, with state-of-the-art performance. In Reference [114], Wang et al. proposed a dynamic 2D/3D registration algorithm for accurate alignment between 2-D and 3-D images for fusion applications.

The model introduced by the author was based on point-to-plane correspondence (PPC) and its dynamic registration procedure was fully capable of recovering 3-D motion from single-2D view images.

5. Challenges and Conclusions

It takes a large number of training samples to train deep learning models [53,115,116]. This is further strengthened by the recent successes of deep learning models trained on large datasets like the ImageNet. However, it is still ambiguous whether deep learning models can successfully work with smaller datasets, as in the case of medical images. The ambiguity is caused by the nature and characteristics of medical images. For example, the images from the ImageNet dataset possess large variations in their appearance (e.g., light, intensity, edges, color, etc.) [14,36,117–119] since the images were taken at different angles and distances, and have several different features that are completely different from medical images. Therefore, networks that need to learn meaningful representations of these images require large training parameters and thus training samples. However, in the case of medical images, there is much less variation in comparison to traditional image datasets [120]. In this regard, the process of fine-tuning of 3D CNN models, which are already trained on natural image datasets, can be applied to medical images [14,36,117–119,121,122]. This process, known as transfer learning, has been successfully applied to many areas of medical imaging.

Regardless of their high computational complexity, 3D deep networks have shown incredible performance in diverse domains. 3D deep networks require a large number of training parameters, especially in the case of 3D medical images, where the depth of the image volume varies from 20 to 400 slices per scan [7,36,79,123], with each scan containing very fine and important information about the patient. Usually, high-resolution scan volumes are of the size 512 × 512, and need to be downsampled before being fed into the 3D network to reduce the computational cost. Researchers generally use interpolation techniques to reduce the overall size of these medical image volumes, but come at the cost of significant information loss. There are also restrictions on the resizing of the medical image volume without the loss of significant information. This is still an unexplored area and there is further research scope.

While the number of trainable parameters of convolutional layers is independent of the input size, the number of trainable parameters in the subsequent fully connected layers depend on the output of the convolution layers. This often leads to intractable models due to a large number of trainable weights when the input images are fed into 3D CNN models without any down-sampling. However, this is not an issue in the case of 2D images, which have smaller latent representations that are learnt by convolution filters. This makes it harder (and more GPU intensive) to train 3D deep networks based on CNNs. The inception module by GoogLeNet can be further explored to address computational complexity in 3D medical image analysis. In recent times, many computational 3D imaging techniques have appeared in the literature where the acquired data is not necessarily a traditional image. Sometimes raw data may be suitable for a few applications in deep learning. For example, single-pixel imaging techniques are popular in unconventional applications, including X-rays. A brief review of various applications of single-pixel imaging in 3D reconstruction can be found in Reference [124]. Ghost imaging is also popular for image reconstruction, such as lens-less imaging and X-ray imaging. In order to enhance the quality of image reconstruction, Wang et al. [125] applied deep learning on the images reconstructed from traditional ghost imaging.

Indeed, in the deep learning context, learning the correct features might sound unconventional because we cannot be sure if the models learn features that are discriminating for the condition or just overfit on some specific features for the given dataset. CNNs can handle raw image data and they do not need to be handcrafted [11,117]. It is the responsibility of CNN to discover the right features from the data. While CNNs have made encoding the raw features in a latent space very convenient, it is important to understand whether the features learned by CNN are generalizable across datasets. Machine learning models often overfit on training samples as they only perform well on the test samples from the training dataset. This issue is acute in the case of medical imaging applications where there are issues with scanner variability, scan acquisition settings, subject demography, and heterogeneity in disease characteristics across subjects. Therefore, it is important to decode the trained network using model interpretability approaches and validate the important features learned by the network [126]. It also becomes important to report testing results with an external dataset whose samples were not used for training. However, this may not always be possible because of the paucity of datasets for training and testing.

Finally, the ultimate challenge is to go beyond a human-level performance. Researchers are working on reaching human-level performance for many tasks (known as Artificial General Intelligence) [35,53,127,128]. However, the lack of labeled images, high costs involved in labeling the datasets and lack of consensus among experts in validating the assigned labels [38,129,130] are some present challenges in the field. These issues force us to consider using reliable data augmentation methods and to generate samples with known ground-truths. In this regard, generative adversarial networks (GAN) [131], especially CycleGANs for cross-modal image synthesis, offer a viable approach for synthesizing data. They are being used to produce pseudo images that are highly similar to the original dataset.

Author Contributions: All authors conceptualized the ideas and conducted the literature search, prepared the figures, tables, and drafted the manuscript. All authors have read and approved the manuscript.

References

1. Doi, K. Computer-Aided Diagnosis in Medical Imaging: Historical Review, Current Status and Future Potential. *Comput. Med. Imaging Graph.* **2007**, *31*, 198–211. [CrossRef]
2. Miller, A.S.; Blott, B.H.; hames, T.K. Review of neural network applications in medical imaging and signal processing. *Med. Biol. Eng. Comput.* **1992**, *30*, 449–464. [CrossRef] [PubMed]
3. Siedband, M.P. Medical imaging systems. *Med. Instrum.-Appl. Des.* **1998**, 518–576.
4. Prince, J.; Links, J. *Medical Imaging Signals and Systems*; Pearson: London, UK, 2006; pp. 315–379.
5. Shapiro, R.S.; Wagreich, J.; Parsons, R.B.; Stancato-Pasik, A.; Yeh, H.C.; Lao, R. Tissue harmonic imaging sonography: Evaluation of image quality compared with conventional sonography. *Am. J. Roentgenol.* **1998**, *171*, 1203–1206. [CrossRef] [PubMed]
6. Matsumoto, K.; Jinzaki, M.; Tanami, Y.; Ueno, A.; Yamada, M.; Kuribayashi, S. Virtual Monochromatic Spectral Imaging with Fast Kilovoltage Switching: Improved Image Quality as Compared with That Obtained with Conventional 120-kVp CT. *Radiology* **2011**, *259*, 257–262. [CrossRef] [PubMed]
7. Thibault, J.-B.; Sauer, K.D.; Bouman, C.A.; Hsieh, J. A three-dimensional statistical approach to improved image quality for multislice helical CT. *Med. Phys.* **2007**, *34*, 4526–4544. [CrossRef]
8. Marin, D.; Nelson, R.C.; Schindera, S.T.; Richard, S.; Youngblood, R.S.; Yoshizumi, T.T.; Samei, E. Low-Tube-Voltage, High-Tube-Current Multidetector Abdominal CT: Improved Image Quality and Decreased Radiation Dose with Adaptive Statistical Iterative Reconstruction Algorithm—Initial Clinical Experience. *Radiology* **2010**, *254*, 145–153. [CrossRef]
9. Ker, J.; Singh, S.P.; Bai, Y.; Rao, J.; Lim, T.; Wang, L. Image Thresholding Improves 3-Dimensional Convolutional Neural Network Diagnosis of Different Acute Brain Hemorrhages on Computed Tomography Scans. *Sensors* **2019**, *19*, 2167. [CrossRef]
10. Parmar, H.S.; Nutter, B.; Long, R.; Antani, S.; Mitra, S. Deep learning of volumetric 3D CNN for fMRI in Alzheimer's disease classification. In *Medical Imaging 2020: Biomedical Applications in Molecular, Structural, and Functional Imaging, Houston, TX, USA, 2020*; Gimi, B.S., Krol, A., Eds.; SPIE: Bellingham, WA, USA, 2020; Volume 11317, p. 11.
11. Shen, D.; Wu, G.; Suk, H.-I. Deep Learning in Medical Image Analysis. *Annu. Rev. Biomed. Eng.* **2017**, *19*, 221–248. [CrossRef]
12. Gruetzemacher, R.; Gupta, A.; Paradice, D. 3D deep learning for detecting pulmonary nodules in CT scans. *J. Am. Med. Inform. Assoc.* **2018**, *25*, 1301–1310. [CrossRef] [PubMed]
13. Wang, S.H.; Phillips, P.; Sui, Y.; Liu, B.; Yang, M.; Cheng, H. Classification of Alzheimer's Disease Based on Eight-Layer Convolutional Neural Network with Leaky Rectified Linear Unit and Max Pooling. *J. Med. Syst.* **2018**, *42*, 85. [CrossRef] [PubMed]
14. Krizhevsky, A.; Sutskever, I.; Hinton, G.E. ImageNet classification with deep convolutional neural networks. *Commun. ACM* **2017**, *60*, 84–90. [CrossRef]
15. Szegedy, C.; Liu, W.; Jia, Y.; Sermanet, P.; Reed, S.; Anguelov, D.; Erhan, D.; Vanhoucke, V.; Rabinovich, A. Going deeper with convolutions. In Proceedings of the IEEE Computer Society Conference on Computer Vision and Pattern Recognition, Boston, MA, USA, 7–12 June 2015.
16. Hoi, S.C.H.; Jin, R.; Zhu, J.; Lyu, M.R. Batch mode active learning and its application to medical image classification. In Proceedings of the 23rd International Conference on Machine Learning, New York, NY, USA, 25–29 June 2006; pp. 417–424.
17. Rahman, M.M.; Bhattacharya, P.; Desai, B.C. A Framework for Medical Image Retrieval Using Machine Learning and Statistical Similarity Matching Techniques With Relevance Feedback. *IEEE Trans. Inf. Technol. Biomed.* **2007**, *11*, 58–69. [CrossRef]
18. Wernick, M.; Yang, Y.; Brankov, J.; Yourganov, G.; Strother, S. Machine Learning in Medical Imaging. *IEEE Signal. Process. Mag.* **2010**, *27*, 25–38. [CrossRef] [PubMed]

19. Criminisi, A.; Shotton, J.; Konukoglu, E. Decision forests: A unified framework for classification, regression, density estimation, manifold learning and semi-supervised learning. *Found. Trends®Comput. Graph. Vis.* **2012**, *7*, 81–227. [CrossRef]
20. Singh, S.P.; Urooj, S. An Improved CAD System for Breast Cancer Diagnosis Based on Generalized Pseudo-Zernike Moment and Ada-DEWNN Classifier. *J. Med. Syst.* **2016**, *40*, 105. [CrossRef]
21. Urooj, S.; Singh, S.P. Rotation invariant detection of benign and malignant masses using PHT. In Proceedings of the 2015 2nd International Conference on Computing for Sustainable Global Development (INDIACom), New Delhi, India, 11–13 March 2015.
22. Ji, S.; Xu, W.; Yang, M.; Yu, K. 3D Convolutional Neural Networks for Human Action Recognition. *IEEE Trans. Pattern Anal. Mach. Intell.* **2013**, *35*, 221–231. [CrossRef]
23. Moher, D.; Liberati, A.; Tetzlaff, J.; Altman, D.G.; Altman, D.; Antes, G.; Atkins, D.; Barbour, V.; Barrowman, N.; Berlin, J.A.; et al. Preferred reporting items for systematic reviews and meta-analyses: The PRISMA statement. *PLoS Med.* **2009**, *6*, e1000097. [CrossRef]
24. Pezeshk, A.; Hamidian, S.; Petrick, N.; Sahiner, B. 3-D Convolutional Neural Networks for Automatic Detection of Pulmonary Nodules in Chest CT. *IEEE J. Biomed. Heal. Inform.* **2019**, *23*, 2080–2090. [CrossRef]
25. Springenberg, J.T.; Dosovitskiy, A.; Brox, T.; Riedmiller, M. Striving for simplicity: The all convolutional net. In Proceedings of the 3rd International Conference on Learning Representations, ICLR 2015–Workshop Track Proceedings, San Diego, CA, USA, 7–9 May 2015.
26. Kukačka, J.; Golkov, V.; Cremers, D. Regularization for Deep Learning: A Taxonomy. *arXiv* **2017**, arXiv:1710.10686.
27. Srivastava, N.; Hinton, G.; Krizhevsky, A.; Salakhutdinov, R. Dropout: A Simple Way to Prevent Neural Networks from Overfitting. *J. Mach. Learn. Res.* **2014**, *15*, 1929–1958.
28. Ioffe, S.; Szegedy, C. Batch normalization: Accelerating deep network training by reducing internal covariate shift. In Proceedings of the 32nd International Conference on Machine Learning, ICML 2015, International Machine Learning Society (IMLS), Lile, France, 6–11 July 2015; Volume 1, pp. 448–456.
29. Simonyan, K.; Zisserman, A. Very deep convolutional networks for large-scale image recognition. In Proceedings of the 3rd International Conference on Learning Representations, ICLR 2015, Conference Track Proceedings, San Diego, CA, USA, 7–9 May 2015.
30. Szegedy, C.; Vanhoucke, V.; Ioffe, S.; Shlens, J.; Wojna, Z. Rethinking the Inception Architecture for Computer Vision. In Proceedings of the IEEE Computer Society Conference on Computer Vision and Pattern Recognition, Las Vegas, NV, USA, 27 June–28 July 2016; Volume 1, pp. 2818–2826.
31. Szegedy, C.; Ioffe, S.; Vanhoucke, V.; Alemi, A.A. Inception-v4, inception-ResNet and the impact of residual connections on learning. In Proceedings of the 31st AAAI Conference on Artificial Intelligence, AAAI 2017, San Francisco, CA, USA, 4–9 February 2017; pp. 4278–4284.
32. He, K.; Zhang, X.; Ren, S.; Sun, J. Deep residual learning for image recognition. In Proceedings of the IEEE Computer Society Conference on Computer Vision and Pattern Recognition, Las Vegas, NV, USA, 27 June–28 July 2016; Volume 1, pp. 770–778.
33. Ronneberger, O.; Fischer, P.; Brox, T. U-net: Convolutional networks for biomedical image segmentation. In *Lecture Notes in Computer Science (Including Subseries Lecture Notes in Artificial Intelligence and Lecture Notes in Bioinformatics)*; Springer: Quebec City, QC, Canada, 2015; Volume 9351, pp. 234–241.
34. Çiçek, Ö.; Abdulkadir, A.; Lienkamp, S.S.; Brox, T.; Ronneberger, O. 3D U-net: Learning dense volumetric segmentation from sparse annotation. In *Lecture Notes in Computer Science (Including Subseries Lecture Notes in Artificial Intelligence and Lecture Notes in Bioinformatics)*; Springer: Quebec City, QC, Canada, 2016; Volume 9901, pp. 424–432.
35. Ker, J.; Wang, L.; Rao, J.; Lim, T. Deep Learning Applications in Medical Image Analysis. *IEEE Access* **2018**, *6*, 9375–9389. [CrossRef]
36. Burt, J. Volumetric Quantification of Cardiovascular Structures from Medical Imaging. U.S. Patent 9,968,257, 15 May 2018.
37. Esteban, O.; Markiewicz, C.J.; Blair, R.W.; Moodie, C.A.; Isik, A.I.; Erramuzpe, A.; Kent, J.D.; Goncalves, M.; DuPre, E.; Snyder, M.; et al. fmriprep: A Robust Preprocessing Pipeline for fMRI Data—Fmriprep version documentation. *Nat. Methods* **2019**, 111–116. [CrossRef] [PubMed]

38. Alansary, A.; Kamnitsas, K.; Davidson, A.; Khlebnikov, R.; Rajchl, M.; Malamateniou, C.; Rutherford, M.; Hajnal, J.V.; Glocker, B.; Rueckert, D.; et al. Fast Fully Automatic Segmentation of the Human Placenta from Motion Corrupted MRI. In *International Conference on Medical Image Computing and Computer-Assisted Intervention*; Springer: Cham, Switzerland, 2016; pp. 589–597.
39. Yang, C.; Rangarajan, A.; Ranka, S. Visual Explanations from Deep 3D Convolutional Neural Networks for Alzheimer's Disease Classification. *AMIA Annu. Symp. Proc. AMIA Symp.* **2018**, *2018*, 1571–1580. [PubMed]
40. Jones, D.K.; Griffin, L.D.; Alexander, D.C.; Catani, M.; Horsfield, M.A.; Howard, R.; Williams, S.C.R. Spatial Normalization and Averaging of Diffusion Tensor MRI Data Sets. *Neuroimage* **2002**, *17*, 592–617. [CrossRef] [PubMed]
41. Jnawali, K.; Arbabshirani, M.; Rao, N. Deep 3D Convolution Neural Network for CT Brain Hemorrhage Classification. In Proceedings of the Medical Imaging 2018: Computer-Aided Diagnosis, International Society for Optics and Photonics, Houston, TX, USA, 10–15 February 2018; p. 105751C.
42. Dubost, F.; Adams, H.; Bortsova, G.; Ikram, M. 3D Regression Neural Network for the Quantification of Enlarged Perivascular Spaces in Brain MRI. *Med. Image Anal.* **2019**, *51*, 89–100. [CrossRef]
43. Lian, C.; Liu, M.; Zhang, J.; Zong, X.; Lin, W.; Shen, D. Automatic Segmentation of 3D Perivascular Spaces in 7T MR Images Using Multi-Channel Fully Convolutional Network. In Proceedings of the International Society for Magnetic Resonance in Medicine, Scientific Meeting and Exhibition, Paris, France, 16–21 June 2018; pp. 5–7.
44. Pauli, R.; Bowring, A.; Reynolds, R.; Chen, G.; Nichols, T.E.; Maumet, C. Exploring fMRI Results Space: 31 Variants of an fMRI Analysis in AFNI, FSL, and SPM. *Front. Neuroinform.* **2016**, *10*. [CrossRef]
45. Parker, D.; Liu, X.; Razlighi, Q.R. Optimal slice timing correction and its interaction with fMRI parameters and artifacts. *Med. Image Anal.* **2017**, *35*, 434–445. [CrossRef]
46. Goebel, R. Brain Voyager—Past, present, future. *Neuroimage* **2012**, *62*, 748–756. [CrossRef]
47. Maes, F.; Collignon, A.; Vandemeulen, D.; Marchal, G.; Suetens, P. Multimodality image registration by maximization of mutual information. *IEEE Trans. Med. Imaging* **1997**, *16*, 187–198. [CrossRef] [PubMed]
48. Maintz, J.A.; Viergever, M.A. A survey of medical image registration. *Med. Image Anal.* **1998**, *2*, 1–36. [CrossRef]
49. Pluim, J.P.W.; Maintz, J.B.A.; Viergever, M.A. Interpolation Artefacts in Mutual Information Based Image Registration. *Comput. Vis. Image Underst.* **2000**, *77*, 211–232. [CrossRef]
50. Penney, G.P.; Weese, J.; Little, J.A.; Desmedt, P.; Hill, D.L.G.; Hawkes, D.J. A comparison of similarity measures for use in 2-D-3-D medical image registration. *Med. Imaging IEEE Trans.* **1998**, *17*, 586–595. [CrossRef] [PubMed]
51. Ahmed, M.N.; Yamany, S.M.; Mohamed, N.; Farag, A.A.; Moriarty, T. A modified fuzzy c-means algorithm for bias field estimation and segmentation of MRI data. *IEEE Trans. Med. Imaging* **2002**, *21*, 193–199. [CrossRef] [PubMed]
52. Li, C.; Xu, C.; Anderson, A.W.; Gore, J.C. MRI tissue classification and bias field estimation based on coherent local intensity clustering: A unified energy minimization framework. In *Lecture Notes in Computer Science (Including Subseries Lecture Notes in Artificial Intelligence and Lecture Notes in Bioinformatics)*; Springer: Quebec City, QC, Canada, 2009; Volume 5636, pp. 288–299.
53. Kamnitsas, K.; Ferrante, E.; Parisot, S.; Ledig, C.; Nori, A.V.; Criminisi, A.; Rueckert, D.; Glocker, B. DeepMedic for Brain Tumor Segmentation. In Proceedings of the International Workshop on Brainlesion: Glioma, Multiple Sclerosis, Stroke and Traumatic Brain Injuries, Athens, Greece, 17 October 2016; pp. 138–149.
54. Kamnitsas, K.; Ledig, C.; Newcombe, V.F.J.; Simpson, J.P.; Kane, A.D.; Menon, D.K.; Rueckert, D.; Glocker, B. Efficient multi-scale 3D CNN with fully connected CRF for accurate brain lesion segmentation. *Med. Image Anal.* **2017**, *36*, 61–78. [CrossRef]
55. Casamitjana, A.; Puch, S.; Aduriz, A.; Vilaplana, V. 3D convolutional neural networks for brain tumor segmentation: A comparison of multi-resolution architectures. In Proceedings of the Lecture Notes in Computer Science (including subseries Lecture Notes in Artificial Intelligence and Lecture Notes in Bioinformatics); Springer: Athens, Greece, 2016; pp. 150–161.
56. Zhou, C.; Ding, C.; Wang, X.; Lu, Z.; Tao, D. One-pass Multi-task Networks with Cross-task Guided Attention for Brain Tumor Segmentation. *IEEE Trans. Image Process.* **2020**, *29*, 4516–4529. [CrossRef]

57. Chen, W.; Liu, B.; Peng, S.; Sun, J.; Qiao, X. S3D-UNET: Separable 3D U-Net for brain tumor segmentation. In *Lecture Notes in Computer Science (Including Subseries Lecture Notes in Artificial Intelligence and Lecture Notes in Bioinformatics)*; Springer: Quebec City, QC, Canada, 2019; Volume 11384, pp. 358–368.
58. Kayalibay, B.; Jensen, G.; van der Smagt, P. CNN-based Segmentation of Medical Imaging Data. *arXiv* **2017**, arXiv:1701.03056.
59. Isensee, F.; Kickingereder, P.; Wick, W.; Bendszus, M.; Maier-Hein, K.H. Brain tumor segmentation and radiomics survival prediction: Contribution to the BRATS 2017 challenge. In *Lecture Notes in Computer Science (Including Subseries Lecture Notes in Artificial Intelligence and Lecture Notes in Bioinformatics)*; Springer: Quebec City, QC, Canada, 2018; Volume 10670, pp. 287–297.
60. Peng, S.; Chen, W.; Sun, J.; Liu, B. Multi-Scale 3D U-Nets: An approach to automatic segmentation of brain tumor. *Int. J. Imaging Syst. Technol.* **2019**, *30*, 5–17. [CrossRef]
61. Milletari, F.; Ahmadi, S.A.; Kroll, C.; Plate, A.; Rozanski, V.; Maiostre, J.; Levin, J.; Dietrich, O.; Ertl-Wagner, B.; Bötzel, K.; et al. Hough-CNN: Deep Learning for Segmentation of Deep Brain Regions in MRI and Ultrasound. *Comput. Vis. Image Underst.* **2017**, *164*, 92–102. [CrossRef]
62. Dolz, J.; Desrosiers, C. 3D fully convolutional networks for subcortical segmentation in MRI: A large-scale study. *Neuroimage* **2018**, *170*, 456–470. [CrossRef] [PubMed]
63. Sato, D.; Hanaoka, S.; Nomura, Y.; Takenaga, T.; Miki, S.; Yoshikawa, T.; Hayashi, N.; Abe, O. A primitive study on unsupervised anomaly detection with an autoencoder in emergency head CT volumes. In Proceedings of the Medical Imaging 2018: Computer-Aided Diagnosis, Houston, TX, USA, 10–15 February 2018; p. 60.
64. Dou, Q.; Yu, L.; Chen, H.; Jin, Y.; Yang, X.; Qin, J.; Heng, P.A. 3D deeply supervised network for automated segmentation of volumetric medical images. *Med. Image Anal.* **2017**, *41*, 40–54. [CrossRef] [PubMed]
65. Zeng, G.; Yang, X.; Li, J.; Yu, L.; Heng, P.A.; Zheng, G. 3D U-net with multi-level deep supervision: Fully automatic segmentation of proximal femur in 3D MR images. In *Lecture Notes in Computer Science (Including Subseries Lecture Notes in Artificial Intelligence and Lecture Notes in Bioinformatics)*; Springer: Quebec City, QC, Canada, 2017; Volume 10541, pp. 274–282.
66. Zhu, Z.; Xia, Y.; Shen, W.; Fishman, E.; Yuille, A. A 3D coarse-to-fine framework for volumetric medical image segmentation. In Proceedings of the 2018 International Conference on 3D Vision, Verona, Italy, 5–8 September 2018; pp. 682–690.
67. Yang, X.; Bian, C.; Yu, L.; Ni, D.; Heng, P.A. Hybrid loss guided convolutional networks for whole heart parsing. In *Lecture Notes in Computer Science (Including Subseries Lecture Notes in Artificial Intelligence and Lecture Notes in Bioinformatics)*; Springer: Quebec City, QC, Canada, 2018; Volume 10663, pp. 215–223.
68. Roth, H.R.; Oda, H.; Zhou, X.; Shimizu, N.; Yang, Y. Computerized Medical Imaging and Graphics An application of cascaded 3D fully convolutional networks for medical image segmentation. *Comput. Med. Imaging Graph.* **2018**, *66*, 90–99. [CrossRef]
69. Yu, L.; Yang, X.; Qin, J.; Heng, P.A. 3D FractalNet: Dense volumetric segmentation for cardiovascular MRI volumes. In *Lecture Notes in Computer Science (Including Subseries Lecture Notes in Artificial Intelligence and Lecture Notes in Bioinformatics)*; Springer: Quebec City, QC, Canada, 2017; Volume 10129, pp. 103–110.
70. Li, X.; Chen, H.; Qi, X.; Dou, Q.; Fu, C.-W.; Heng, P.A. H-DenseUNet: Hybrid Densely Connected UNet for Liver and Liver Tumor Segmentation from CT Volumes. *IEEE Trans. Med. Imaging* **2018**, *37*, 2663–2674. [CrossRef] [PubMed]
71. Ambellan, F.; Tack, A.; Ehlke, M.; Zachow, S. Automated segmentation of knee bone and cartilage combining statistical shape knowledge and convolutional neural networks: Data from the Osteoarthritis Initiative. *Med. Image Anal.* **2019**, *52*, 109–118. [CrossRef]
72. Chen, L.; Shen, C.; Li, S.; Albuquerque, K.; Folkert, M.R.; Wang, J.; Maquilan, G. Automatic PET cervical tumor segmentation by deep learning with prior information. In Proceedings of the Physics in Medicine and Biology, Houston, TX, USA, 10–15 February 2018; p. 111.
73. Heinrich, M.P.; Oktay, O.; Bouteldja, N. OBELISK-Net: Fewer layers to solve 3D multi-organ segmentation with sparse deformable convolutions. *Med. Image Anal.* **2019**, *54*, 1–9. [CrossRef]
74. Chen, S.; Zhong, X.; Hu, S.; Dorn, S.; Kachelrieß, M.; Lell, M.; Maier, A. Automatic multi-organ segmentation in dual-energy CT (DECT) with dedicated 3D fully convolutional DECT networks. *Med. Phys.* **2020**, *47*, 552–562. [CrossRef]
75. Kruthika, K.R.; Rajeswari; Maheshappa, H.D. CBIR system using Capsule Networks and 3D CNN for Alzheimer's disease diagnosis. *Inform. Med. Unlocked* **2019**, *14*, 59–68. [CrossRef]

76. Feng, C.; Elazab, A.; Yang, P.; Wang, T.; Zhou, F.; Hu, H.; Xiao, X.; Lei, B. Deep Learning Framework for Alzheimer's Disease Diagnosis via 3D-CNN and FSBi-LSTM. *IEEE Access* **2019**, *7*, 63605–63618. [CrossRef]
77. Wegmayr, V.; Aitharaju, S.; Buhmann, J. Classification of brain MRI with big data and deep 3D convolutional neural networks. In Proceedings of the Medical Imaging 2018: Computer-Aided Diagnosis, Houston, TX, USA, 10–15 February 2018. [CrossRef]
78. Gao, X.; Hui, R.; Biomedicine, Z.T. Classification of CT brain images based on deep learning networks. *Omput. Methods Prog. Biomed. Elsevier* **2017**, *138*, 49–56. [CrossRef]
79. Nie, D.; Zhang, H.; Adeli, E.; Liu, L.; Shen, D. 3D deep learning for multi-modal imaging-guided survival time prediction of brain tumor patients. In Proceedings of the International Conference on Medical Image Computing and Computer-Assisted Intervention, Athens, Greece, 17–21 October 2016; Springer: Quebec City, QC, Canada, 2016; pp. 212–220.
80. Zhou, J.; Luo, L.; Dou, Q.; Chen, H.; Chen, C.; Li, G.; Jiang, Z.; Heng, P. Weakly supervised 3D deep learning for breast cancer classification and localization of the lesions in MR images. *J. Magn. Reson. Imaging* **2019**, *50*, 1144–1151. [CrossRef] [PubMed]
81. Ha, R.; Chang, P.; Mema, E.; Mutasa, S.; Karcich, J.; Wynn, R.T.; Liu, M.Z.; Jambawalikar, S. Fully Automated Convolutional Neural Network Method for Quantification of Breast MRI Fibroglandular Tissue and Background Parenchymal Enhancement. *J. Digit. Imaging* **2019**, *32*, 141–147. [CrossRef] [PubMed]
82. Chen, L.; Zhou, Z.; Sher, D.; Zhang, Q.; Shah, J.; Pham, N.-L.; Jiang, S.B.; Wang, J. Combining many-objective radiomics and 3-dimensional convolutional neural network through evidential reasoning to predict lymph node metastasis in head and neck cancer. *Phys. Med. Biol.* **2019**, *64*, 075011. [CrossRef]
83. Shaish, H.; Mutasa, S.; Makkar, J.; Chang, P.; Schwartz, L.; Ahmed, F. Prediction of lymph node maximum standardized uptake value in patients with cancer using a 3D convolutional neural network: A proof-of-concept study. *Am. J. Roentgenol.* **2019**, *212*, 238–244. [CrossRef] [PubMed]
84. Oh, K.; Chung, Y.C.; Kim, K.W.; Kim, W.S.; Oh, I.S. Classification and Visualization of Alzheimer's Disease using Volumetric Convolutional Neural Network and Transfer Learning. *Sci. Rep.* **2019**, *9*, 1–16. [CrossRef]
85. Amidi, A.; Amidi, S.; Vlachakis, D.; Megalooikonomou, V.; Paragios, N.; Zacharaki, E. EnzyNet: Enzyme classification using 3D convolutional neural networks on spatial representation. *PeerJ* **2018**, *6*, e4750. [CrossRef]
86. Dou, Q.; Chen, H.; Yu, L.; Zhao, L.; Qin, J.; Wang, D.; Mok, V.C.; Shi, L.; Heng, P.A. Automatic detection of cerebral microbleeds from MR images via 3D convolutional neural networks. *IEEE Trans. Med. Imaging* **2016**, *35*, 1182–1195. [CrossRef]
87. Standvoss, K.; Goerke, L.; Crijns, T.; van Niedek, T.; Alfonso Burgos, N.; Janssen, D.; van Vugt, J.; Gerritse, E.; Mol, J.; van de Vooren, D.; et al. Cerebral microbleed detection in traumatic brain injury patients using 3D convolutional neural networks. In Proceedings of the Medical Imaging 2018: Computer-Aided Diagnosis, Houston, TX, USA, 10–15 February 2018; p. 48.
88. Wolterink, J.M.; van Hamersvelt, R.W.; Viergever, M.A.; Leiner, T.; Išgum, I. Coronary Artery Centerline Extraction in Cardiac CT Angiography. *Med. Image Anal.* **2019**, *51*, 46–60. [CrossRef]
89. Anirudh, R.; Thiagarajan, J.J.; Bremer, T.; Kim, H. Lung nodule detection using 3D convolutional neural networks trained on weakly labeled data. In Proceedings of the Medical Imaging 2016: Computer-Aided Diagnosis, San Diego, CA, USA, 27 February–3 March 2016; Volume 9785, p. 978532.
90. Dou, Q.; Chen, H.; Yu, L.; Qin, J.; Heng, P.A. Multilevel Contextual 3-D CNNs for False Positive Reduction in Pulmonary Nodule Detection. *IEEE Trans. Biomed. Eng.* **2017**, *64*, 1558–1567. [CrossRef]
91. Huang, X.; Shan, J.; Vaidya, V. Lung nodule detection in CT using 3D convolutional neural networks. In Proceedings of the International Symposium on Biomedical Imaging, Melbourne, Australia, 18–21 April 2017; pp. 379–383.
92. Gu, Y.; Lu, X.; Yang, L.; Zhang, B.; Yu, D.; Zhao, Y.; Gao, L.; Wu, L.; Zhou, T. Automatic lung nodule detection using a 3D deep convolutional neural network combined with a multi-scale prediction strategy in chest CTs. *Comput. Biol. Med.* **2018**, *103*, 220–231. [CrossRef]
93. Winkels, M.; Cohen, T.S. Pulmonary nodule detection in CT scans with equivariant CNNs. *Med. Image Anal.* **2019**, *55*, 15–26. [CrossRef] [PubMed]
94. Gong, L.; Jiang, S.; Yang, Z.; Zhang, G.; Wang, L. Automated pulmonary nodule detection in CT images using 3D deep squeeze-and-excitation networks. *Int. J. Comput. Assist. Radiol. Surg.* **2019**, *14*, 1969–1979. [CrossRef] [PubMed]

95. Wolterink, J.; Leiner, T.; Viergever, M.A.; Išgum, I. *Automatic Coronary Calcium Scoring in Cardiac CT Angiography Using Convolutional Neural Networks*; Springer: Munich, Germany, 2015; Volume 9349.
96. De Vos, B.D.; Wolterink, J.M.; De Jong, P.A.; Leiner, T.; Viergever, M.A.; Išgum, I. ConvNet-Based Localization of Anatomical Structures in 3-D Medical Images. *IEEE Trans. Med. Imaging* **2017**, *36*, 1470–1481. [CrossRef]
97. Huo, Y.; Xu, Z.; Xiong, Y.; Aboud, K.; Parvathaneni, P.; Bao, S.; Bermudez, C.; Resnick, S.M.; Cutting, L.E.; Landman, B.A. 3D whole brain segmentation using spatially localized atlas network tiles. *Neuroimage* **2019**, *194*, 105–119. [CrossRef] [PubMed]
98. Huang, R.; Xie, W.; Alison Noble, J. VP-Nets: Efficient automatic localization of key brain structures in 3D fetal neurosonography. *Med. Image Anal.* **2018**, *47*, 127–139. [CrossRef] [PubMed]
99. O'Neil, A.Q.; Kascenas, A.; Henry, J.; Wyeth, D.; Shepherd, M.; Beveridge, E.; Clunie, L.; Sansom, C.; Šeduikytė, E.; Muir, K.; et al. Attaining human-level performance with atlas location autocontext for anatomical landmark detection in 3D CT data. In *Lecture Notes in Computer Science (Including Subseries Lecture Notes in Artificial Intelligence and Lecture Notes in Bioinformatics)*; Springer: Quebec City, QC, Canada, 2019; Volume 11131, pp. 470–484.
100. Mohseni Salehi, S.S.; Khan, S.; Erdogmus, D.; Gholipour, A. Real-Time Deep Pose Estimation With Geodesic Loss for Image-to-Template Rigid Registration. *IEEE Trans. Med. Imaging* **2019**, *38*, 470–481. [CrossRef]
101. Li, X.; Dou, Q.; Chen, H.; Fu, C.W.; Qi, X.; Belavý, D.L.; Armbrecht, G.; Felsenberg, D.; Zheng, G.; Heng, P.A. 3D multi-scale FCN with random modality voxel dropout learning for Intervertebral Disc Localization and Segmentation from Multi-modality MR Images. *Med. Image Anal.* **2018**, *45*, 41–54. [CrossRef]
102. Vesal, S.; Maier, A.; Ravikumar, N. Fully Automated 3D Cardiac MRI Localisation and Segmentation Using Deep Neural Networks. *J. Imaging* **2020**, *6*, 65. [CrossRef]
103. Sokooti, H.; de Vos, B.; Berendsen, F.; Lelieveldt, B.P.F.; Išgum, I.; Staring, M. Nonrigid image registration using multi-scale 3D convolutional neural networks. In *Lecture Notes in Computer Science (Including Subseries Lecture Notes in Artificial Intelligence and Lecture Notes in Bioinformatics)*; Springer: Quebec City, QC, Canada, 2017; Volume 10433, pp. 232–239.
104. Torng, W.; Altman, R.B. 3D deep convolutional neural networks for amino acid environment similarity analysis. *BMC Bioinform.* **2017**, *18*, 302. [CrossRef]
105. Blendowski, M.; Heinrich, M.P. Combining MRF-based deformable registration and deep binary 3D-CNN descriptors for large lung motion estimation in COPD patients. *Int. J. Comput. Assist. Radiol. Surg.* **2019**, *14*, 43–52. [CrossRef]
106. Lowekamp, B.C.; Chen, D.T.; Ibáñez, L.; Blezek, D. The Design of SimpleITK. *Front. Neuroinform.* **2013**, *7*, 45. [CrossRef] [PubMed]
107. Avants, B.; Tustison, N.; Song, G. Advanced Normalization Tools (ANTS). *Insight J.* **2009**, *2*, 1–35.
108. Chee, E.; Wu, Z. AIRNet: Self-Supervised Affine Registration for 3D Medical Images using Neural Networks. *arXiv* **2018**, arXiv:1810.02583.
109. Huang, G.; Liu, Z.; van der Maaten, L.; Weinberger, K.Q. Densely Connected Convolutional Networks. In Proceedings of the IEEE Conference on Computer Vision and Pattern Recognition (CVPR), Honolulu, HI, USA, 21–26 July 2017; pp. 2261–2269.
110. Zhou, S.; Xiong, Z.; Chen, C.; Chen, X.; Liu, D.; Zhang, Y.; Zha, Z.J.; Wu, F. Fast and accurate electron microscopy image registration with 3D convolution. In *Lecture Notes in Computer Science (Including Subseries Lecture Notes in Artificial Intelligence and Lecture Notes in Bioinformatics)*; Springer: Quebec City, QC, Canada, 2019; Volume 11764, pp. 478–486.
111. Zhao, S.; Lau, T.; Luo, J.; Chang, E.I.C.; Xu, Y. Unsupervised 3D End-to-End Medical Image Registration with Volume Tweening Network. *IEEE J. Biomed. Heal. Inform.* **2020**, *24*, 1394–1404. [CrossRef]
112. Klein, S.; Staring, M.; Murphy, K.; Viergever, M.A.; Pluim, J.P.W. Elastix: A toolbox for intensity-based medical image registration. *IEEE Trans. Med. Imaging* **2010**, *29*, 196–205. [CrossRef]
113. Balakrishnan, G.; Zhao, A.; Sabuncu, M.R.; Dalca, A.V.; Guttag, J. An Unsupervised Learning Model for Deformable Medical Image Registration. In Proceedings of the IEEE Computer Society Conference on Computer Vision and Pattern Recognition, Salt Lake City, UT, USA, 18–23 June 2018; pp. 9252–9260.
114. Wang, J.; Schaffert, R.; Borsdorf, A.; Heigl, B.; Huang, X.; Hornegger, J.; Maier, A. Dynamic 2-D/3-D rigid registration framework using point-to-plane correspondence model. *IEEE Trans. Med. Imaging* **2017**, *36*, 1939–1954. [CrossRef]

115. Najafabadi, M.M.; Villanustre, F.; Khoshgoftaar, T.M.; Seliya, N.; Wald, R.; Muharemagic, E. Deep learning applications and challenges in big data analytics. *J. Big Data* **2015**, *2*, 1. [CrossRef]
116. Chen, X.W.; Lin, X. Big data deep learning: Challenges and perspectives. *IEEE Access* **2014**, *2*, 514–525. [CrossRef]
117. Vedaldi, A.; Lenc, K. MatConvNet–Convolutional Neural Networks for MATLAB. In Proceedings of the 23rd ACM international Conference on Multimedia, Brisbane, Australia, 12–16 October 2015; pp. 689–692.
118. Duncan, J.; Ayache, N. Medical image analysis: Progress over two decades and the challenges ahead. *IEEE Trans. Pattern Anal. Mach. Intell.* **2000**, *22*, 85–106. [CrossRef]
119. Iglehart, J.K. Health Insurers and Medical-Imaging Policy—A Work in Progress. *N. Engl. J. Med.* **2009**, *360*, 1030–1037. [CrossRef]
120. Wang, L.; Wang, Y.; Chang, Q. Feature selection methods for big data bioinformatics: A survey from the search perspective. *Methods* **2016**, *111*, 21–31. [CrossRef] [PubMed]
121. Prasoon, A.; Petersen, K.; Igel, C.; Lauze, F.; Dam, E.; Nielsen, M. Deep feature learning for knee cartilage segmentation using a triplanar convolutional neural network. In *Lecture Notes in Computer Science (Including Subseries Lecture Notes in Artificial Intelligence and Lecture Notes in Bioinformatics)*; Springer: Quebec City, QC, Canada, 2013; Volume 8150, pp. 246–253.
122. Hinton, G.E.; Osindero, S.; Teh, Y.-W. A Fast Learning Algorithm for Deep Belief Nets. *Neural Comput.* **2006**, *18*, 1527–1554. [CrossRef] [PubMed]
123. Frackowiak, R.S.J. Functional brain imaging. In Proceedings of the Radiation Protection Dosimetry; Oxford University Press: New York, NY, USA, 1996; pp. 55–61.
124. Sun, M.J.; Zhang, J.M. Single-pixel imaging and its application in three-dimensional reconstruction: A brief review. *Sensors* **2019**, *19*, 732. [CrossRef] [PubMed]
125. Lyu, M.; Wang, W.; Wang, H.; Wang, H.; Li, G.; Chen, N.; Situ, G. Deep-learning-based ghost imaging. *Sci. Rep.* **2017**, *7*, 17865. [CrossRef]
126. Gupta, S.; Chan, Y.H.; Rajapakse, J.C. Decoding brain functional connectivity implicated in AD and MCI. *bioRxiv* **2019**, 697003. [CrossRef]
127. Seward, J. Artificial General Intelligence System and Method for Medicine that Determines a Pre-Emergent Disease State of a Patient Based on Mapping a Topological Module. U.S. Patent 9,864,841, 9 January 2018.
128. Huang, T. Imitating the brain with neurocomputer a "new" way towards artificial general intelligence. *Int. J. Autom. Comput.* **2017**, *14*, 520–531. [CrossRef]
129. Shigeno, S. Brain evolution as an information flow designer: The ground architecture for biological and artificial general intelligence. In *Brain Evolution by Design*; Springer: Tokyo, Japan, 2017; pp. 415–438.
130. Mehta, N.; Devarakonda, M.V. Machine Learning, Natural Language Programming, and Electronic Health Records: The next step in the Artificial Intelligence Journey? *J. Allergy Clin. Immunol.* **2018**, *141*, 2019–2021. [CrossRef]
131. Goodfellow, I.J.; Pouget-Abadie, J.; Mirza, M.; Xu, B.; Warde-Farley, D.; Ozair, S.; Courville, A.; Bengio, Y. Generative adversarial nets. In Proceedings of the Advances in Neural Information Processing Systems, Montreal, QC, Canada, 8–13 December 2014; Volume 3, pp. 2672–2680.

3

Bone Age Assessment Empowered with Deep Learning: A Survey, Open Research Challenges and Future Directions

Muhammad Waqas Nadeem [1,2,*], Hock Guan Goh [1,*], Abid Ali [2], Muzammil Hussain [3], Muhammad Adnan Khan [2] and Vasaki a/p Ponnusamy [1]

1 Faculty of Information and Communication Technology (FICT), Universiti Tunku Abdul Rahman (UTAR), Kampar 31900, Perak, Malaysia; vasaki@utar.edu.my
2 Department of Computer Science, Lahore Garrison University, Lahore 54000, Pakistan; abidali.cs17@gmail.com (A.A.); madnankhan@lgu.edu.pk (M.A.K.)
3 Department of Computer Science, School of Systems and Technology, University of Management and Technology, Lahore 54000, Pakistan; muzammil.hussain@umt.edu.pk
* Correspondence: waqasnadeem1995@gmail.com (M.W.N.); gohhg@utar.edu.my (H.G.G.)

Abstract: Deep learning is a quite useful and proliferating technique of machine learning. Various applications, such as medical images analysis, medical images processing, text understanding, and speech recognition, have been using deep learning, and it has been providing rather promising results. Both supervised and unsupervised approaches are being used to extract and learn features as well as for the multi-level representation of pattern recognition and classification. Hence, the way of prediction, recognition, and diagnosis in various domains of healthcare including the abdomen, lung cancer, brain tumor, skeletal bone age assessment, and so on, have been transformed and improved significantly by deep learning. By considering a wide range of deep-learning applications, the main aim of this paper is to present a detailed survey on emerging research of deep-learning models for bone age assessment (e.g., segmentation, prediction, and classification). An enormous number of scientific research publications related to bone age assessment using deep learning are explored, studied, and presented in this survey. Furthermore, the emerging trends of this research domain have been analyzed and discussed. Finally, a critical discussion section on the limitations of deep-learning models has been presented. Open research challenges and future directions in this promising area have been included as well.

Keywords: bone age; deep learning; image processing; health care; survey; segmentation; magnetic resonance images (MRIs)

1. Introduction

The advancement in medical technologies gives more effective and efficient e-health care systems to the medical industry to facilitate the clinical experts for better treatments for patients. E-health care systems are beneficial in various medical domains [1]. Since more computer vision-based biomedical imaging application has gained more importance because these applications provide recognizable information to the radiologists for better treatment [2,3].

Skeletal bone age assessment (BAA) is a mechanism that used for therapeutic investigation [4] and diagnostic of endocrinology problems such as genetic disorders and children's growth [5], in the field of pediatric radiology [6]. The BAA method is commonly performed by radiological examination of the left hand, due to the discriminant nature of bone ossification stages of the non-dominant hand, and afterward it is compared with chronological age. Magnetic resonance images (MRIs), computed tomography (CT), and X-ray images are most commonly used for the analysis of bone maturity and age. The analysis of bone age from these images modalities is widely used due to simplicity, minimum radiation, and availability of multiple ossification centers. Two clinical methods such as Greulich and Pyle (G&P) and Tanner–Whitehouse (TW) are most commonly employed for BAA [5]. The G&P method used by the 76% radiologists, due to its speed and simplicity, it compares a reference atlas and a whole X-ray scan. This method suffers significantly form inter-observer and intra variabilities [7]. The TW based methods and approaches such as TW2 and TW3 have been used for the analysis of particular bones rather than of whole-body bones as in the G&P method.

In particular, the TW based methods take a set of specific region of interest (ROIs) and then divided it into carpal ROIs and metaphysis/epiphysis ROIs. The ROIs are also divided into discrete stages and each stage is represented with a letter (A, B, C, D, . . . , I) along with a corresponding numerical score which varies according to sex and race. Afterward, by adding the score of all ROIs the final bone maturity score is obtained. The TW methods used less because they need more time as compared to G&P methods to perform bone age analysis. However, the TW methods give a more effective and accurate performance as compared to G&P methods [8]. The TW methods are also suitable for automation due to their modular structure. Somehow these are automatic medical image analysis methods but need domain expert feedback for a clinical report [9].

Numerous image-processing approaches and techniques have been used for bone age assessment. Segmentation is a basic step in image processing applications that extract the ROIs from different image modalities like MRI, CT, and X-rays [10–13]. Segmentation of ROIs is an important task for BAA. MRI and X-ray have different features that are used for BAA that includes local histograms [14,15], image textures [16,17], and structure tensor eigenvalues [18–20].

Deep learning (DL) has gained attention for medical imaging problems. DL-based models and architectures are prominent in bone age segmentation, prediction, and classification. It has performed effectively in the field of medical image analysis, object detection and recognition [21], medical image classification [22–24], medical image processing and segmentation [25–27]. The deep learning-based models efficiently resolved the problems related to automatic segmentation, classification, and prediction by using MRI and X-ray images. The convolutional neural network (CNN), deep belief network (DBN), and recurrent neural network (RNN) are powerful deep-learning models for image recognition, segmentation, prediction, and classification. The CNN model is most commonly used for segmentation and classification of bone age. Among all the deep learning models, CNN gives effective performance for image segmentation, prediction, and classification. Two-dimensional CNNs (2D-CNNs) and 3D-CNNs [28–33] are both used for bone age segmentation.

The development of deep-learning models and applications toward bone age assessment encouraged us to present an extensive survey on different categories of BAA such as segmentation, classification, and prediction, from applications and methodology-driven perspectives. The survey also describes the summary of large research publications related to BAA in tabular form that help researchers and readers to speedily evaluate the field. The survey also presents a discussion section that covers the successful deep learning development, research challenges, and a summary for future research directions. This survey covers a wide number of recent publications and presents a variety of DL models and applications for BAA. For identification of the most relevant recent contribution "Deep Learning" AND "Bone Age Assessment" query in the title and abstract is performed. In short, the objectives of the presented survey are (a) to present recent deep learning development for bone age assessment, (b) an overview of open research challenges for successful deep-learning models related to BAA, and (c) to highlight the successful and effective DL contribution for BAA.

2. Typical Deep-Learning Models

Deep learning is a tremendously hot research area in the community of machine learning that has been presented in science magazines since 2006. Different deep-learning models and techniques have been developed in the last few years. The most typical deep-learning models include CNN, RNN, and DBN that are most commonly used in various fields. Most of the other DL models can be derived from these deep architectures. In this section, these models are briefly reviewed.

2.1. *Convolutional Neural Network (CNN)*

The convolutional neural network is a powerful and commonly useable model that learns the features from a large scale image to perform recognition and classification [34–39]. The CNN model has three basic layers such as convolutional, pooling, and fully-connected layers respectively as shown in Figure 1.

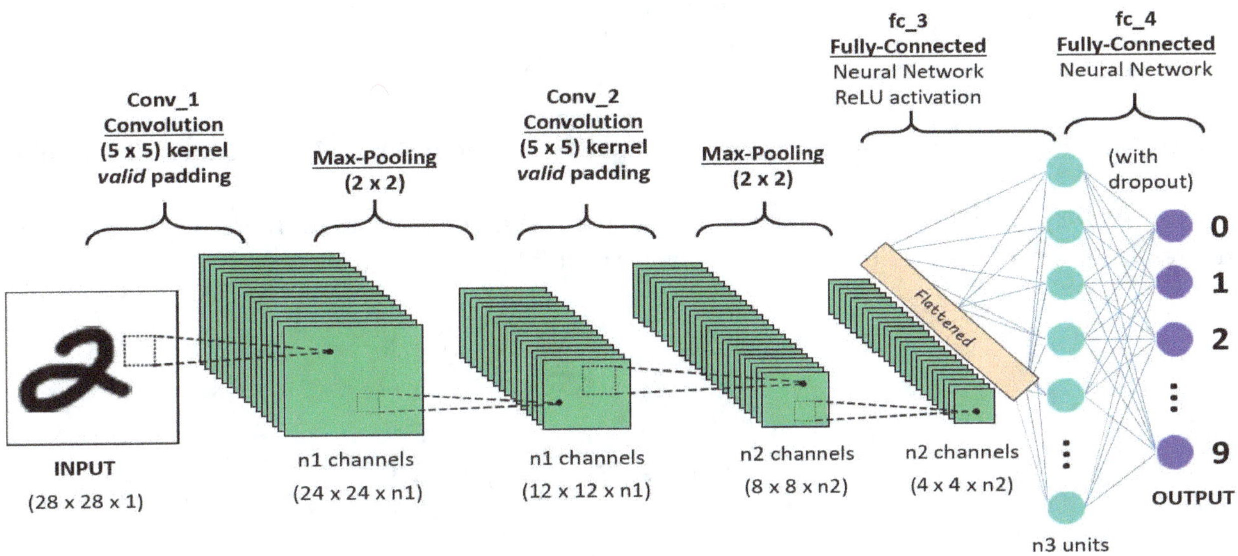

Figure 1. Convolutional neural network [40].

The convolutional layer, share the weights by performing convolution operations the weight and the pooling layer reduce the dimensions. For example, suppose x is a two-dimensional image. Firstly, the image x is divided into a sequential input $x = \{x_1, x_2 \ldots x_n\}$. The convolutional layer to share the weights is defined as:

$$y_j = f\left(\Sigma_i k_{ij} \otimes x_i + b_j\right) \tag{1}$$

The above equation y_j denotes the jth output of the convolution layer and k_{ij} indicates the kernel size with the ith input map x_i $\otimes$ indicates the discrete convolutional operator and b_j represents the bias. Additionally, f is a non-linear activation function, and it is called a scaled hyperbolic tangent. The pooling layer reduces the dimension of the features map. Average pooling or max pooling operations are typically implemented by the pooling layer. Afterward, a softmax and fully-connected layers are deployed on the top of the layer for recognition and classification. Consequently, the deep convolutional neural network (DCNN) usually consists of many pooling and convolutional layers. In the last few years, the DCNN has achieved an effective performance in various domains such as speech recognition, language processing, and so on [40–45].

2.2. *Deep Belief Network (DBN)*

The deep belief network was the first deep-learning model that was trained successfully [46,47]. The DBN is a different form of stacked auto-encoder, and this network is stacked through various restricted Boltzmann machines (RBM). The restricted Boltzmann machine has two layers that include the hidden layer h and visible layer v, as shown in Figure [48,49]. Gibbs samples are used to train parameters by the restricted Boltzmann machine. In particular, conditional probability P (h|v) is utilized in the restricted Boltzmann machine at the hidden layer to compute the value of the respective unit as well as at the visible layer the value of each unit also calculated by conditional probability P (h|v); this mechanism is continuous until the convergence is achieved. RBM has joint distribution for all its units which is defined as:

$$p(v,h;\theta) = \frac{\exp(-E(v,h;\theta)}{z} \tag{2}$$

where $Z = \Sigma_V \Sigma_H \exp(-E(v,h;\theta)$ is utilized for normalization and E is an energy function that used with Bernoulli distribution and computed as:

$$E(v,h;\theta) = -\sum_{i=1}^{I}\sum_{j=1}^{J} w_{ij}v_i h_j - \sum_{i=1}^{I} b_i v_i - \sum_{j=1}^{J} a_j h_j \tag{3}$$

In the above equation, *i* represents the number of visible units and *j* indicates the number of hidden units.

$\theta = \{W, b, a\}$ indicates the set of parameters of the RBM. The computation of sampling probability for the respective unit is described in Equations (4) and (5):

$$P\left(h_j = 1\middle|v;\theta\right) = f\left(\sum_{i=1}^{I} w_{ij}v_i + a_j\right) \tag{4}$$

$$P\left(h_j = 1\middle|v;\theta\right) = f\left(\sum_{j=1}^{J} w_{ij}v_i + b_j\right) \tag{5}$$

where *f* indicates a sigmoid function. The energy function of Gauss–Bernoulli distribution is also used for variation in RBM, which is computed as in [50]:

$$E(v,h;\theta) = -\sum_{i=1}^{I}\sum_{j=1}^{J} w_i v_i h_i + \frac{1}{2}\sum_{i=1}^{I}(v_i - b_i) - \sum_{j=1}^{J} a_j h_j \tag{6}$$

Equation (7) computes the conditional probability of every visible unit.

$$p(v_i = 1|h;\theta) = N\left(\sum_{j=1}^{J} w_{ij}h_j + b_j, 1\right) \tag{7}$$

In the above equation v_i denotes the real value, and the mean value of $\Sigma_{j=1}^{J} w_{ij}h_j + b_j$ along with variance 1 is used for the satisfaction of Gauss distribution. The transformation of a real variable into a binary variable is performed by RBM with Gauss–Bernoulli distribution. Various RBMs are stacked into a model that is called DBN as shown in Figure 2. The two-stage strategy is used to train the DBN. To train the initial parameters, the pre-training phase is used as an unsupervised manner; a supervised training strategy is used to tune the parameters in the fine-tuning phase to the labeled samples; and a softmax-layer is added on the top of layers. DBN has an extensive range of applications in acoustic modeling [51] and image classification [52,53], and so on [54–56].

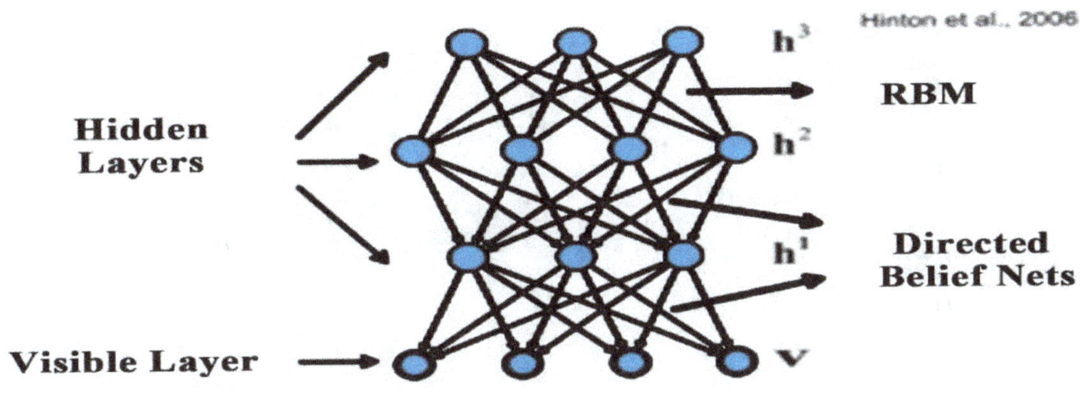

Figure 2. Deep belief network [51].

2.3. *Recurrent Neural Network (RNN)*

DBN, stacked auto-encoders, and CNN do not deal with problems that are related to time series, so these models are not capable of learning features from time-series data. One natural language sentence is an example of time-series data. Hence, in a sentence every word has a close correlation with other words so, to predict the next word the current word and one or more previous words should be used as input. The feed-forward models do not have the capabilities to store the information of the previous input and these models cannot be performed well for these types of tasks. RNN can learn sequentially form data. The internal state of the neural network store the data of the previous inputs and the RNN model learns the features from that series data. Figure 3 presents the directed cycle which is useful for the construction of a connection between different neurons.

A recurrent neural network consists of input units $\{x_o, x_1 \ldots\ldots x_t \ldots\ldots x_{t+1}\}$, output units $\{y_o, y_1 \ldots\ldots y_t \ldots\ldots y_{t+1}\}$, and hidden units $\{s_o, s_1 \ldots\ldots s_t \ldots\ldots s_{t+1}\}$. Figure 3 is shown that at time step t, the RNN takes a current sample x_t and the previously hidden representation s_{t-1} as input to achieve the currently hidden representation s_t:

$$s_t = f(x_t, s_{t-1}) \tag{8}$$

In the above equation, f is an encoder function. One most commonly useable vanilla of RNN for a time step t is described as:

$$s_t = f\big(W_{sx}, x_t + w_{ys} s_{t-1} + b_s\big) \tag{9}$$

$$y_t = g\big(w_{ys} s_{t-1} + b_y\big) \tag{10}$$

where f and g indicate the encoder and decoder, respectively, and $\theta = \{W_{sx}, W_{ss}, b_s, W_{ys}, b_y\}$ denotes the parameter set. Therefore, the RNN captures the dependencies between the current samples x_t with the previous one sample x_{t-1} through the integration of the previously hidden demonstration s_{t-1} into the forward pass. From the theoretical point of view, arbitrary-length dependencies can be capture by RNN. However, the capturing of long-term dependencies by the RNN is a difficult task because of the training of parameters complete by backpropagation with a gradient vanishing strategy. Some other models that prevent a form of gradient exploding or gradient vanishing have been presented to tackle this problem such as long short-term memory (LSTM) [57–60]. The RNN and its variants have attained great performance in various applications such as machine translation, natural language processing, and speech recognition [61–65].

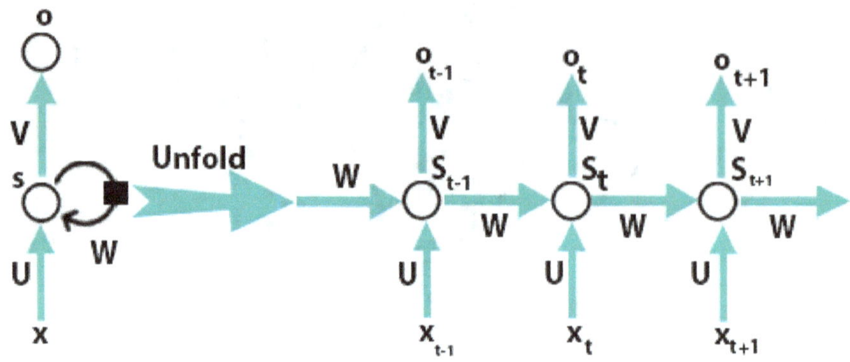

Figure 3. Recurrent neural network [57].

3. Deep-Learning Models for Bone Age Assessment

The bone age assessment process is decided into three stages: segmentation, prediction, and classification. In this section, a comprehensive review of deep-learning models for bone age assessment is presented according to three aspects, i.e., deep-learning models for segmentation, prediction, and classification.

3.1. Deep-Learning Models for Bone Segmentation

Bone segmentation is a separation of weak and diffused boundaries of bones that have strong interaction between their adjacent surfaces. Various image modalities such as CT, MRIs, and ultrasound images are used for the segmentation of bones. A 3D surface voxel-based technique is proposed in [66] for the segmentation. This technique consists of three-phase and uses 3D CT images. In Phase-1 the Gaussian standard deviation (GSD) method is applied to locate joined corrector of the bone surface that increases the regular directions of the bone image. In the second phase, the correction of the regular direction is enhanced by updating the values of different parameters of the GSD. In the 3rd phase, the irregular boundaries of the image are modified. This technique is more powerful for tight joint and noisy images. The ultrasound gives real-time, two or three-dimensional images. The interpretation of Ultra Sound (US) based images is hard because of high-level noise, various imaging artifacts, and a very small thickness of the bone surface. Therefore, the segmentation of US-based images is important for bone age assessment. In recent years, a filter-layer-guided CNN is proposed that uses US-based images for the segmentation of bone surface. This method use fusion of feature maps to decrease the variation in the sensitivity of the multi-modal images affected by the artifacts and low image boundary of the bone. Furthermore, the encoders in the CNN-based architecture maps the input image into the low-dimensional latent space and the decoder maps the latent picture into to original space. Firstly, the architecture resizes the US (x, y) input image and its complementary local phase to a standardized 256×256 size. In fusion-based CNN the every input image would connect with the independent primary and secondary network. Convolutional blocks process the image in each network and every block consist of many convolutional layers. The architecture divides into four distinct blocks as shown in Figure 4. The d1 and d2 blocks represent the depth of each convolutional layer and blocks represent stride. Furthermore, the skip connection block is used to reduce and restore the channel dimensions. The aforementioned convolutions concatenate with its image to obtain the output of the skip connection block. Finally, in the decoder of each network transpose convolution blocks were implemented to up-sample the feature maps. Similarly, as in the other deep-learning models, the fusion CNN architecture uses batch normalization and rectified linear unit (ReLU) activation at each convolutional layer. Finally, to generate the final segmentation probability distribution sigmoid activation function is used at the output layer [29].

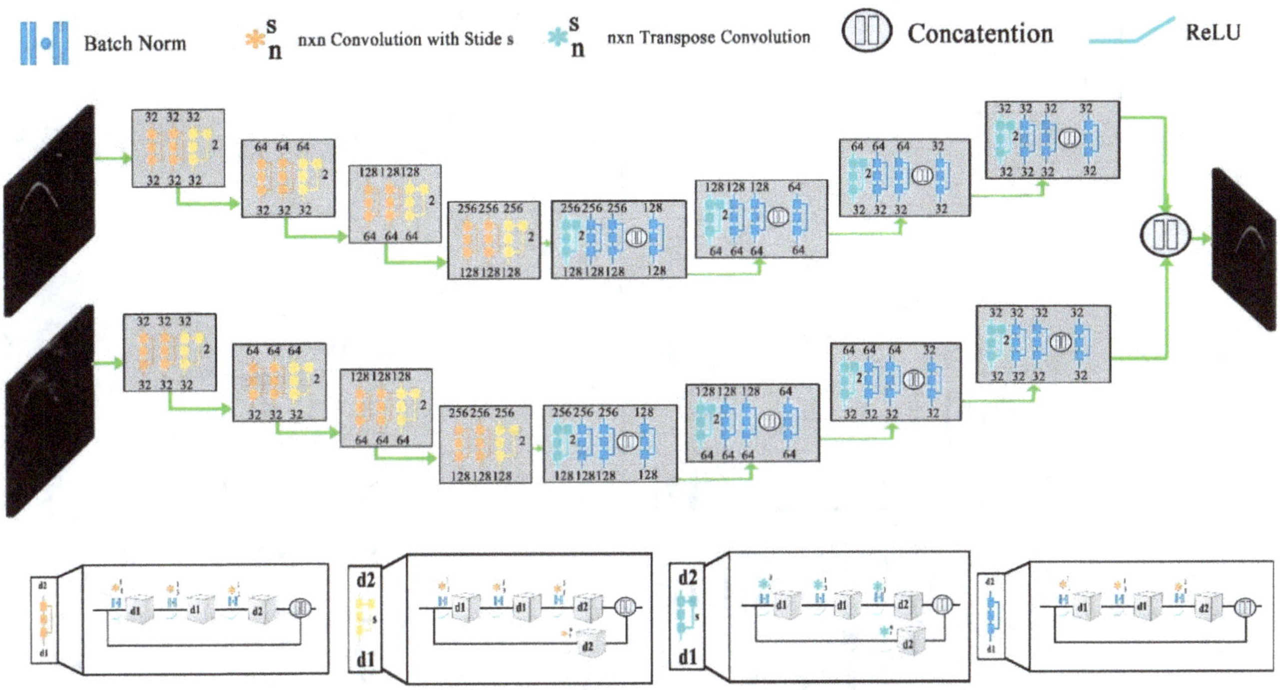

Figure 4. Structure of filter-layer-guided convolutional neural network (CNN) [29].

Furthermore, another U-net based encoder-decoder architecture that uses ultrasound images for the segmentation of bone is presented in recent years. This architecture has several contracting convolution layers that are followed by various expanding de-convolutional layers along with a skip connections layer that make the architecture more efficient and effective for the segmentation [67]. Furthermore, the segmentation of the vertebral osteoporosis bones is difficult due to the complexity of the bone shape. A robust FU-net based model was proposed in [68] for the segmentation of vertebral bone. The U-net model is a U-shaped deep learning model that has contraction on the left side and expansion on the right side. This model adds padding in the convolutional layers and uses uniform dimension images for input and output. On the contraction side, the batch normalization and ReLU activation function are applied on each convolutional layer. The architecture takes an overall image of size 128×128 of the same dimension and segments the image into two output channels in a probabilistic way.

Another, U-net CNN as shown in Figure 5 architecture developed by the researchers for the segmentation of bone images. The architecture consists of five convolution layers which accept 512×512 input image with four down-sampling layers that convert the image into $32 \times 32 \times 512$ representation along with four up-sampling layers. The dropout 0.20 is applied in down-sizing along with 3×3 padded convolutions. At each layer max-pooling with 2×2 kernel size and ReLU also applied. The output layer consisted of 1×1 convolution that followed by a sigmoid activation function that gives the output score for each class. The U-net CNN is effective and efficient when the size of the data set is limited [69].

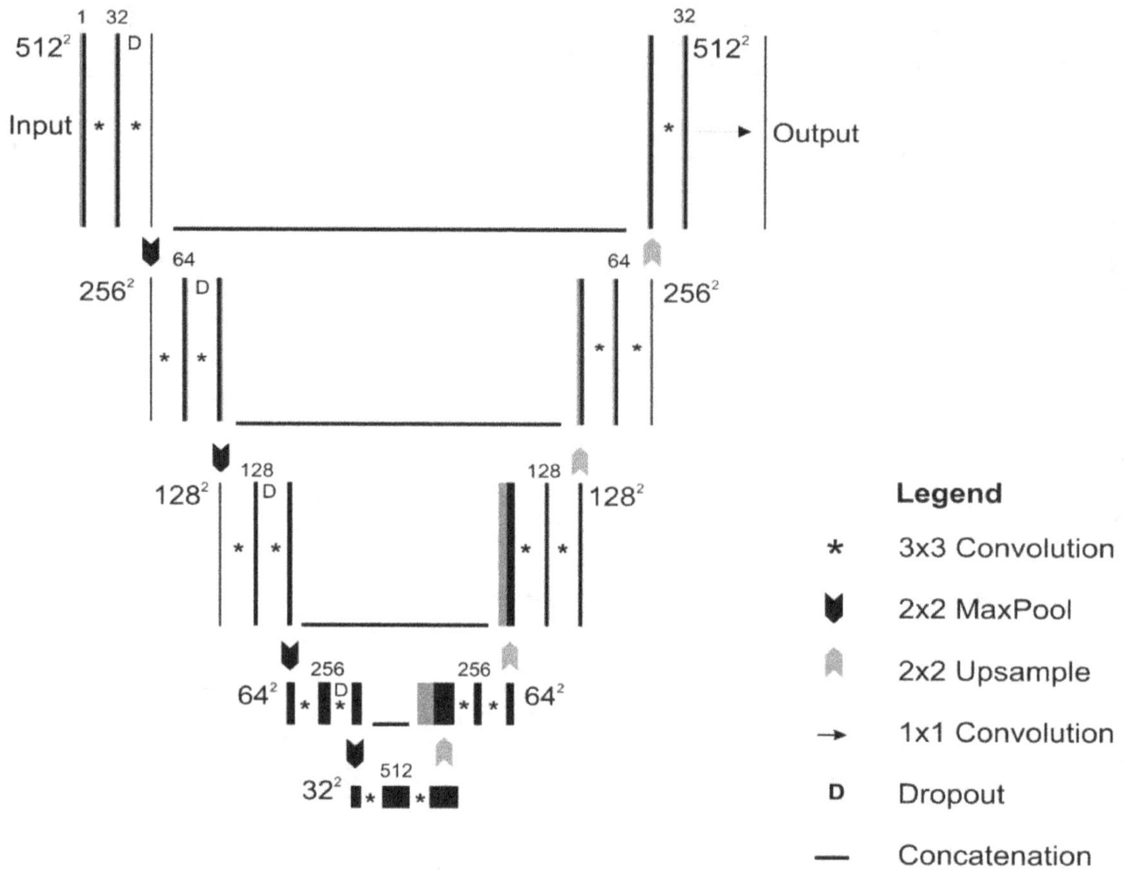

Figure 5. Schematic of the U-net model [69].

In recent years, a fully connected CNN (F-CNN) has been presented for the automatic segmentation of bones instead of manual segmentation. This architecture performs three tasks; firstly, the F-CNN detects the anatomical landmarks of each bone by using the shape model. Then the identified anatomical landmarks are fed to CNN as input for final segmentation. The proposed architecture does not depend on any pre-conceived features or an extensive range of data for training and improvement. It just depends on the size and quality of data that is being fed into the F-CNN. Furthermore, the F-CNN uses CT scans with heterogeneous characteristics form the patients that increase the training performance of the model in recognizing various skeletal patterns [70]. Consequently, another fully convolutional network (FCN) is described in [71] for the automatic localization of bone surface. The FCN model accepts the colored image as input by three different red, green and blue (RGB) channels. The individual channel accepts the original and confident map of the image. The FCN model operates the convolutional filters homogeneously on these three channels. The FCN model is most effective for the segmentation of inter and intra-variation bone surfaces.

Similarly, a multi-feature guided CNN that uses US data was presented in [72]. The model has a pre-enhancing net and modified U-net. The pre-enhancing net phase concatenates the B-mode US input image and three filtered image features to enhance the bone surface, after that U-net performs the segmentation process. Furthermore, the pre-enhancing net enhances the surface of the bone image for better segmentation by performing three tasks that include: (i) local phase tensor image, (ii) local phase bone image, and (iii) bone shadow enhancement. The local phase tensor $(LPT(x,y)) : LPT(x,y)$ image is computed by performing even and odd filter response as

$$\begin{aligned} T_{even} &= [\mathbf{H}(US_{DB}(x,y))][\mathbf{H}(US_{DB}(x,y))]^T \\ T_{odd} &= -0.5 \times \left([\nabla US_{DB}(x,y)]\left[\nabla\nabla^2 US_{DB}(x,y)\right]^T + [\nabla\nabla^2 US_{DB}(x,y)]\left[\nabla US_{DB}(x,y)\right]^T\right) \end{aligned} \quad (11)$$

In the above equation the T_{odd} and T_{even} represent the asymmetric and symmetric features of $US(x,y)$. ∇^2 and $\mathbf{H}$, ∇ represent the Laplacian and gradient operations respectively. Furthermore, to enhance the surface of the bone Log-Gabor filter along with the distance map is also used. $US_{DB}(x,y)$ represents the resulting image obtained from this operation. The final $LPT(x,y)$ image is obtained using $LPT(x,y) = \sqrt{T_{even}^2 + T_{odd}^2} \times \cos(\varnothing)$ where $\varnothing$ represents the instantaneous phase obtained from asymmetric and symmetric features of the input image [5]. Furthermore, the local phase of the bone $(LP(x,y)) : LP(x,y)$ image is computed using: $(LP(x,y)) = LPT(x,y) \times LPE(x,y) \times LwPA(x,y)$ where $LPE(x,y)$ represents local phase energy features and $LwPA(x,y)$ demonstrates local weighted mean phase angle image features. The monogenic signal theory is used to compute these two features such as $LPE(x,y) = \Sigma_{SC}|US_{M1}(x,y)| - \sqrt{US_{M2}^2(x,y) + US_{M2}^3(x,y)}$

$$LwPA(x,y) = arctan \frac{\Sigma_{SC}\, US_{M1}(x,y)}{\sqrt{\Sigma_{SC}\, US_{M1}^2 + \Sigma_{SC}\, US_{M2}^2(x,y)}}$$

where $US_{M1}, US_{M2}, US_{M3}$ denote the three different components of the monogenic signal image $US_M(x,y)$ that measures from $LPT(x,y)$ the image and sc represent the number of filters.

The model also enhanced the shadow of a bone $(BSE(x,y)) : BSE(x,y)$ image by modeling the interaction of the US signal within tissue as attenuation and scattering.

$$BSE(x,y) = [(CM_{LP}(x,y) - \rho)] / \left[\max(US_A(x,y), \varepsilon)]^{\delta}\right] + \rho \quad (12)$$

where $CM_{LP}(x,y)$ represents the confident map of the US image and $US_A(x,y)$ maximizes the visibility of the bone features. δ and ρ represent tissue attenuation coefficient and tissue echogenicity respectively. ε is a small constant that is used to escape division by zero.

Finally, the integration of cU-net + PE with the original U-net model gives more effective results as compared to the simple U-net model. The cU-net + PE take more running time because the convolutional layers of the model performed more computation to learn features. Hence the cU-Net + PE for online and off-line applications.

In recent years, an encoder–decoder network (IE2D-net) also presented for segmentation. The IE2D-net imitates the encoding behavior of the convolutional auto-encoder (CAE) in the latent space that uses ground truth as an input to make sure they use of CAE U-net improved decoder component. The enhancement in the U-net architecture and imitation of prior knowledge is better to improve localization capabilities. The IE2D-net consists of three major modules that include U-net subnetwork, CAE, and IE2D-net. The U-net subnetwork extracts the pertinent hierarchical features from the input images. The CAE module enhances the components of the decoder. The IE2D-net combines the imitating encoders that aim to mirror the CAE generated features in latent space, and the CAE decoders improve the hierarchical features for better segmentation. The IE2D-net achieves better accuracy than simple U-net architecture [73]. Table 1 describes the recent deep-learning development for segmentation.

Table 1. Overview of recent studies for segmentation using deep learning.

Study	Data Set	Method/Model	Proposed Solution	Languages/Libraries/Frameworks/Tools/Software's for Implementation and Simulation	Evaluation
Faisal Rehman et al. [68]	CSI 2014 and xVertSeg.v1	U-Net	FU-Net based Model	Python using Tensor flow on windows desktop system Intel-(R) i-7 Central Processing Unit (CPU) and 1080 GTX graphics card with GPU memory 8 GB.	Dice Score = 96.4 ± 0.8 ASD (mm) = 0.1 ± 0.05
Ahmed Z. Alsinan et al. [29]	B-mode US images ClariusC3	Convolutional Neural Network	Filter-Layer-Guided CNN	Keras framework and Tensor flow, Intel Xeon CPU at 3.00 GHz, and Nvidia Titan-X GPU with 8 GB of memory, Sonix-Touch	F-Score = 95% Bone Surface Localization Error = 0.2 mm
Robert Hemke et al. [74]	Custom Developed (200 Samples)	Convolutional Neural Network	Deep Convolutional Neural Network-based Model	Python 3.7, Keras library (V2.2.4, https://keras.io), Tensorflow 1.13.1, Multi-GPU (4× NVIDIA Titan Xp units)	Dice score = 0.92 Mean Time to segment one CT image = 0.07 s (GPU), 2.51 s (CPU)
Asaduz Zaman et al. [67]	Custom Developed (1950 Samples)	U-Net	U-Net based Encoder–Decoder Model	Not Mentioned	Dice Score = 0.692 ± 0.011
Sarah Lindgren Belala et al. [70]	Custom Developed at Sahlgrenska University Hospital, Goteborg, Sweden (100 Samples)	CNN	Fully Convolutional Neural Network	Not Mentioned	Sorensen-Dice index (SDI) for Sacrum bone = 0.88%
D. D. Pham et al. [73]	Custom Developed	U-Net	2D Encoder-Decoder based U-Net Model	Tensor flow, GTX 1080 GPU	Dice Score = 73.45 ± 5.93
Haoyan Guo et al. [66]	Custom Developed (212 Samples)	Not Mention	Gaussian Standard Deviation (GSD)	C++, Ubuntu platform, PC with a 2.33 GHz Intel quad-core processor, 8 GB RAM	Dice Overlap Coefficient = 98.06 ± 0.58%
M. Villa et al. [71]	Custom developed US images based (3692 Samples)	Fully Convolutional Networks (FCN)	FCN based Model	Python, Caffe framework	RMSE = 1.32 ± 3.70 mm Mean Recall = 62% Precision = 64% F1 Score = 57% Accuracy = 80% Specificity = 83%
Andre Klein et al. [75]	Custom-developed (6000 Samples)	U-Net	U-Net with Padded Convolutions based Model	MITK, NVIDIA Titan X GPU.	Dice Score = 0.96
Puyang Wang et al. [72]	Custom developed US images based (519 Samples)	CNN	Multi-Feature Guided Convolutional Neural Network (CNN)	MATLAB	Recall = 0.97 Precision = 0.965 F-score = 0.968

3.2. Deep-Learning Models for Prediction of Bone Age

Bone age assessment (BAA) is a fundamental process that is used to evaluate the states of many diseases. The actual BAA process has not significantly changed since the publication of the groundbreaking atlas in 1950 by Greulich and Pyle [76] that was developed between 1931 and 1942 by studying children in Ohio. The BAA process can be implemented by using either the Tanner–Whitehouse (TW2) [77] or Greulich and Pyle (GP) [76] methods. The GP method determines bone age by comparing the patient's radiograph with an atlas descriptive age. While the TW2 method is based on the scoring mechanism that examines 20 specific bones. In both cases, the BAA process needs considerable time and comprises substantial interrater variabilities, that lead toward clinical challenges when therapy decisions are made based on changes in patients' BAA. DL [78] gives powerful and efficient models for BAA that overcome these challenges. The DL models replace the conventional models that use manually crafted features for BAA in an automated manner. This section describes the recent devilment in deep learning for BAA.

A fully automated deep-learning model that segments the region of interest, standardizes the image, and processes the input radiographs for the BAA process is presented in [79]. This architecture consists of two parts that include ImageNet pre-trained and a fine-tuned CNN. This model also uses the input occlusion method which creates the attention maps of the input image that reveal which features are used for the training of the model for the BAA process. Finally, the proposed model is deployed in the clinical environment in real-time that gives a much faster interpretation time instead of conventional methods.

Furthermore, skeletal bone age assessment is an extensively famous standard procedure that is used for both growth and disease prediction in the endocrinology area. Furthermore, a CNN and multiple kernel learning (MKL)-based deep automated bone age assessment framework was presented in recent years. The model exploiting the heterogeneous features of the image for bone assessment. Firstly, the visual geometry group (VGG-net) [39] is used to refine the features of the input image. Then the refined features of the image are combined with some other heterogeneous features to make a fused description for the under test object. Support vector regression (SVR) uses the aforementioned heterogeneous features for the estimation of bone age. In the SVR process, the combination of optimal MKL algorithms is used for learning of the model instead of the fixed kernel. This is because the heterogeneous features are from different sources with different similarity notions. The CNN and SVR-based model is effective and gives better performance for the estimation of bone age when the data are in the heterogeneous form [80].

Another, deep-learning based automated bone age estimation model is presented. The model consists of two phases: the features extraction and bone age classification method. The depth neural network (DNN) is utilized to extract local binary pattern (LBP) features and the glutamate cysteine ligase modifier subunit (GCLM) features of the input image. Along with DNN, RCNNs also utilize to locate the key position by creating a sliding window on the input image, the movement of the sliding window along the image gets the potential target areas of the image. The RCNN extract the standard features of the target area and then produces a fixed dimensions output. Finally, the spatial transformer res-net (ST-res net) uses the standard features that produce by RCNN to predict the bone age [81]. In recent years, Greulich–Pyle-based deep learning model developed in [82] for the estimation of bone age, as well as this model, have also validated its feasibility in clinical practice.

Furthermore, a DL and Gaussian process regression (GPR)-based model that observe inter and intra variation in the features of the image for bone age estimation. First, the radiographs are re-scaled to the size of 224 × 224 pixels to train the deep-learning visual geometry group (VGG16) [39] model. During the rescaling process, the aspect ratios of the input image are not altered because they are padded with black pixels. Subsequently, to highlight the surface of the bones in the radiographs, edge enhancement techniques ware also applied in the proposed model. The convolutional layers of the model enhance the pixels of the image where the given matrix E represents the enhancement and e represents the strength of enhancement.

$$E = \begin{pmatrix} -1 & -1 & -1 \\ -1 & e & -1 \\ -1 & -1 & -1 \end{pmatrix}$$

Afterward, the enhanced image pass-through data augmentation phase which is mandatory to train deep-learning networks because deep learning models require a large amount of data for their training [79]. The model rotates a single radiograph 18 times at [−90, 90] degrees. Hence the sensitivity of the model is enhanced due to rotation and flips of the input image that increases the overall prediction performance of the model instead of using a simple deep-learning model [83]. Another CaffeNet-based Convolution Neural Network model that has low complexity compared to other deep learning models is presented in [84]. The CaffeNet model has numerous edges that are connecting with its neurons, and fixed values of neurons are used. CaffeNet-CNN gives more accuracy when the size of the training data is far smaller.

Furthermore, the LeNet-5 network based on CNN architectures is presented in [85] that accepts a 32 × 32 input image instead of 512 × 512 images to estimate the age of bone. First, the architecture converts the input data into a tf-record format which is faster than the original method. Sliding window operation that may include multiple windows is used by the model to scan the standardized image. Lastly, the maximum connected region algorithm is adopted by the LeNet-5 CNN network to determine the age of the bone. Table 2 describes the recent deep-learning development for prediction.

Table 2. Overview of recent deep-learning development for prediction.

Study	Data Set	Method/Model	Proposed Solution	Languages/Libraries/ Frameworks/ Tools/Software's Used for Implementation and Simulation	Evaluation
Xu Chen et al. [81]	Custom Developed at Shengjing Hospital of China Medical University (Samples)	Convolutional Neural Network (CNN)	Depth Neural Network, Local Binary Patterns (LBP) features and Glutamate Cysteine Ligase Modifier subunit (GCLM)	Tensor flow	Average Absolute Error = 0.455
Chao Tong et al. [80]	Public Database Digital Hand-Atlas (Samples)	Convolutional Neural Networks (CNNs)	Convolutional Neural Networks (CNNs) and Support Vector Regression (SVR) based Model	Matlab, Keras framework with Tensor Flow	Mean Absolute Error (MAE) = 0.547
Jang Hyung Lee et al. [84]	Radiological Society of North America (RSNA) challenge dataset	CNN	CNN and CaffeNet based Model	Caffe, Tensorflow, Keras, Theano and Torch, Linux Ubuntu OS, NVIDIA GTX 1060 GPU, CUDA library, and CUDNN library.	Concordance Correlation Coefficient = 0.78
Tom Van Steenkiste et al. [83]	Radiological Society of North America challenge dataset (Samples)	Visual Geometry Group (VGG16)	Visual Geometry Group (VGG16) and Gaussian Process Regression (GPR) based Model	Not Mention	Mean Absolute Difference = 6.80 (−0.94)
Hyunkwang Lee et al. [79]	Custom-developed using open-source software OsiriX and DICOM images (Samples)	CNN	ImageNet pre-trained, fine-tuned convolutional neural network (CNN)	GoogLeNet and Caffe Zoo	Accuracy = 98.56%
Jeong Rye Kim et al. [82]	Custom Developed (Samples)	Deep Neural Network	Greulich-Pyle and Deep Neural Network-Based Model	Not Mention	Root Mean Square Error = 0.42

3.3. Deep-Learning Models for Classification

The Greulich and Pyle (GP) and Tanner–Whitehouse (TW2) are traditional clinical methods that are commonly used for BAA and classification. These methods use radiological images for visual examination and classification, and the performance of the examination highly depends on practitioners' experiences. In recent years, numerous techniques, models, and algorithms are developed that use images-processing techniques to extract explicit features for bone age classification. For example, 15 short bones to encode features of the bone for age estimation. Similarly, in [86] extract features of the bone from seven regions of the interest that includes the carpal bone region and six phalangeal regions for the classification of bone age. However, all these methods and techniques need much effort and are time-consuming. Consequently, the performance of classification extremely depends on hand-crafted features. Therefore, the deep-learning models show prominent performance in bone age classification.

This section briefly describes the recent development in the field of deep learning for bone age classification. DCNNs have had much success in different computer vision problems [87,88]. In [89] a DCNNs model is described for the classification of bone. The DCNNs model extracts the task-relevant, layered and data-driven features automatically from the training data without any feature engineering technique [90]. Due to relatively small samples of training data the DCNN does not give potential solutions. Furthermore, transfer learning is used to train the DCNNs when the size of the data is limited to obtain better performance. First, the DCNNs model use domain knowledge to define different ROIs. Finally, the extracted ROIs and transfer learning are used to perform bone age classification. Similarly, in another study a deep neural network-based model use for the classification of bone. The DNN model to classify the bone on presence skull features on curved maximum intensity projections (CMIP).

A customized CNN that uses a relatively large amount of data as compared to other models is presented in [91]. The model trained from random weight initializations for evaluation and classification of bone age. The customized CNN model consists of a series of convolution matrices that accept vectorized input images and iteratively separate the input image into the target vector space. The main goal of this model is to balance the training parameters for the small size of datasets. The customized CNN model incorporates a combination of residual connections, inception block, and explicit spatial transformation modules. After the initialization of the convolutional layer, a series of residual layers are used in the first portion of the network. The originally residual layers are described in [92,93]; the residual neural networks used by the model to stabilize the gradients during backpropagation, improved the optimization and facilitating greater network depth. Secondly, the inception block introduced by Szegedy et al. [94] also used the customized CNN model to select the optimal filter for input feature maps, and improved the learning rates. The model with residual layers and inception block improve the overall performance of the basic CNN model. Furthermore, a faster-RCNN model with inception-v4 networks is presented in [95,96]. The model is the integration of Tanner–Whitehouse (TW3) and Deep Convolutional Neural Network that used to extract Region of Interest (ROI) for classification. The model explores the expert knowledge from the TW3 method and features engineering from DNN to enhance the accuracy of bone age classification.

Furthermore, most of the studies use transfer learning for bone age classification. A Google Net deep network with a depth of 22 layers was used in [85] for classification. The network was already trained on ImageNet which accepts the final input image and then simply classifies it. The deep convolutional neural with an inception block is used for the training of the classification model. The model reduces the requirement of parameters and increases the number of layers and neurons for effective performance. Table 3 describes the recent deep-learning development for classification.

Table 3. Overview of recent deep-learning development for classification.

Study	Data Set	Method/Model	Proposed Solution	Languages/Libraries/ Frameworks/ Tools/Software's Used for Implementation and Simulation	Evaluation
Jakob Heime et al. [89]	Custom-developed (150 Samples)	Deep Neural Network	Deep Neural Network-based Customized Model	VIDI, COGNEX, Natick, MA, USA	Accuracy = 0.965% Threshold = 0.79% Sensitivity = 91.4% Specificity = 87.5%
Simukayi Mutasa et al. [91]	Digital Hand-Atlas (Samples)	Convolutional Neural Networks (CNNs)	Customized Convolutional Neural Networks with Inception Block	Python Tensor Flow v1.1 library, Ubuntu 16.04 workstation, NVIDIA TITAN X Pascal GPU.	Mean Absolute Error (MAE) = 0.536
Yagang WANG et al. [85]		GoogLeNet		Matlab	Accuracy = 94.4%
Toan Duc Bui et al. [95]	Public Dataset Digital Hand-Atlas (DHA) (1375 Samples)	Deep Convolutional Networks (DNNs)	Deep Convolutional Networks (DNNs) and Tanner Whitehouse (TW3) based Model	Not Mentioned	MAE = 0.59 RMS = 0.76
Jianlong Zhou et al. [97]	Digital Hand-Atlas	Convolutional Neural Networks	Convolutional Neural Networks and Transfer Learning Based Model	Not Mentioned	MAE = 0.72

4. Discussion

4.1. Overview

A large number of scientific research publications were studied and covered by this survey to elaborate on how DL models achieved effective performance in the field of medical image processing and analysis especially in bone age assessment, segmentation, prediction, and classification. Several deep-learning models are discussed in this research. The CNN is used as a feature extractor in numerous publications. The DCNN- and RNN-based models are also used by [31,39] for BAA. The pre-trained deep learning models are available on different archives and these models download from the repository easily and use for different image modalities. Furthermore, the current models most commonly used hand-crafted image features. In recent years, the researchers preferred end-to-end trained models for medical image processing and analysis. It is also reported that deep-learning models such as CNN, DCNN, and RNN have replaced the traditional hand-crafted ML models and integrated these models into present medical images processing and analysis pipelines. Nemours publications that were covered in this survey follow this mechanism and are being practiced in current standards.

4.2. Key Aspects of Successful Deep-Learning Models

After studying a large number of papers, one would expect to be adept to condense the perfect DL model for application areas or individual tasks. The CNN-based models give efficient performance in most bone age assessment applications. We can draw one prominent assumption that is the exact architecture of any model is not a significant determinant for obtaining an effective solution. We have perceived, in various papers i.e., [39,95] that authors have used the same architecture in the model but obtained different results. Furthermore, in [61,85] researchers add more layers in the network of models such as CNN to enhance the performance of the DL model, which is a key aspect that is overlooked in expert knowledge. The authors obtained efficient performance, implement novel preprocessing, and data augmentation techniques along with deep-learning models. In several studies i.e., [83,85], researchers improved the accuracy of the model by adding some normalized pre-processing steps that effectively improved the generalize capabilities of the model without changing the architecture of the model. Consequently, most of the researchers focus on the use of data augmentation strategies and techniques to make the network of models, e.g., the network of the CNN model becomes more robust by using these techniques and improve the performance model. The pre-processing and data augmentation strategies become a key contributor to the effective performance of DL models. Researchers also observed that the designing of a model for a specific task attain betters results as compared to "straightforward" architectures. Multi-scale and multi-view both are cases of the task-specific models. The receptive fields and network input size are fundamental components for designing a network. The increment in patch size should not be changed without the change in receptive fields of the network. If the researchers are domain experts and the model does not give effective performance then there is a need for modification in the network architecture. Furthermore, the performance of the model is also affected by the optimization of different hyper-parameters (e.g., learning rate, dropout rate). There is no best method or technique that currently exists that evaluates the best set of features for empirical exercise. Research also performed and implemented various Bayesian methods that are used for the optimization of hyper-parameters in many medical fields but there is a skill gap in the field of BAA.

4.3. Open Research Challenges, Limitations, and Future Directions

The DL models have various unique challenges in the domain of BAA. Firstly, the deep-learning model required large datasets for their training which is a challenging obstacle. In recent years, several X-rays, MRIs, CT, and Premature Atrial Complexes (PACs) systems (i.e., WebPT, MedEZ, Centricity PACs, ImageGrid, and iQ-4CLOUD) have been installed in hospitals that produce a large number of medical images. Digital archives that have image data in well-structured form have been used for a precise goal. It is also perceived that the number of available public datasets for BAA will increase day-to-day. Sophisticated text-mining methods are mandatory while writing reports on structured labels when the automated method is performed. The process of writing reports using automatic structured labeling in the domain of health care, especially in BAA, will become easier in the future. It is also predicted in the future that the use of structured and text-free reports for the training of the models will increase, especially in the field of bone age assessment. The researchers have asked by domain specialists (e.g., radiologists, pathologists) to make task-specific (e.g., segmentation, classification, and prediction) and text–free reports from image data for training DL models. The labeling of bone images requires a high level of expertise and more time and that is why it is a challenging task in the field of BAA. In the training of a 3D network-based model, slice-by-slice annotations are performed by the network which is a challenging and time-consuming task. Effective and efficient training of a model from a limited amount of data is a major limitation of DL models. The additional pre-processing step that includes modeling uncertainty and noise removal is also performed on data before training the model. Some research incorporates label uncertainties directly into loss function, but this is still a challenge. In [30] researchers use 2D segmented data for the training of 3D segmentation models because of the limited amount of training data. Class-imbalance is another problem that is related to training data. For example, several data-augmentation approaches (additive noise, brightness adjustment, image flipping, image cropping, etc.) were used to generate new lesions from the bone image by rotation and scaling the image which may cause class-imbalance. However, most of the DL models in bone age assessment deal with patch-classification, where the network remains unknown as regards the anatomical location of the patch. To solve this problem a solution is for the full image to be stacked into the network of the model and different methods to be used to achieve the learning process of the network, for example, a dice coefficient-based loss function. Since more, if a model has small receptive fields for full image data then this is not beneficent for a model. Due to some limitations such as bandwidth, Graphics Processing Unit (GPU), and limited memory, the feeding of the full image into the network is not feasible because the size of bone images generally in the giga-pixels range. Another challenge for the DL models is that most of the researchers slice the bone input image using the fixed size of the kernel, the results of which may hide or ignore some useful information by the kernel of the model. Very few researchers i.e., [29] used variable kernel size instead of the fix for slicing of the bone image but there is more work needed in this domain for better performance of deep-learning models toward bone age assessment.

Author Contributions: M.W.N. and A.A. have collected data from different resources, M.W.N. and M.H. performed formal analysis, M.W.N. and A.A. contributed in writing—original draft preparation, M.W.N. and M.A.K.; writing—review and editing, H.G.G. and V.P.; performed supervision, H.G.G., and M.A.K.; drafted pictures and tables, M.H. and V.P.; performed revision and improve the quality of the draft. All authors have read and agreed to the published version of the manuscript.

References

1. Zhao, X.; Wu, Y.; Song, G.; Li, Z.; Zhang, Y.; Fan, Y. A deep learning model integrating FCNNs and CRFs for brain tumor segmentation. *Med. Image Anal.* **2017**, *43*, 98–111. [CrossRef] [PubMed]
2. Singh, N.; Jindal, A. Ultra sonogram images for thyroid segmentation and texture classification in diagnosis of malignant (cancerous) or benign (non-cancerous) nodules. *Int. J. Eng. Innov. Technol.* **2012**, *1*, 202–206.
3. Christ, J.; Sivagowri, S.; Babu, G. Segmentation of Brain Tumors using Meta Heuristic Algorithms. *Open J. Commun. Softw.* **2014**, *2014*, 1–10. [CrossRef]
4. White, H. Radiography of infants and children. *JAMA* **1963**, *185*, 223. [CrossRef]
5. Carty, H. Assessment of skeletal maturity and prediction of adult height (TW3 method). *J. Bone Jt. Surgery. Br. Vol.* **2002**, 310–311. [CrossRef]
6. Poznanski, A.K.; Hernandez, R.J.; Guire, K.E.; Bereza, U.L.; Garn, S.M. Carpal Length in Children—A Useful

Measurement in the Diagnosis of Rheumatoid Arthritis and Some Congenital Malformation Syndromes. *Radiology* **1978**, *129*, 661–668. [CrossRef]

7. Berst, M.J.; Dolan, L.; Bogdanowicz, M.M.; Stevens, M.A.; Chow, S.; Brandser, E.A. Effect of Knowledge of Chronologic Age on the Variability of Pediatric Bone Age Determined Using the Greulich and Pyle Standards. *Am. J. Roentgenol.* **2001**, *176*, 507–510. [CrossRef]
8. King, D.G.; Steventon, D.M.; O'Sullivan, M.P.; Cook, A.M.; Hornsby, V.P.L.; Jefferson, I.G.; King, P.R. Reproducibility of bone ages when performed by radiology registrars: An audit of Tanner and Whitehouse IIversusGreulich and Pyle methods. *Br. J. Radiol.* **1994**, *67*, 848–851. [CrossRef]
9. Spampinato, C.; Palazzo, S.; Giordano, D.; Aldinucci, M.; Leonardi, R. Deep learning for automated skeletal bone age assessment in X-ray images. *Med. Image Anal.* **2017**, *36*, 41–51. [CrossRef]
10. Eckstein, F.; Burstein, D.; Link, T.M. Quantitative MRI of cartilage and bone: Degenerative changes in osteoarthritis. *NMR Biomed.* **2006**, *19*, 822–854. [CrossRef]
11. Daffner, R.; Lupetin, A.; Dash, N.; Deeb, Z.; Sefczek, R.; Schapiro, R. MRI in the detection of malignant infiltration of bone marrow. *Am. J. Roentgenol.* **1986**, *146*, 353–358. [CrossRef]
12. Karampinos, D.C.; Ruschke, S.; Dieckmeyer, M.; Diefenbach, M.; Franz, D.; Gersing, A.S.; Krug, R.; Baum, T. Quantitative MRI and spectroscopy of bone marrow. *J. Magn. Reson. Imaging* **2017**, *47*, 332–353. [CrossRef]
13. Jerban, S.; Ma, Y.; Wong, J.H.; Nazaran, A.; Searleman, A.; Wan, L.; Williams, J.; Du, J.; Chang, E.Y. Ultrashort echo time magnetic resonance imaging (UTE-MRI) of cortical bone correlates well with histomorphometric assessment of bone microstructure. *Bone* **2019**, *123*, 8–17. [CrossRef]
14. Carrion, C.; Guérin, E.; Gachard, N.; Le Guyader, A.; Giraut, S.; Feuillard, J. Adult Bone Marrow Three-Dimensional Phenotypic Landscape of B-Cell Differentiation. *Cytom. Part. B Clin. Cytom.* **2018**, *96*, 30–38. [CrossRef]
15. Zimmermann, E.A.; Riedel, C.; Schmidt, F.N.; Stockhausen, K.E.; Chushkin, Y.; Schaible, E.; Gludovatz, B.; Vettorazzi, E.; Zontone, F.; Püschel, K.; et al. Mechanical Competence and Bone Quality Develop during Skeletal Growth. *J. Bone Miner. Res.* **2019**, *34*, 1461–1472. [CrossRef]
16. Rafałko, G.; Borowska, M.; Szarmach, J. Statistical Analysis of Radiographic Textures Illustrating Healing Process after the Guided Bone Regeneration Surgery. In *Proceedings of the Advances in Intelligent Systems and Computing*; Springer Science and Business Media LLC: Berlin, Germany, 2018; pp. 217–226.
17. Toghyani, S.; Nasseh, I.; Aoun, G.; Noujeim, M. Effect of Image Resolution and Compression on Fractal Analysis of the Periapical Bone. *Acta Inform. Medica* **2019**, *27*, 167–170. [CrossRef]
18. Baltina, T.; Sachenkov, O.; Gerasimov, O.; Baltin, M.; Fedyanin, A.; Lavrov, I. The Influence of Hindlimb Unloading on the Bone Tissue's Structure. *BioNanoScience* **2018**, *8*, 864–867. [CrossRef]
19. Karamov, R.; Martulli, L.M.; Kerschbaum, M.; Sergeichev, I.; Swolfs, Y.; Lomov, S.V. Micro-CT based structure tensor analysis of fibre orientation in random fibre composites versus high-fidelity fibre identification methods. *Compos. Struct.* **2020**, *235*, 111818. [CrossRef]
20. Gerasimov, O.; Yaikova, V.; Baltina, T.; Baltin, M.; Fedyanin, A.; Zamaliev, R.; Sachenkov, O. Modeling the change in the stiffness parameters of bone tissue under the influence of external loads. *J. Phys. Conf. Ser.* **2019**, *1158*, 022045. [CrossRef]
21. Ren, Y.; Zhu, C.; Xiao, S. Small Object Detection in Optical Remote Sensing Images via Modified Faster R-CNN. *Appl. Sci.* **2018**, *8*, 813. [CrossRef]
22. Li, S.; Song, W.; Fang, L.; Chen, Y.; Ghamisi, P.; Benediktsson, J.A. Deep Learning for Hyperspectral Image Classification: An Overview. *IEEE Trans. Geosci. Remote. Sens.* **2019**, *57*, 6690–6709. [CrossRef]
23. Talo, M.; Baloglu, U.B.; Yildirim, O.; Acharya, U.R. Application of deep transfer learning for automated brain abnormality classification using MR images. *Cogn. Syst. Res.* **2019**, *54*, 176–188. [CrossRef]
24. Yang, X.; Ye, Y.; Li, X.; Lau, R.Y.; Zhang, X.; Huang, X. Hyperspectral Image Classification with Deep Learning Models. *IEEE Trans. Geosci. Remote. Sens.* **2018**, *56*, 5408–5423. [CrossRef]
25. Sun, W.; Wang, R. Fully Convolutional Networks for Semantic Segmentation of Very High Resolution Remotely Sensed Images Combined With DSM. *IEEE Geosci. Remote. Sens. Lett.* **2018**, *15*, 474–478. [CrossRef]
26. Monteiro, M.; Figueiredo, M.A.T.; Oliveira, A.L. Conditional Random Fields as Recurrent Neural Networks for 3D Medical Imaging Segmentation. *arXiv* **2018**, arXiv:1807.07464.
27. Yang, T.; Wu, Y.; Zhao, J.; Guan, L. Semantic segmentation via highly fused convolutional network with multiple soft cost functions. *Cogn. Syst. Res.* **2019**, *53*, 20–30. [CrossRef]

28. Ambellan, F.; Tack, A.; Ehlke, M.; Zachow, S. Automated segmentation of knee bone and cartilage combining statistical shape knowledge and convolutional neural networks: Data from the Osteoarthritis Initiative. *Med. Image Anal.* **2019**, *52*, 109–118. [CrossRef]
29. Alsinan, A.Z.; Patel, V.M.; Hacihaliloglu, I. Automatic segmentation of bone surfaces from ultrasound using a filter-layer-guided CNN. *Int. J. Comput. Assist. Radiol. Surg.* **2019**, *14*, 775–783. [CrossRef]
30. Fu, J.; Yang, Y.; Singhrao, K.; Ruan, D.; Low, D.A.; Lewis, J.H. Male pelvic synthetic CT generation from T1-weighted MRI using 2D and 3D convolutional neural networks. *arXiv* **2018**, arXiv:1803.00131.
31. Liu, F.; Zhou, Z.; Jang, H.; Samsonov, A.; Zhao, G.; Kijowski, R. Deep convolutional neural network and 3D deformable approach for tissue segmentation in musculoskeletal magnetic resonance imaging. *Magn. Reson. Med.* **2017**, *79*, 2379–2391. [CrossRef]
32. Deniz, C.M.; Xiang, S.; Hallyburton, R.S.; Welbeck, A.; Babb, J.S.; Honig, S.; Cho, K.; Chang, G. Segmentation of the Proximal Femur from MR Images using Deep Convolutional Neural Networks. *Sci. Rep.* **2018**, *8*, 16485. [CrossRef] [PubMed]
33. Noguchi, S.; Nishio, M.; Yakami, M.; Nakagomi, K.; Togashi, K. Bone segmentation on whole-body CT using convolutional neural network with novel data augmentation techniques. *Comput. Biol. Med.* **2020**, *121*, 103767. [CrossRef] [PubMed]
34. Ajayakumar, R.; Rajan, R. Predominant Instrument Recognition in Polyphonic Music Using GMM-DNN Framework. In Proceedings of the 2020 International Conference on Signal. Processing and Communications (SPCOM), Bangalore, India, 20–23 July 2020; pp. 1–5.
35. Lunga, D.; Yang, H.L.; Reith, A.E.; Weaver, J.; Yuan, J.; Bhaduri, B.L. Domain-Adapted Convolutional Networks for Satellite Image Classification: A Large-Scale Interactive Learning Workflow. *IEEE J. Sel. Top. Appl. Earth Obs. Remote. Sens.* **2018**, *11*, 962–977. [CrossRef]
36. Zhang, C.; Li, G.; Du, S. Multi-Scale Dense Networks for Hyperspectral Remote Sensing Image Classification. *IEEE Trans. Geosci. Remote. Sens.* **2019**, *57*, 9201–9222. [CrossRef]
37. Karpathy, A.; Toderici, G.; Shetty, S.; Leung, T.; Sukthankar, R.; Fei-Fei, L.; Shetty, S.; Leung, T. Large-Scale Video Classification with Convolutional Neural Networks. In Proceedings of the 2014 IEEE Conference on Computer Vision and Pattern Recognition, Columbus, OH, USA, 23–28 June 2014; pp. 1725–1732.
38. Tur, G.; Celikyilmaz, A.; He, X.; Hakkani-Tür, D.; Deng, L. Deep Learning in Conversational Language Understanding. In *Deep Learning in Natural Language Processing*; Springer Science and Business Media LLC: Singapore, 2018; pp. 23–48.
39. Simonyan, K.; Zisserman, A. Very deep convolutional networks for large-scale image recognition. Sep. 4, 2014. *arXiv* **2019**, arXiv:1409.1556.
40. Abdel-Hamid, O.; Mohamed, A.-R.; Jiang, H.; Deng, L.; Penn, G.; Yu, D. Convolutional Neural Networks for Speech Recognition. *IEEE/ACM Trans. Audio Speech Lang. Process.* **2014**, *22*, 1533–1545. [CrossRef]
41. Qian, Y.; Bi, M.; Tan, T.; Yu, K. Very Deep Convolutional Neural Networks for Noise Robust Speech Recognition. *IEEE/ACM Trans. Audio Speech Lang. Process.* **2016**, *24*, 2263–2276. [CrossRef]
42. Abdel-Hamid, O.; Mohamed, A.-R.; Jiang, H.; Penn, G. Applying Convolutional Neural Networks concepts to hybrid NN-HMM model for speech recognition. In Proceedings of the 2012 IEEE International Conference on Acoustics, Speech and Signal Processing (ICASSP), Kyoto, Japan, 25–30 March 2012; pp. 4277–4280.
43. Shi, H.; Ushio, T.; Endo, M.; Yamagami, K.; Horii, N. A multichannel convolutional neural network for cross-language dialog state tracking. In Proceedings of the 2016 IEEE Spoken Language Technology Workshop (SLT), San Diego, CA, USA, 13–16 December 2016; pp. 559–564. [CrossRef]
44. Mane, D.T.; Kulkarni, U.V. A Survey on Supervised Convolutional Neural Network and Its Major Applications. In *Deep Learning and Neural Networks*; IGI Global: Hershey, PA, USA, 2020; pp. 1058–1071.
45. Świętojański, P.; Ghoshal, A.; Renals, S. Convolutional Neural Networks for Distant Speech Recognition. *IEEE Signal. Process. Lett.* **2014**, *21*, 1120–1124. [CrossRef]
46. Hinton, G.E.; Salakhutdinov, R.R. Reducing the Dimensionality of Data with Neural Networks. *Science* **2006**, *313*, 504–507. [CrossRef]
47. Hinton, G.E.; Osindero, S.; Teh, Y.-W. A Fast Learning Algorithm for Deep Belief Nets. *Neural Comput.* **2006**, *18*, 1527–1554. [CrossRef]
48. Larochelle, H.; Mandel, M.; Pascanu, R.; Bengio, y. Learning algorithms for the classification restricted boltzmann machine. *J. Mach. Learn. Res.* **2012**, *13*, 643–669.

49. Salakhutdinov, R.; Mnih, A.; Hinton, G. Restricted Boltzmann machines for collaborative filtering. In Proceedings of the 24th International Conference on Machine learning, Corvalis, OR, USA, 20–24 June 2007; pp. 791–798.
50. Cho, K.; Ilin, A.; Raiko, T. Improved Learning of Gaussian-Bernoulli Restricted Boltzmann Machines. In *Proceedings of the Haptics: Science, Technology, Applications*; Springer Science and Business Media LLC: Berlin, Germany, 2011; Volume 6791, pp. 10–17.
51. Mohamed, A.-R.; Dahl, G.; Hinton, G. Acoustic Modeling Using Deep Belief Networks. *IEEE Trans. Audio Speech Lang. Process.* **2011**, *20*, 14–22. [CrossRef]
52. Li, T.; Zhang, J.; Zhang, Y. Classification of hyperspectral image based on deep belief networks. In Proceedings of the 2014 IEEE International Conference on Image Processing (ICIP), Paris, France, 27–30 October 2014; pp. 5132–5136.
53. Jie, N.; Xiongzhu, B.; Zhong, L.; Yao, W. An Improved Bilinear Deep Belief Network Algorithm for Image Classification. In Proceedings of the 2014 Tenth International Conference on Computational Intelligence and Security, Kunming, China, 15–16 November 2014; pp. 189–192.
54. Huang, W.; Song, G.; Hong, H.; Xie, K. Deep Architecture for Traffic Flow Prediction: Deep Belief Networks with Multitask Learning. *IEEE Trans. Intell. Transp. Syst.* **2014**, *15*, 2191–2201. [CrossRef]
55. Zhang, X.-L.; Wu, J. Deep Belief Networks Based Voice Activity Detection. *IEEE Trans. Audio Speech Lang. Process.* **2012**, *21*, 697–710. [CrossRef]
56. Sarikaya, R.; Hinton, G.E.; Deoras, A. Application of Deep Belief Networks for Natural Language Understanding. *IEEE/ACM Trans. Audio Speech Lang. Process.* **2014**, *22*, 778–784. [CrossRef]
57. Chung, J.; Gulcehre, C.; Cho, K.; Bengio, Y. Empirical evaluation of gated recurrent neural networks on sequence modeling. *arXiv* **2014**, arXiv:1412.3555.
58. Gers, F.A.; Schraudolph, N.N.; Schmidhuber, J. Learning precise timing with LSTM recurrent networks. *J. Mach. Learn. Res.* **2002**, *3*, 115–143.
59. Gers, F.A.; Schmidhuber, J.; Cummins, F. Learning to Forget: Continual Prediction with LSTM. *Neural Comput.* **2000**, *12*, 2451–2471. [CrossRef]
60. Wang, Y.; Chen, Q.; Ding, M.; Li, J. High Precision Dimensional Measurement with Convolutional Neural Network and Bi-Directional Long Short-Term Memory (LSTM). *Sensors* **2019**, *19*, 5302. [CrossRef]
61. Hermanto, A.; Adji, T.B.; Setiawan, N.A. Recurrent neural network language model for English-Indonesian Machine Translation: Experimental study. In Proceedings of the 2015 International Conference on Science in Information Technology (ICSITech), Yogyakarta, Indonesia, 27–28 October 2015; pp. 132–136.
62. Fu, T.; Han, Y.; Li, X.; Liu, Y.; Wu, X. Integrating prosodic information into recurrent neural network language model for speech recognition. In Proceedings of the 2015 Asia-Pacific Signal and Information Processing Association Annual Summit and Conference (APSIPA), Hong Kong, China, 16–19 December 2015; pp. 1194–1197.
63. Chen, X.; Liu, X.; Wang, Y.; Gales, M.J.F.; Woodland, P.C. Efficient Training and Evaluation of Recurrent Neural Network Language Models for Automatic Speech Recognition. *IEEE/ACM Trans. Audio Speech Lang. Process.* **2016**, *24*, 2146–2157. [CrossRef]
64. Chien, J.-T.; Ku, Y.-C. Bayesian Recurrent Neural Network for Language Modeling. *IEEE Trans. Neural Networks Learn. Syst.* **2015**, *27*, 361–374. [CrossRef] [PubMed]
65. Zhang, X.-Y.; Xie, G.-S.; Liu, C.-L.; Bengio, Y. End-to-End Online Writer Identification with Recurrent Neural Network. *IEEE Trans. Human-Mach. Syst.* **2016**, *47*, 285–292. [CrossRef]
66. Guo, H.; Song, S.; Wang, J.; Guo, M.; Cheng, Y.; Wang, Y.; Tamura, S. 3D surface voxel tracing corrector for accurate bone segmentation. *Int. J. Comput. Assist. Radiol. Surg.* **2018**, *13*, 1549–1563. [CrossRef]
67. Zaman, A.; Park, Y.; Park, C.; Park, I.; Joung, S. Deep Learning-based Bone Contour Segmentation from Ultrasound Images. *대한전자공학회 학술대회* **2019**, 1341–1342.
68. Rehman, F.; Shah, S.I.A.; Riaz, M.N.; Gilani, S.O.; Faiza, R. A Region-Based Deep Level Set Formulation for Vertebral Bone Segmentation of Osteoporotic Fractures. *J. Digit. Imaging* **2019**, 33, 191–203. [CrossRef] [PubMed]
69. Ronneberger, O.; Fischer, P.; Brox, T. U-net: Convolutional networks for biomedical image segmentation. In *International Conference on Medical Image Computing and Computer-Assisted Intervention*; Springer: New York, NY, USA, 2015; pp. 234–241.

70. Belal, S.L.; Sadik, M.; Kaboteh, R.; Enqvist, O.; Ulén, J.; Poulsen, M.H.; Simonsen, J.A.; Hoilund-Carlsen, P.F.; Edenbrandt, L.; Trägårdh, E. Deep learning for segmentation of 49 selected bones in CT scans: First step in automated PET/CT-based 3D quantification of skeletal metastases. *Eur. J. Radiol.* **2019**, *113*, 89–95. [CrossRef] [PubMed]
71. Villa, M.; Dardenne, G.; Nasan, M.; LeTissier, H.; Hamitouche, C.; Stindel, E. FCN Based Approach for the Automatic Segmentation of Bone Surfaces in Ultrasound Images. In Proceedings of the CAOS the 18th Annual Meeting of the International Society for Computer Assisted Orthopaedic Surgery, Beijing, China, 6–9 June 2018; Volume 13, pp. 1707–1716. [CrossRef]
72. Wang, P.; Patel, V.M.; Hacihaliloglu, I. Simultaneous Segmentation and Classification of Bone Surfaces from Ultrasound Using a Multi-feature Guided CNN. In *Proceedings of the Agreement Technologies*; Springer Science and Business Media LLC: Berlin, Germany, 2018; pp. 134–142.
73. Pham, D.D.; Dovletov, G.; Warwas, S.; Landgraeber, S.; Jager, M.; Pauli, J. Deep Learning with Anatomical Priors: Imitating Enhanced Autoencoders in Latent Space for Improved Pelvic Bone Segmentation in MRI. In Proceedings of the 2019 IEEE 16th International Symposium on Biomedical Imaging (ISBI 2019), Venice, Italy, 8–11 April 2019; pp. 1166–1169. [CrossRef]
74. Hemke, R.; Buckless, C.G.; Tsao, A.; Wang, B.; Torriani, M. Deep learning for automated segmentation of pelvic muscles, fat, and bone from CT studies for body composition assessment. *Skelet. Radiol.* **2019**, *49*, 387–395. [CrossRef]
75. Klein, A.; Warszawski, J.; Hillengaß, J.; Maier-Hein, K.H. Towards Whole-body CT Bone Segmentation. In *Informatik Aktuell*; Springer Science and Business Media LLC: Berlin, Germany, 2018; pp. 204–209.
76. Greulich, W.W.; Pyle, S.I. Radiographic atlas of skeletal development of the hand and wrist. *Am. J. Med. Sci.* **1959**, *238*, 393. [CrossRef]
77. Garn, S.M.; Tanner, J.M. Assessment of Skeletal Maturity and Prediction of Adult Height (TW2 Method). *Man* **1986**, *21*, 142. [CrossRef]
78. Nadeem, M.W.; Al Ghamdi, M.A.; Hussain, M.; Khan, M.A.; Masood, K.; AlMotiri, S.H.; Butt, S.A. Brain Tumor Analysis Empowered with Deep Learning: A Review, Taxonomy, and Future Challenges. *Brain Sci.* **2020**, *10*, 118. [CrossRef]
79. Lee, H.; Tajmir, S.; Lee, J.; Zissen, M.; Yeshiwas, B.A.; Alkasab, T.K.; Choy, G.; Do, S. Fully Automated Deep Learning System for Bone Age Assessment. *J. Digit. Imaging* **2017**, *30*, 427–441. [CrossRef] [PubMed]
80. Tong, C.; Liang, B.; Li, J.; Zheng, Z. A Deep Automated Skeletal Bone Age Assessment Model with Heterogeneous Features Learning. *J. Med. Syst.* **2018**, *42*, 249. [CrossRef] [PubMed]
81. Chen, X.; Li, J.; Zhang, Y.; Lu, Y.; Liu, S.-Y. Automatic feature extraction in X-ray image based on deep learning approach for determination of bone age. *Futur. Gener. Comput. Syst.* **2020**, *110*, 795–801. [CrossRef]
82. Kim, J.R.; Yoon, H.M.; Hong, S.H.; Kim, S.; Shim, W.H.; Lee, J.S.; Cho, Y.A. Computerized Bone Age Estimation Using Deep Learning Based Program: Evaluation of the Accuracy and Efficiency. *Am. J. Roentgenol.* **2017**, *209*, 1374–1380. [CrossRef]
83. Van Steenkiste, T.; Ruyssinck, J.; Janssens, O.; Vandersmissen, B.; Vandecasteele, F.; Devolder, P.; Achten, E.; Van Hoecke, S.; Deschrijver, D.; Dhaene, T. Automated Assessment of Bone Age Using Deep Learning and Gaussian Process Regression. In Proceedings of the 2018 40th Annual International Conference of the IEEE Engineering in Medicine and Biology Society (EMBC), Honolulu, HI, USA, 17–21 July 2018; pp. 674–677.
84. Lee, J.H.; Kim, K.G. Applying Deep Learning in Medical Images: The Case of Bone Age Estimation. *Health Inform. Res.* **2018**, *24*, 86–92. [CrossRef]
85. Wang, Y.; Zhang, Q.; Han, J.; Jia, Y. Application of Deep learning in Bone age assessment. *IOP Conf. Series: Earth Environ. Sci.* **2018**, *199*, 032012.
86. Wang, S.; Summers, R.M. Machine learning and radiology. *Med. Image Anal.* **2012**, *16*, 933–951. [CrossRef] [PubMed]
87. Litjens, G.; Kooi, T.; Bejnordi, B.E.; Setio, A.A.A.; Ciompi, F.; Ghafoorian, M.; Van Der Laak, J.A.; Van Ginneken, B.; Sánchez, C.I. A survey on deep learning in medical image analysis. *Med. Image Anal.* **2017**, *42*, 60–88. [CrossRef] [PubMed]
88. Myers, J.C.; Okoye, M.I.; Kiple, D.; Kimmerle, E.H.; Reinhard, K.J. Three-dimensional (3-D) imaging in post-mortem examinations: Elucidation and identification of cranial and facial fractures in victims of homicide utilizing 3-D computerized imaging reconstruction techniques. *Int. J. Leg. Med.* **1999**, *113*, 33–37. [CrossRef]

89. Heimer, J.; Thali, M.J.; Ebert, L. Classification based on the presence of skull fractures on curved maximum intensity skull projections by means of deep learning. *J. Forensic Radiol. Imaging* **2018**, *14*, 16–20. [CrossRef]
90. Connor, S.; Tan, G.; Fernando, R.; Chaudhury, N. Computed tomography pseudofractures of the mid face and skull base. *Clin. Radiol.* **2005**, *60*, 1268–1279. [CrossRef] [PubMed]
91. Mutasa, S.; Chang, P.D.; Ruzal-Shapiro, C.; Ayyala, R. MABAL: A Novel Deep-Learning Architecture for Machine-Assisted Bone Age Labeling. *J. Digit. Imaging* **2018**, *31*, 513–519. [CrossRef]
92. He, K.; Zhang, X.; Ren, S.; Sun, J. Deep Residual Learning for Image Recognition. In Proceedings of the 2016 IEEE Conference on Computer Vision and Pattern Recognition (CVPR), Las Vegas, NV, USA, 27–30 June 2016; pp. 770–778.
93. Szegedy, C.; Ioffe, S.; Vanhoucke, V.; Alemi, A.A. Inception-v4, inception-resnet and the impact of residual connections on learning. In Proceedings of the Thirty-first AAAI Conference on Artificial Intelligence, San Francisco, CA, USA, 4–9 February 2017.
94. Szegedy, C.; Liu, W.; Jia, Y.; Sermanet, P.; Reed, S.; Anguelov, D.; Erhan, D.; Vanhoucke, V.; Rabinovich, A. Going deeper with convolutions. In Proceedings of the 2015 IEEE Conference on Computer Vision and Pattern Recognition (CVPR), Boston, MA, USA, 7–12 June 2015; pp. 1–9.
95. Bui, T.D.; Lee, J.-J.; Shin, J. Incorporated region detection and classification using deep convolutional networks for bone age assessment. *Artif. Intell. Med.* **2019**, *97*, 1–8. [CrossRef] [PubMed]
96. Khalid, H.; Hussain, M.; Al Ghamdi, M.A.; Khalid, T.; Khalid, K.; Khan, M.A.; Fatima, K.; Masood, K.; AlMotiri, S.H.; Farooq, M.S.; et al. A Comparative Systematic Literature Review on Knee Bone Reports from MRI, X-rays and CT Scans Using Deep Learning and Machine Learning Methodologies. *Diagnostics* **2020**, *10*, 518. [CrossRef]
97. Zhou, J.; Li, Z.; Zhi, W.; Liang, B.; Moses, D.; Dawes, L. Using Convolutional Neural Networks and Transfer Learning for Bone Age Classification. In Proceedings of the 2017 International Conference on Digital Image Computing: Techniques and Applications (DICTA), Sydney, Australia, 29 November–1 December 2017; pp. 1–6.

4

Musculoskeletal Images Classification for Detection of Fractures using Transfer Learning

Ibrahem Kandel [1,*], Mauro Castelli [1] and Aleš Popovič [1,2]

1 Nova Information Management School (NOVA IMS), Universidade Nova de Lisboa, Campus de Campolide, 1070-312 Lisboa, Portugal; mcastelli@novaims.unl.pt (M.C.); ales.popovic@ef.uni-lj.si (A.P.)

2 School of Economics and Business, University of Ljubljana, Kardeljeva Ploščad 17, 1000 Ljubljana, Slovenia

* Correspondence: D20181143@novaims.unl.pt

Abstract: The classification of the musculoskeletal images can be very challenging, mostly when it is being done in the emergency room, where a decision must be made rapidly. The computer vision domain has gained increasing attention in recent years, due to its achievements in image classification. The convolutional neural network (CNN) is one of the latest computer vision algorithms that achieved state-of-the-art results. A CNN requires an enormous number of images to be adequately trained, and these are always scarce in the medical field. Transfer learning is a technique that is being used to train the CNN by using fewer images. In this paper, we study the appropriate method to classify musculoskeletal images by transfer learning and by training from scratch. We applied six state-of-the-art architectures and compared their performance with transfer learning and with a network trained from scratch. From our results, transfer learning did increase the model performance significantly, and, additionally, it made the model less prone to overfitting.

Keywords: transfer learning; computer vision; convolutional neural networks; image classification; musculoskeletal images; deep learning; medical images

---

1. Introduction

Bone fractures are among the most common conditions that are treated in emergency rooms [1]. Bone fractures represent a severe condition that could result from an accident or a disease like osteoporosis. The fractures can lead to permanent damage or even death in severe cases. The most common way of detecting bone fractures is by investigating an X-ray image of the suspected organ. Reading an X-ray is a complex task, especially in emergency rooms, where the patient is usually in severe pain, and the fractures are not always visible to doctors. Musculoskeletal images are a subspecialty of radiology, which includes several techniques like X-ray, Computed Tomography (CT), and Magnetic Resonance Imaging (MRI), among others. For detecting fractures, the most commonly used method is the musculoskeletal X-ray image [2]. This process involves the radiologists, who are the doctors responsible for classifying the musculoskeletal images, and the emergency physicians, who are the doctors present in the emergency room where any patient with a sudden injury is admitted once arrived at the hospital. Emergency physicians are not very experienced in reading X-ray images like the radiologists, and they are prone to errors and misclassifications [3,4]. Image-classification software can help emergency physicians to accurately and rapidly diagnose a fracture [5], especially in emergency rooms, where a second opinion is much needed and, usually, is not available.

Deep learning is a recent breakthrough in the field of artificial intelligence, and it has demonstrated its potential in learning and prioritizing essential features of a given dataset without being explicitly programmed to do so. The autonomous behavior of deep learning makes it particularly suitable in the field of computer vision. The area of computer vision includes several tasks, like image segmentation, image detection, and image classification. Deep learning was successfully applied in many computer vision tasks, like in retinal image segmentation [6], histopathology image classification [7], and MRI image classification [8], among others.

Focusing on image classification, in 2012, Krizhevsky et al. [9] proposed a convolutional neural network CNN-based model, and they won a very popular image classification challenge called ILSVRC. Afterward, CNNs gained popularity in the area of computer vision, and it is nowadays considered the state-of-the-art technique for image classification. The process of training a classifier is time-consuming and requires large datasets to be correctly trained. In the medical field, there is always a scarcity of images that can be used to train a classifier, mainly due to the regulations implemented in the medical field. Transfer learning is a technique that is usually used to train CNNs, when there are not enough images available or when obtaining new images is particularly difficult. Transfer learning is about training a CNN to classify large non-medical datasets and then use the weights of such a CNN as a starting point for classifying other target images, in our case, X-ray images.

Several studies addressed the classification of musculoskeletal images using deep learning techniques. Rajpurkar et al. [10] introduced a novel dataset called MURA dataset that contains 40,005 musculoskeletal images. The authors used DenseNet169 CNN to compare the performance of the CNN against three radiologists. The model achieved an acceptable performance compared to the predictions of the radiologists. Chada [11] investigated the performance of three state-of-the-art CNNs, namely DenseNet169, DenseNet201, and InceptionResNetV2, on the MURA dataset. The author fine-tuned the three architectures using Adam optimizer with a learning rate of 0.0001. Fifty epochs were used with a batch size of eight images to train the model. The author reported that DenseNet201 achieved the best performance for the humerus images, with a Kappa score of 0.764, and InceptionResNetV2 achieved the best performance for the finger images, with a Kappa score of 0.555.

To demonstrate the importance of deep learning in the emergency room for fracture detections, Lindsey et al. [5] investigated the usage of CNNs to detect wrist fractures. Subsequently, they measured the radiologists' performance of detecting fractures with and without the help of CNN. The authors reported that, by using a CNN, the performance of the radiologists increased significantly. Kitamura et al. [12] studied the possibility of detecting ankle fractures with CNNs, using InceptionV3, ResNet, and Xception networks for their experiments. The authors trained a CNN from scratch without any transfer learning, and they used a private dataset and an ensemble of the three architectures and reported an accuracy of 81%.

In this paper, we are extending the work of Rajpurkar et al. [10] and Chada [11] by investigating the usage of transfer learning of a CNN to classify X-ray images to detect bone fractures. To do so, we used six state-of-the-art CNN architectures that were previously trained on the ImageNet dataset (an extensive non-medical dataset). To the best of our knowledge, this is the first paper that performs a rigorous investigation on the use of transfer learning in the context of musculoskeletal image classification. More in detail, we investigate the following:

1. The effect of transfer learning on image classification performance. To do that, we compare the performance of six CNN architectures that were trained on ImageNet to classify fractures images. Then, we train the same datasets with the same networks, but without the ImageNet weights.
2. The best classifier that achieves the best results on the musculoskeletal images.
3. The effect of the fully connected layers on the performance of the network. To do that, two fully connected layers were added after each network, and then we recorded their performance. Subsequently, the layers are removed, and the performance of the networks is recorded as well.

The paper is organized as follows: In Section 2, we present the methodology used. In Section 3, we present the results achieved by training the MURA dataset on the considered CNNs. In Section 4, we present a discussion about the results obtained, and we compare them to other state-of-the-art results. In Section 5, we conclude the paper by summarizing the main findings of this work.

2. Methodology

In this section, we briefly describe the main methods used in this paper.

2.1. *Convolutional Neural Networks and Transfer Learning*

A convolutional neural network is a feed-forward neural network with at least one convolution layer. A convolution layer is a hidden neural network layer that has a convolution operation, where the convolution operation is a mathematical operation that is used to make use of the spatial information presented in images. Training a CNN requires a significant amount of images, and this is one of the most severe limitations in deep learning. In particular, deep learning has a very strong dependence on massive training data compared to traditional machine learning methods because it needs a large amount of data to understand the latent patterns of data. Unfortunately, there are problems in which insufficient training data are an inescapable issue. This may happen in domains in which obtaining new observations are either expensive, time-consuming, or impossible. In these situations, transfer learning provides a suitable way for training a CNN. More in detail, transfer learning is a technique used in the deep learning field to make use of knowledge that can be shared by different domains. According to Pan and Yang [13], transfer learning can be defined as improving the predictive function, $f_T(.)$ by using the knowledge acquired from the source domain, D_S, into the target domain, D_T. Transfer learning relaxes the hypothesis that the training data must be independent and identically distributed with the test data. This allows us to use transfer learning for training CNNs in a given domain and to use them to subsequently address a problem in which data scarcity is a significant limitation. For more details on transfer learning, the interested reader is referred to Pan and Yang [13].

2.2. *State-of-the-Art Architectures*

Many CNNs were introduced to participate in the ILSVRC challenge. In this section, we present different CNNs that are considered in this study.

2.2.1. VGG

Simonyan et al. [14] introduced the VGG network in 2014. The VGG was implemented in many variations like VGG16 and VGG19, which only differ in the number of convolution layers used in each. In this paper, we use VGG19 because it is the largest one, and it usually produces better performance than VGG16. VGG19 consists of 19 convolution layers and one dense layer with 4096 neurons to classify the ImageNet images. For more information, the reader is referred to the corresponding paper [14].

2.2.2. Xception

Chollet [15] introduced a novel architecture called Xception (extreme inception), where the author replaced the conventional convolutional layers with depthwise separable convolutional layers. These modified layers decreased the network parameters without decreasing its capacity, which yielded a robust network with fewer parameters and so less computational resources needed for training. For more information, the reader is referred to the corresponding paper [15].

2.2.3. ResNet

ResNet architecture was introduced by He et al. [16] in 2015. ResNet was developed by exploiting the concept of residual connections. The authors introduced the concept of a residual connection to minimize the effect of the vanishing gradient. The ResNet architecture comes in many variants. In this paper, we use the ResNet50 network, which contains 50 layers. For more information, the reader is referred to the corresponding paper [16].

2.2.4. GoogLeNet

GoogLeNet architecture was introduced by Szegedy et al. [17] in 2014. The authors proposed a novel idea called the inception module, which takes the aspect ratio of each image into account. There are many variants for GoogLeNet architecture, and we use the InceptionV3 network. For more information, the reader is referred to the corresponding paper [17].

2.2.5. InceptionResNet

Längkvist et al. [18] created a novel architecture called InceptionResNet, where the authors combined the inception module idea from GoogLeNet architecture [17] with the residual idea from ResNet architecture [16]. InceptionResNet is more computationally efficient than both ResNet and Inception architectures and achieved higher results than both on the ImageNet dataset. For more information, the reader is referred to the corresponding paper [18].

2.2.6. DenseNet

Huang et al. [19] introduced a novel architecture called DenseNet. In this architecture, the convolution blocks are densely connected to each other, and the convolution blocks are concatenated to each other instead of being added like in the ResNet network. For more information, the reader is referred to the corresponding paper [19].

2.3. *Evaluation Metrics*

Two evaluation metrics are being used to assess the performance of each network. Accuracy and Kappa. Below, we briefly summarize each metric:

2.3.1. Accuracy

This metric quantifies how accurate the classifier is. It is calculated as the number of correctly classified data points divided by the total number of the data points. The formula is shown in Equation (1).

$$\text{Accuracy} = \frac{\text{TN} + \text{TP}}{\text{TP} + \text{TN} + \text{FP} + \text{FN}} \tag{1}$$

where TP stands for true positive, TN stands for true negative, FP stands for false positive, and FN stands for false negative. In the context of this study, images without fractures belong to the negative class, whereas images with a bone fracture belong to the positive class.

2.3.2. Kappa

This is an evaluation metric that is usually used to take into account the probability of selecting by chance, especially in cases of unbalanced datasets, and it was introduced by Cohen [20]. The upper limit of the Kappa metric is 1, which means that the classifier classified everything correctly. At the same time, the lower bound can go below zero, which indicates the classifier is just classifying by luck. The Kappa formula is presented in Equation (2).

$$\text{Kappa} = \frac{\text{Agreement}_{\text{Observed}} - \text{Agreement}_{\text{Expected}}}{1 - \text{Agreement}_{\text{Expected}}} \tag{2}$$

2.4. *Statistical Analysis*

A statistical analysis was performed to assess the statistical significance of the results. We considered a confidence interval with a 95% error rate (95% CI) and a hypothesis test. Two hypothesis tests can be used: ANOVA or Kruskal–Wallis test. The choice of the test mainly depends on the normality of the data under observation. The ANOVA test is a parametric test that assumes that the data have a normal distribution. The null hypothesis of the ANOVA test is that the considered samples have the same mean, and the alternative hypothesis is that the samples have a different mean.

The non-parametric test is the Kruskal–Wallis hypothesis test [21]. This test does not make any assumption on the normality of the data, and it compares the medians of different samples. The null and alternative hypotheses tested are the following:

Hypothesis 0 (H0). *The populations medians are all equal.*

Hypothesis 1 (H1). *The populations medians are not all equal.*

In this paper, we first tested the normality assumption by using the Shapiro–Wilk test. Considering that the test does not allow to reject the alternative hypothesis (i.e., data not normally distributed), the Kruskal–Wallis test was used to test the significance of the results obtained. To make the hypothesis test and to report means and significance errors, each setting was repeated 30 times using different seeds and different validation split. In this way, each approach's stability can be assessed by also mitigating the effect of lucky seeds [22].

2.5. Dataset

The dataset used in this paper is the publicly available MURA dataset [10]. The dataset consists of seven different skeletal bones: elbow, finger, forearm, hand, humerus, shoulder, and wrist. Each category has a binary label, indicating if the image presents a broken bone or not. The dataset contains a total of 40,005 images. The authors of the dataset split it into training and test sets. The train set included 21,935 images without fractures (54.83% of the dataset) and 14,873 images with fractures (37.17% of the dataset), and the test set contained 1667 images without fractures (4.16% of the dataset) and 1530 images with fractures (3.84% of the dataset).

All in all, 92% of the dataset is used for training, and 8% of the dataset is used for testing the results. The summary of the dataset is presented in Table 1. A sample of the MURA dataset is presented in Figure 1.

Table 1. MURA dataset summary.

Category	Training Dataset		Test Dataset	
	Normal	Fractured	Normal	Fractured
Elbow	2925	2006	235	230
Finger	3138	1968	214	247
Hand	4059	1484	271	189
Humerus	673	599	148	140
Forearm	1164	661	150	151
Shoulder	4211	4168	285	278
Wrist	5765	3987	364	295
Total	21,935	14,873	1667	1530

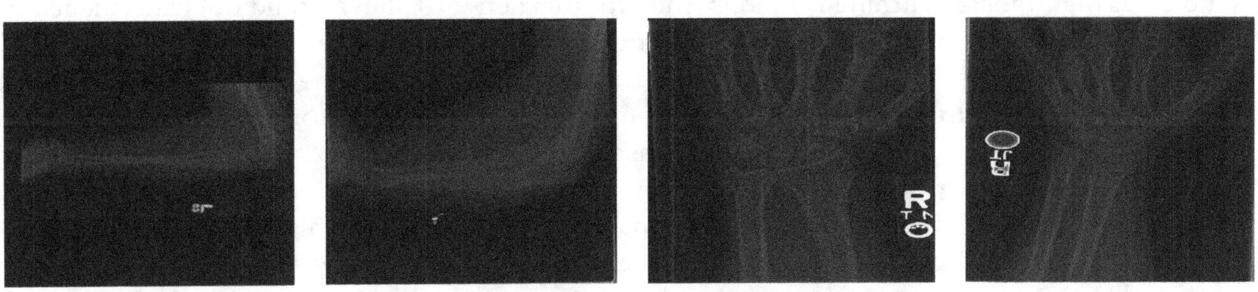

Broken Forearm | Normal Forearm | Broken Wrist | Normal Wrist

Figure 1. A sample of the MURA dataset.

3. Results

Throughout the experiments, all the hyperparameters were fixed. All the networks were either fine-tuned completely or trained from scratch. Adam optimizer [21] was used in all the experiments. As noted by studies [22,23], the learning rate should be low to avoid dramatically changing the original weights, so we set the learning rate to be 0.0001. All the images were resized to 96×96 pixels. Binary cross-entropy was used as the loss function because the images are binary classified. An early stopping criterion of 50 epochs would be used to stop the algorithms if no updates happened to the validation score. The batch size was selected to be 64, and the training dataset was split into 80% to train and 20% to validate the results during training. Four image augmentation techniques were used to increase the training dataset's size and make the network more robust against overfitting; the augmentation techniques used are horizontal and vertical flips, 180 rotations, and zooming.

Additionally, image augmentation is performed to balancing the number of images in the two target classes, thus achieving 50% of images without fractures and 50% of images with fractures in the training set. After the training, each network's performance was tested using the dataset that was supplied by the owner and creator of the dataset. The test dataset was not used during the training phase, but only in the final testing phase. The hyperparameters used are presented in Table 2. In the following sections, Kappa is the metric considered for comparing the performance of the different architectures.

Table 2. The hyperparameters were used for all the experiments.

Framework	Keras with Python
Optimizer	Adam
Learning Rate	0.0001
Loss Function	Binary Cross-entropy
Early Stopping	50 epochs
Batch Size	64
Validation Split	20%
Image Augmentation	Horizontal flips Vertical flips 180 rotations Zooming

3.1. *Wrist Images Classification Results*

Two main sets of experiments were performed: the first consists of adding two fully connected layers after each architecture to act as a classifier block. The second consists of adding only a sigmoid layer after the network. Both the results of the first set and the second set are presented in Table 3.

In the first set of experiments, the fine-tuned VGG19 network had a Kappa score of 0.5989, while the network that was trained from scratch had a score of 0.5476. For the Xception network, the transfer learning score was higher than the one trained from scratch by a large margin. The ResNet50 network performance improved significantly by using transfer learning rather than training it from scratch. This indicates that transfer learning is fundamental for this network, that it could not learn the features of the images from scratch. Both the fine-tuned InceptionV3, InceptionResNetV2, and DenseNet121 networks have a higher score than training them from scratch. Overall, fine-tuning the networks did yield better results than training the networks from scratch. The best performance for the first set of experiments was achieved by fine-tuning the DenseNet121 network.

In the second set of experiments, all the networks' performance increased by fine-tuning than by training from scratch. The ResNet network was the network with the highest difference between fine-tuning and training from scratch. Overall, the best performance for the second set of experiments was achieved by fine-tuning the Xception network. Comparing the first set of experiments to the second set, we see that the best performance for classifying wrist images was the fine-tuned DenseNet121 network with fully connected layers. The presence of fully connected layers did not have any noticeable increase in performance; however, it is worth noting that the ResNet network with fully connected layers did not converge when trained from scratch.

Table 3. Accuracy and Kappa scores of classifying wrist images with and without fully connected layers (±95% CI).

Network	Method	With FC		Without FC	
		Mean Accuracy	Mean Kappa	Mean Accuracy	Mean Kappa
VGG19	TL	80.45% ± 1.26%	0.5989 ± 2.39%	80.63% ± 1.64%	0.6035 ± 3.33%
	Scratch	78.07% ± 0.94%	0.5476 ± 2.11%	79.89% ± 1.84%	0.5846 ± 3.74%
InceptionV3	TL	79.92% ± 2.07%	0.5886 ± 3.61%	79.94% ± 1.46%	0.5876 ± 2.77%
	Scratch	77.01% ± 2.98%	0.5241 ± 6.49%	77.59% ± 1.51%	0.5389 ± 3.03%
ResNet	TL	78.76% ± 0.88%	0.5647 ± 2.04%	80.85% ± 1.70%	0.6046 ± 3.63%
	Scratch	58.65% ± 8.70%	0.0836 ± 21.31%	70.99% ± 4.20%	0.4018 ± 8.27%
Xception	TL	80.93% ± 0.88%	0.6098 ± 1.69%	81.18% ± 0.47%	0.6133 ± 0.94%
	Scratch	77.44% ± 1.99%	0.5333 ± 4.41%	77.14% ± 1.86%	0.5318 ± 3.32%
DenseNet	TL	81.71% ± 0.94%	0.6245 ± 1.98%	78.76% ± 2.27%	0.5663 ± 4.29%
	Scratch	76.40% ± 2.30%	0.5083 ± 5.17%	76.68% ± 3.62%	0.5214 ± 7.25%
InceptionResNet	TL	80.1% ± 1.66%	0.5917 ± 3.32%	80.55% ± 1.06%	0.6010 ± 2.25%
	Scratch	77.77% ± 1.59%	0.5450 ± 2.85%	78.55% ± 1.70%	0.5580 ± 3.48%

3.2. *Hand Images Classification Results*

As done with the wrist images, two sets of experiments were performed. Both the results of the first set and the second set are presented in Table 4.

In the first set of experiments, for the VGG19 and the ResNet networks, fine-tuning the networks resulted in significantly higher performance than training the networks from scratch. The networks trained from scratch did not converge to an acceptable result. This fact highlights that the importance of transfer learning for these networks, that are not able to learn the images' features from scratch. For the remaining networks, fine-tuning achieved significantly better performance than by training the networks from scratch. Overall, all the fine-tuned networks achieved better results than by training from scratch. The best performance of the first set of experiments was obtained with the fine-tuned Xception network.

Table 4. Accuracy and Kappa scores of classifying hand images with and without fully connected layers (±95% CI).

Network	Method	With FC		Without FC	
		Mean Accuracy	Mean Kappa	Mean Accuracy	Mean Kappa
VGG19	TL	70.11% ± 9.23%	0.3089 ± 25.42%	73.04% ± 1.27%	0.3960 ± 3.23%
	Scratch	58.91% ± 0%	0 ± 0%	63.22% ± 5.90%	0.1312 ± 15.90%
InceptionV3	TL	70.25% ± 1.34%	0.3261 ± 3.57%	72.10% ± 0.79%	0.3829 ± 2.15%
	Scratch	66.38% ± 3.80%	0.2382 ± 9.76%	66.56% ± 2.48%	0.2361 ± 6.07%
ResNet	TL	72.25% ± 1.25%	0.3754 ± 3.55%	71.12% ± 1.94%	0.3503 ± 5.44%
	Scratch	59.28% ± 0.93%	0.0103 ± 2.65%	62.10% ± 1.21%	0.0971 ± 3.26%
Xception	TL	75.36% ± 2.56%	0.4621 ± 6.27%	72.50% ± 2.0%	0.3778 ± 5.41%
	Scratch	66.74% ± 2.58%	0.2277 ± 7.20%	66.81% ± 3.60%	0.2334 ± 10.05%
DenseNet	TL	72.21% ± 1.69%	0.3746 ± 4.33%	70.22% ± 3.28%	0.3243 ± 9.03%
	Scratch	63.33% ± 1.16%	0.1308 ± 3.47%	62.79% ± 1.50%	0.1231 ± 4.39%
InceptionResNet	TL	71.96% ± 1.80%	0.3709 ± 4.33%	71.81% ± 1.91%	0.3670 ± 4.65%
	Scratch	68.48% ± 1.53%	0.2788 ± 4.36%	69.09% ± 1.04%	0.3071 ± 2.43%

In the second set of experiments, the performance of all the networks increased by fine-tuning than by training from scratch. The ResNet network was the network with the highest difference between fine-tuning and training from scratch. Overall, the best network was the VGG19 network. Comparing the first set of experiments to the second set, we see that the best performance for classifying hand images was the fine-tuned Xception network with fully connected layers. The presence of fully connected layers did not significantly increase the performance; however, it is important to point out that the VGG19 network with fully connected layers did not converge when it was trained from scratch.

3.3. Humerus Images Classification Results

For the humerus images, the results of both the first and second sets of experiments are presented in Table 5. In the first set of experiments, fine-tuning VGG19 architecture did not converge to any acceptable results, while training the VGG19 from scratch did yield higher performance. For the rest of the networks, fine-tuning did achieve better results than training the networks from scratch. The highest difference was between fine-tuning the ResNet network and training it from scratch. Overall, the best network in the first sets of experiments was the fine-tuned DenseNet network, with a Kappa score of 0.6260.

In the second set of experiments, fine-tuning did achieve better results for all the networks than training the networks from scratch. The best-achieved network was the VGG19 network, with a Kappa score of 0.6333. Comparing the first set of experiments to the second set, we see that the best performance for classifying humerus images was the fine-tuned VGG19 network without fully connected layers. Just as in the previous experiments, the fully connected layers' presence did not provide any significant performance improvement; however, fine-tuning the VGG19 with fully connected layers did not converge compared to fine-tuning the same network without any fully connected layers.

Table 5. Accuracy and Kappa scores of classifying humerus images with and without fully connected layers (±95% CI).

Network	Method	With FC		Without FC	
		Mean Accuracy	Mean Kappa	Mean Accuracy	Mean Kappa
VGG19	TL	51.39% ± 0%	0 ± 0%	81.66% ± 2.74%	0.6333 ± 5.43%
	Scratch	62.04% ± 3.67%	0.239 ± 8.01%	69.44% ± 8.28%	0.3893 ± 16.77%
InceptionV3	TL	80.32% ± 2.74%	0.6070 ± 5.51%	80.56% ± 1.48%	0.6114 ± 2.94%
	Scratch	67.77% ± 3.12%	0.3603 ± 6.08%	64.06% ± 3.51%	0.2879 ± 6.81%
ResNet	TL	80.38% ± 2.55%	0.6084 ± 5.03%	78.18% ± 2.20%	0.5647 ± 4.31%
	Scratch	54.28% ± 7.46%	0.0849 ± 14.97%	65.63% ± 5.19%	0.3171 ± 10.26%
Xception	TL	80.03% ± 1.92%	0.6010 ± 3.81%	79.75% ± 1.67%	0.5942 ± 3.40%
	Scratch	66.55% ± 2.84%	0.3386 ± 5.46%	66.32% ± 4.72%	0.3334 ± 9.11%
DenseNet	TL	81.31% ± 1.88%	0.6260 ± 3.81%	77.84% ± 1.52%	0.5563 ± 3.16%
	Scratch	70.54% ± 5.85%	0.4134 ± 11.37%	71.93% ± 2.74%	0.4406 ± 5.35%
InceptionResNet	TL	78.41% ± 1.84%	0.5697 ± 3.61%	78.76% ± 2.56%	0.5761 ± 5.07%
	Scratch	65.34% ± 3.89%	0.3135 ± 7.61%	65.34% ± 4.37%	0.3139 ± 8.47%

3.4. Elbow Images Classification Results

For the elbow images, we performed the same two sets of experiments performed with the previously analyzed datasets. Both the results of the first set and the second set are presented in Table 6. In the first set of experiments, the fine-tuned VGG19 score was less than training the same network from scratch. For the rest of the networks, fine-tuning did achieve higher performance than training the networks from scratch. The ResNet network achieved the highest difference between fine-tuning and training from scratch. Overall, the best network was the fine-tuned DenseNet121, with a Kappa score of 0.6510.

In the second set of experiments, no fully connected layers were added. For all the networks, fine-tuning did achieve higher results than training from scratch. Overall, the best network was the fine-tuned Xception network, with a Kappa score of 0.6711. Comparing the first set of experiments to the second set, we see that the best performance for classifying elbow images was the fine-tuned Xception network without fully connected layers.

Table 6. Accuracy and Kappa scores of classifying elbow images with and without fully connected layers (±95% CI).

Network	Method	With FC Mean Accuracy	With FC Mean Kappa	Without FC Mean Accuracy	Without FC Mean Kappa
VGG19	TL	71.36% ± 16.95%	0.4232 ± 13.01%	81.61% ± 1.56%	0.6316 ± 3.12%
	Scratch	75.81% ± 34.45%	0.5136 ± 26.45%	76.52% ± 13.45%	0.5279 ± 27.33%
InceptionV3	TL	81.72% ± 0.91%	0.6339 ± 1.84%	80.93% ± 2.3%	0.6180 ± 4.6%
	Scratch	77.96% ± 2.92%	0.5583 ± 5.84%	76.09% ± 4.29%	0.5208 ± 8.6%
ResNet	TL	81.79% ± 3.28%	0.6351 ± 6.61%	81.9% ± 2.22%	0.6374 ± 4.44%
	Scratch	56.20% ± 9.60%	0.1161 ± 19.68%	71.04% ± 4.02%	0.4191 ± 8.09%
Xception	TL	82.15% ± 1.21%	0.6425 ± 2.42%	83.58% ± 1.64%	0.6711 ± 3.31%
	Scratch	78.21% ± 2.83%	0.5631 ± 5.70%	78.49% ± 1.88%	0.5690 ± 3.75%
DenseNet	TL	82.58% ± 1.97%	0.6510 ± 3.92%	81.08% ± 2.23%	0.6208 ± 4.47%
	Scratch	75.38% ± 3.36%	0.5060 ± 6.82%	73.84% ± 4.70%	0.4754 ± 9.49%
InceptionResNet	TL	80.82% ± 0.61%	0.6159 ± 1.21%	80.47% ± 1.68%	0.6087 ± 3.37%
	Scratch	79.82% ± 1.45%	0.5955 ± 2.91%	78.49% ± 1.28%	0.5694 ± 2.58%

3.5. *Finger Images Classification Results*

As with the previous datasets, two main sets of experiments were performed. Both the results of the first set and the second set are presented in Table 7. In the first set of experiments, fine-tuning achieved better results than training the networks from scratch for all the networks. The best-achieved network was the fine-tuned VGG19, with a Kappa score of 0.4379. In the second set of experiments, fine-tuning produced better results than training from scratch for all the six networks. The best network was the fine-tuned InceptionResNet network, with a Kappa score of 0.4455. Comparing the first set of experiments to the second set, we see that the best performance for classifying finger images was the fine-tuned InceptionResNet network without fully connected layers. Moreover, in this case, the presence of the fully connected layers did not provide any significant advantage in terms of performance.

Table 7. Accuracy and Kappa scores of classifying finger images with and without fully connected layers (±95% CI).

Network	Method	With FC Mean Accuracy	With FC Mean Kappa	Without FC Mean Accuracy	Without FC Mean Kappa
VGG19	TL	71.4% ± 1.84%	0.4379 ± 3.59%	68.44% ± 2.76%	0.3847 ± 5.10%
	Scratch	66.78% ± 2.83%	0.3505 ± 5.22%	66.16% ± 3.10%	0.3413 ± 5.26%
InceptionV3	TL	67.68% ± 2.15%	0.3686 ± 3.87%	68.55% ± 3.19%	0.3834 ± 5.97%
	Scratch	63.52% ± 2.66%	0.2911 ± 4.82%	63.88% ± 2.15%	0.2916 ± 4.09%
ResNet	TL	70.17% ± 1.16%	0.4129 ± 2.17%	69.02% ± 2.52%	0.3900 ± 4.44%
	Scratch	60.34% ± 8.07%	0.2341 ±13.90%	66.41% ± 2.98%	0.3431 ± 5.68%
Xception	TL	71.37% ± 2.43%	0.4369 ± 4.42%	70.64% ± 2.27%	0.4234 ± 4.28%
	Scratch	64.75% ± 2.79%	0.3109 ± 5.33%	64.57% ± 2.72%	0.3055 ± 5.31%
DenseNet	TL	66.78% ± 2.64%	0.3552 ± 4.66%	66.81% ± 1.92%	0.3512 ± 3.61%
	Scratch	62.18% ± 2.10%	0.2692 ± 3.60%	64.32% ± 3.16%	0.3051 ± 5.64%
InceptionResNet	TL	70.97% ± 2.05%	0.4294 ± 3.80%	71.8% ± 1.49%	0.4455 ± 2.88%
	Scratch	64.64% ± 3.07%	0.3112 ± 5.70%	65.29% ± 3.09%	0.3204 ± 5.72%

3.6. *Forearm Images Classification Results*

As with the previous datasets, two sets of experiments were performed on the forearm images dataset. Both the results of the first set and the second set are presented in Table 8. In the first set of experiments, fine-tuning all the networks produced better results than training from scratch. Training of ResNet network from scratch did not yield any satisfactory results, which can imply that fine-tuning this network was crucial for obtaining a good result. The best network was the DenseNet121 network, with a Kappa score of 0.5851. Moreover, in the second set of experiments, fine-tuning achieved better results than training from scratch. The best network was the fine-tuned ResNet network, with a Kappa score of 0.5673. Comparing the first set of experiments to the second set, we see that the best performance for classifying forearm images was the fine-tuned DenseNet network with fully connected layers. As observed in other datasets, the presence of the fully connected layers did not have any significant advantage in terms of performance.

Table 8. Accuracy and Kappa scores of classifying forearm images with and without fully connected layers (±95% CI).

Network	Method	With FC		Without FC	
		Mean Accuracy	**Mean Kappa**	**Mean Accuracy**	**Mean Kappa**
VGG19	TL	77.02% ± 1.27%	0.5408 ± 2.54%	76.3% ± 2.16%	0.5264 ± 4.31%
	Scratch	64.29% ± 9.50%	0.2870 ± 18.91%	71.15% ± 6.41%	0.4237 ± 12.75%
InceptionV3	TL	76.52% ± 1.46%	0.5308 ± 2.91%	77.46% ± 1%	0.5496 ± 1.99%
	Scratch	64.84% ± 5.50%	0.2973 ± 11.01%	65.84% ± 4.95%	0.3171 ± 9.89%
ResNet	TL	74.7% ± 1.20%	0.4943 ± 2.38%	78.35% ± 3.46%	0.5673 ± 6.92%
	Scratch	50.11% ± 0.56%	0.0055 ± 1.11%	63.79% ± 3.58%	0.2764 ± 7.12%
Xception	TL	75.08% ± 1.84%	0.5022 ± 3.69%	76.08% ± 1.66%	0.5222 ± 3.32%
	Scratch	66.00% ± 2.54%	0.3204 ± 5.08%	65.73% ± 5.31%	0.3148 ± 10.64%
DenseNet	TL	79.24% ± 0.53%	0.5851 ± 1.05%	76.14% ± 2.32%	0.5232 ± 4.63%
	Scratch	68.77% ± 3.75%	0.3755 ± 7.51%	69.66% ± 3.12%	0.3935 ± 6.25%
InceptionResNet	TL	74.7% ± 2.64%	0.4945 ± 5.27%	74.86% ± 1.98%	0.4977 ± 3.95%
	Scratch	65.45% ± 3.36%	0.3096 ± 6.69%	69.1% ± 6.07%	0.3824 ± 12.12%

3.7. *Shoulder Images Classification Results*

In the first set of experiments, the VGG19 network did not converge to an acceptable result by using both methods. For the rest of the networks, fine-tuning the networks achieved better results than training the networks from scratch. The best network was the fine-tuned Xception network, with a Kappa score of 0.4543. Both the results of the first set and the second set are presented in Table 9. In the second set of experiments, training the ResNet network from scratch achieved slightly better results than fine-tuning. For the rest of the networks, fine-tuning achieved better results. The best network was the fine-tuned VGG19, with a Kappa score of 0.4502. Comparing the first set of experiments to the second set, we see that the best performance for classifying shoulder images was the fine-tuned Xception network with fully connected layers. The presence of the fully connected layers did not show any significant advantage in terms of performance. Anyhow, the VGG19 network with fully connected layers did not converge to any satisfactory result compared to the same network without any fully connected layers.

3.8. *Kruskal–Wallis Results*

We applied the Kruskal–Wallis test to assess the statistical significance of different settings. The Kruskal–Wallis test yielded a p-value < 0.05 for all the results, which indicates to reject the null hypothesis that the settings have the same median and to accept the alternative hypothesis that there is a statistically significant difference between different settings (transfer learning "with and without fully connected layers" vs. training from scratch "with and without fully connected layers").

Table 9. Accuracy and Kappa scores of classifying shoulder images with and without fully connected layers (±95% CI).

Network	Method	With FC Mean Accuracy	With FC Mean Kappa	Without FC Mean Accuracy	Without FC Mean Kappa
VGG19	TL	77.02% ± 1.27%	0.5408 ± 2.54%	76.3% ± 2.16%	0.5264 ± 4.31%
	Scratch	64.29% ± 9.50%	0.2870 ± 18.91%	71.15% ± 6.41%	0.4237 ± 12.75%
InceptionV3	TL	76.52% ± 1.46%	0.5308 ± 2.91%	77.46% ± 1%	0.5496 ± 1.99%
	Scratch	64.84% ± 5.50%	0.2973 ± 11.01%	65.84% ± 4.95%	0.3171 ± 9.89%
ResNet	TL	74.7% ± 1.20%	0.4943 ± 2.38%	78.35% ± 3.46%	0.5673 ± 6.92%
	Scratch	50.11% ± 0.56%	0.0055 ± 1.11%	63.79% ± 3.58%	0.2764 ± 7.12%
Xception	TL	75.08% ± 1.84%	0.5022 ± 3.69%	76.08% ± 1.66%	0.5222 ± 3.32%
	Scratch	66.00% ± 2.54%	0.3204 ± 5.08%	65.73% ± 5.31%	0.3148 ± 10.64%
DenseNet	TL	79.24% ± 0.53%	0.5851 ± 1.05%	76.14% ± 2.32%	0.5232 ± 4.63%
	Scratch	68.77% ± 3.75%	0.3755 ± 7.51%	69.66% ± 3.12%	0.3935 ± 6.25%
InceptionResNet	TL	74.7% ± 2.64%	0.4945 ± 5.27%	74.86% ± 1.98%	0.4977 ± 3.95%
	Scratch	65.45% ± 3.36%	0.3096 ± 6.69%	69.1% ± 6.07%	0.3824 ± 12.12%

4. Discussion

In this paper, we compared the performance of fine-tuning on six state-of-the-art CNNs to classify musculoskeletal images. Training a CNN network from scratch can be very challenging, especially in the case of data scarcity. Transfer learning can help solve this problem by initiating the weights with values learned from a large dataset instead of initializing the weights from scratch. Musculoskeletal images play a fundamental role in classifying fractures. However, these images are always challenging to be analyzed, and a second opinion is often required, which will not always be available, especially in the emergency room. As pointed out by Lindsey et al. [5], the presence of an image classifier in the emergency room can significantly increase physicians' performance in classifying fractures.

For the first research question, about the effect of transfer learning, we noted that transfer learning produced better results than training the networks from scratch. For our second research question, the classifier that achieved the best result for wrist images was the fine-tuned DenseNet121 with fully connected layers; the classifier that achieved the best performance for elbow images was the fine-tuned Xception network without fully connected layers; for finger images, the best classifier was the fine-tuned InceptionResNetV2 network without fully connected layers; for forearm images, the best classifier was the fine-tuned DenseNet network with fully connected layers; for hand images, the best classifier was a fine-tuned Xception network with fully connected layers; the best classifier for humerus images was the fine-tuned VGG19 network without fully connected layers; finally, the best classifier for classifying the shoulder images was the fine-tuned Xception network with fully connected layers. A summary of the best CNNs is presented in Table 10. Concerning the third research question, the fully connected layers had a negative effect on the performance of the considered CNNs. In particular, in many cases, it decreased the performance of the network. Further research is needed to study, in more detail, the impact of fully connected layers, especially in the case of transfer learning.

The authors of the MURA dataset [10] assessed the performance of three radiologists on the dataset and compared their performance against the one of a CNN. In Table 11, we present their results, along with our best scores.

For classifying elbow images, the first radiologist achieved the best score, and our score was comparable to other radiologists [10]. For finger images, our score was higher than the three radiologists. For forearm images, our score was lower than the radiologists. For hand images, our score was the lowest. For humerus images, shoulder images, and wrist images, our score was lower than the radiologists. We still believe that the scores achieved in this paper are promising, keeping in mind that these scores came from off-the-shelf models that were not designed for medical images in the first place and that the images were resized to be 96 × 96 pixels due to hardware limitations. Nevertheless, additional efforts are needed to outperform the performance of experienced radiologists.

Table 10. The best convolutional neural network (CNN) for each image category.

Fracture	CNN
Wrist	DenseNet
Elbow	Xception
Finger	InceptionResNetV2
Forearm	DenseNet121
Hand	Xception
Humerus	VGG19
Shoulder	Xception

Table 11. Kappa scores of three radiologists reported in Reference [10] compared to our results.

Fracture	1st Radiologist	2nd Radiologist	3rd Radiologist	Our Score
Elbow	0.850	0.710	0.719	0.671
Finger	0.304	0.403	0.410	0.445
Forearm	0.796	0.802	0.798	0.585
Hand	0.661	0.927	0.789	0.462
Humerus	0.867	0.733	0.933	0.633
Shoulder	0.864	0.791	0.864	0.454
Wrist	0.791	0.931	0.931	0.625

On the other side of the spectrum, there is the study of Raghu et al. [24], where the authors argued that transfer learning is not good enough for medical images and will be less accurate compared to training from scratch or compared to novel networks explicitly designed for the problem at hand. The authors studied the effect of transfer learning on two medical datasets, namely, retina images and chest X-ray images. The authors stated that designing a lightweight CNN can be more accurate than using transfer learning. In our study, we did not consider "small" CNNs trained from scratch. Thus, it is not possible to directly compare the results obtained to the ones presented in Raghu et al. [24]. Anyway, more studies are needed to better understand the effect of transfer learning on medical-image classification.

5. Conclusions

In this paper, we investigated the effect of transfer learning on classifying musculoskeletal images. We find that, out of the 168 results obtained that were performed by using six different CNN architectures and seven different bone types, transfer learning achieved better results than training a CNN from scratch. Only in 3 out of the 168 results did training from scratch achieve slightly better results than transfer learning. The weaker performance of the training-from-scratch approach could be related to the number of images in the considered dataset, as well as to the choice of the hyperparameters. In particular, the CNNs taken into account are characterized by the presence of a large number of trainable parameters (i.e., weights), and the number of images used to train these networks is too small to build a robust model. Concerning the hyperparameters, we highlight the importance of the learning rate. While we used a small value of the learning rate in the fine-tuning approach, to avoid changing the architectures' original weights dramatically, the training-from-scratch approach could require a higher value of the learning rate. A complete study on the hyperparameters' effect will be considered in future work, aiming to fully understand the best approach to be used when dealing with fracture images. Focusing on this study's results, it is possible to state that transfer learning is recommended in the context of fracture images. In our future work, we plan to introduce a novel CNN to classify musculoskeletal images, aiming at outperforming fine-tuned CNNs. This would be the first step towards the design of a CNN-based system, which classifies the image and provides the probable position of the fracture if the fracture is present in the image.

Author Contributions: Conceptualization, I.K. and M.C.; methodology, I.K.; software, I.K.; validation, I.K., M.C. and A.P.; writing—original draft preparation, I.K.; writing—review and editing, M.C. and A.P.; supervision, M.C.; project administration, A.P.; funding acquisition, M.C. and A.P. All authors have read and agreed to the published version of the manuscript.

References

1. CDC. *National Hospital Ambulatory Medical Care Survey: 2017 Emergency Department Summary Tables*; CDC: Atlanta, GA, USA, 2017.
2. Tanzi, L.; Vezzetti, E.; Moreno, R.; Moos, S. X-Ray Bone Fracture Classification Using Deep Learning: A Baseline for Designing a Reliable Approach. *Appl. Sci.* **2020**, *10*, 1507.
3. Hallas, P.; Ellingsen, T. Errors in fracture diagnoses in the emergency deparment—Characteristics of patients and diurnal variation. *BMC Emerg. Med.* **2006**, *6*, 4.
4. Moonen, P.-J.; Mercelina, L.; Boer, W.; Fret, T. Diagnostic error in the Emergency Department: Follow up of patients with minor trauma in the outpatient clinic. *Scand. J. Trauma. Resusc. Emerg. Med.* **2017**, *25*, 13. [PubMed]
5. Lindsey, R.; Daluiski, A.; Chopra, S.; Lachapelle, A.; Mozer, M.; Sicular, S.; Hanel, D.; Gardner, M.; Gupta, A.; Hotchkiss, R.; et al. Deep neural network improves fracture detection by clinicians. *Proc. Natl. Acad. Sci. USA* **2018**, *115*, 11591–11596. [PubMed]
6. Almubarak, H.; Bazi, Y.; Alajlan, N. Two-Stage Mask-RCNN Approach for Detecting and Segmenting the Optic Nerve Head, Optic Disc, and Optic Cup in Fundus Images. *Appl. Sci.* **2020**, *10*, 3833.
7. Kandel, I.; Castelli, M. A novel architecture to classify histopathology images using convolutional neural networks. *Appl. Sci.* **2020**, *10*, 2929.
8. Farooq, A.; Anwar, S.; Awais, M.; Rehman, S. A deep CNN based multi-class classification of Alzheimer's disease using MRI. In Proceedings of the 2017 IEEE International Conference on Imaging Systems and Techniques (IST), Beijing, China, 18–20 October 2017; pp. 1–6.
9. Krizhevsky, A.; Sutskever, I.; Hinton, G.E. ImageNet Classification with Deep Convolutional Neural Networks. In Proceedings of the Neural Information Processing Systems, Lake Tahoe, NV, USA, 3–6 December 2012; Volume 25.
10. Rajpurkar, P.; Irvin, J.; Bagul, A.; Ding, D.Y.; Duan, T.; Mehta, H.; Yang, B.J.; Zhu, K.; Laird, D.; Ball, R.L.; et al. MURA: Large Dataset for Abnormality Detection in Musculoskeletal Radiographs. *arXiv* **2017**, arXiv:1712.06957.
11. Chada, G. Machine Learning Models for Abnormality Detection in Musculoskeletal Radiographs. *Reports* **2019**, *2*, 26.
12. Kitamura, G.; Chung, C.Y.; Moore, B.E. Ankle Fracture Detection Utilizing a Convolutional Neural Network Ensemble Implemented with a Small Sample, De Novo Training, and Multiview Incorporation. *J. Digit. Imaging* **2019**, *32*, 672–677. [PubMed]
13. Pan, S.; Yang, Q. A Survey on Transfer Learning. *IEEE Trans. Knowl. Data Eng. Knowl. Data Eng.* **2010**, *22*, 1345–1359.
14. Simonyan, K.; Zisserman, A. Very Deep Convolutional Networks for Large-Scale Image Recognition. *arXiv* **2014**, arXiv:1409.1556.
15. Chollet, F. Xception: Deep Learning with Depthwise Separable Convolutions. In Proceedings of the IEEE Conference on Computer Vision and Pattern Recognition (CVPR), Honolulu, HI, USA, 21–26 July 2017.
16. He, K.; Zhang, X.; Ren, S.; Sun, J. Deep Residual Learning for Image Recognition. In Proceedings of the 2016 IEEE Conference on Computer Vision and Pattern Recognition (CVPR), Las Vegas, NV, USA, 27–30 June 2016; pp. 770–778.
17. Szegedy, C.; Liu, W.; Jia, Y.; Sermanet, P.; Reed, S.; Anguelov, D.; Erhan, D.; Vanhoucke, V.; Rabinovich, A. Going deeper with convolutions. In Proceedings of the 2015 IEEE Conference on Computer Vision and Pattern Recognition (CVPR), Boston, MA, USA, 7–12 June 2015; pp. 1–9.
18. Längkvist, M.; Karlsson, L.; Loutfi, A. Inception-v4, Inception-ResNet and the Impact of Residual Connections on Learning. *Pattern Recognit. Lett.* **2014**, *42*, 11–24.

19. Huang, G.; Liu, Z.; Van der Maaten, L.; Weinberger, K.Q. Densely Connected Convolutional Networks. In Proceedings of the 2017 IEEE Conference on Computer Vision and Pattern Recognition (CVPR), Honolulu, HI, USA, 21–26 July 2017; pp. 2261–2269.
20. Cohen, J. A Coefficient of Agreement for Nominal Scales. *Educ. Psychol. Meas.* **1960**, *20*, 37–46.
21. Kruskal, W.H.; Wallis, W.A. Use of Ranks in One-Criterion Variance Analysis. *J. Am. Stat. Assoc.* **1952**, *47*, 583–621.
22. Schmidt, R.; Schneider, F.; Hennig, P. Descending through a Crowded Valley—Benchmarking Deep Learning Optimizers. *arXiv* **2020**, arXiv:2007.01547.
23. Kingma, D.; Ba, J. Adam: A Method for Stochastic Optimization. In Proceedings of the International Conference on Learning Representations (ICLR), Banff, AB, Canada, 14–16 April 2014.
24. Raghu, M.; Zhang, C.; Kleinberg, J.; Bengio, S. Transfusion: Understanding Transfer Learning with Applications to Medical Imaging. *arXiv* **2019**, arXiv:1902.07208.

5

Deep Multimodal Learning for the Diagnosis of Autism Spectrum Disorder

Michelle Tang [1], Pulkit Kumar [2], Hao Chen [2] and Abhinav Shrivastava [2,*]

1 Science, Math, and Computer Science Magnet Program, Montgomery Blair High School, Silver Spring, MD 20901, USA; mtang@umiacs.umd.edu
2 Institute for Advanced Computer Studies, University of Maryland College Park, College Park, MD 20742, USA; pulkit@cs.umd.edu (P.K.); chenh@cs.umd.edu (H.C.)
* Correspondence: abhinav@cs.umd.edu

Abstract: Recent medical imaging technologies, specifically functional magnetic resonance imaging (fMRI), have advanced the diagnosis of neurological and neurodevelopmental disorders by allowing scientists and physicians to observe the activity within and between different regions of the brain. Deep learning methods have frequently been implemented to analyze images produced by such technologies and perform disease classification tasks; however, current state-of-the-art approaches do not take advantage of all the information offered by fMRI scans. In this paper, we propose a deep multimodal model that learns a joint representation from two types of connectomic data offered by fMRI scans. Incorporating two functional imaging modalities in an automated end-to-end autism diagnosis system will offer a more comprehensive picture of the neural activity, and thus allow for more accurate diagnoses. Our multimodal training strategy achieves a classification accuracy of 74% and a recall of 95%, as well as an F1 score of 0.805, and its overall performance is superior to using only one type of functional data.

Keywords: deep learning; multimodal learning; convolutional neural networks; autism; fMRI

---

1. Introduction

Autism spectrum disorder (ASD) is a lifelong neurological condition characterized by repetitive, restricted behavior as well as limitations in communication and social abilities, manifesting in a wide range of sensorimotor deficits [1]. Diagnostic processes for ASD are based on the assessment of social behaviors and language skills; however, there is limited understanding of the neural patterns behind the spectrum of autism behavior and the severity of the disease [2]. Recently, noninvasive brain imaging techniques have allowed for a better understanding of the neural circuitry underlying neurodeficiency disorders and their associated symptoms, such as ASD and its behavioral deficits. Specifically, functional magnetic resonance imaging (fMRI) allows physicians and medical experts to visually evaluate the functional characteristics or properties of a brain. This radioimaging procedure is able to assist neuroscientists in acquiring valuable and precise information on different neurological disorders [3]. For instance, in the diagnosis of ASD, instead of solely relying on observation and speaking with the patient, physicians analyze neuroimages for anomalies in brain activity, helping them more efficiently and precisely identify differences in their patients' neural pathways. Identifying the neural patterns of activation for ASD and associating these patterns with physiological and psychological features will aid scientists and medical practitioners in gaining more insight into the etiology of mental disorders [4].

Computational diagnosis: However, even with high-quality images, manual analysis is inefficient and at risk of human error, due to the variation between both doctors and patients. In an effort to make this process more objective, machine learning and computer vision techniques have frequently been applied in medical imaging problems to construct computer-assisted diagnosis systems [5]. State-of-the-art neuroimaging analysis uses activation maps, alternatively known as correlation matrices, which are constructed from the radiology scans. Activation maps provide information regarding the interaction between different areas of the brain by describing the relationship between their corresponding neural activity [6]. In doing so, the activation maps allow scientists to localize abnormal neural activity to specific regions of the brain and focus on those regions when manually analyzing the scans for anomalies.

Traditional machine learning in computer vision relies heavily on features pre-selected by medical experts. Early machine learning algorithms, e.g., support vector machines (SVM), k-nearest neighbors (KNN), decision trees, etc., analyze raw image data without any learning of hidden representations. On the other hand, deep learning (DL) algorithms in computer vision has shown significant advantage in capturing hidden representations and automatically extracting features from the given image data. Based on artificial neural networks structures, DL algorithms have multiple stages of non-linear feature transformation, which leads to hierarchical representations from pixels to edge, motif, part, and the entire object. State-of-the-art deep learning algorithms include convolutional neural networks (CNNs), recurrent neural networks (RNNs), long short term memory (LSTM) networks, generative adversarial networks (GANs), etc., which do not require manual processing or feature selection on raw data.

Related Work

The Autism Brain Imaginge Data Exchange (ABIDE) is a public, anonymized neuroimaging dataset that has been analyzed extensively in the past using various different techniques. Nielsen [7] analyzed ABIDE data to classify autism versus control subjects based on brain connectivity measurements. The study replicated earlier methods and implemented them on point-to-point connectivity data, and achieved roughly 60% accuracy with whole-brain classification.

Connectivity maps. The most common approach to fMRI analysis focuses on ROI mean time series data, since it is a representation of brain activity in distinct regions of the brain. Prior to analysis, pair-wise correlations are calculated between ROIs to form a functional connectivity matrix—each element of the matrix is a Pearson correlation coefficient representing the level of co-activation between the signals in the two ROI based on the time series data. The resulting matrix, also known as an activation map, is reshaped into a feature vector and then used as input into a classification algorithm [8,9].

Full-brain connectivity fingerprints. There are several arguments against exclusively using ROI time series data to analyze fMRI scans. The original form of each functional scan is a complete 3D scan of the brain across time (i.e., 4D matrix); thus, averaged ROI signal intensities only offers a partial representation of the fMRI scan, since by condensing the correlation matrix, one effectively loses the spatial structure of the connectome [10]. Khosla et. al. (2017) [9] proposed an alternative to relying exclusively on ROI data—instead of only computing the correlation between each region's signal intensities, they construct a full-brain connectivity "fingerprint" consisting of correlation coefficients between voxels from the fMRI scan and signal intensities from ROIs, incorporating both the spatial information offered by the original functional image volume along with the averaged time series data. The connectivity fingerprint is then used as input into a simple CNN architecture [8].

Multimodal learning. Computer vision and deep learning have been used extensively to achieve automatic disease diagnosis with medical imaging analysis [11,12]. Specifically, many machine learning problems involve the analysis of different forms of data to arrive at a result; as part of the classification problem, it is important to understand the relationship between these different data types, or modalities of data. Zhang et. al. (2018) [13] use generative adversarial networks (GANs) to translate between computed tomography (CT) and magnetic resonance imaging (MRI) data. Fukui et. al. (2016) [14] propose a new method for multimodal compact bilinear (MCB) pooling by computing the outer product of the different feature vectors from multiple modalities. MCB is based on previous compact bilinear pooling methods and allows for a more expressive and also efficient way of constructing a joint representation of both inputs [15]. The model was used to solve visual question answering (VQA) and visual grounding problems and outperforms state-of-the-art methods.

Our Approach. Previous studies on functional neuroimaging analysis use only one type of activation map in their evaluation [8,9,16]. In this study, we propose to include both activation maps in our analysis, and that by using two modalities instead of one, we will be able to create a more accurate and holistic representation of the functional imaging data, and thus achieve more accurate diagnoses. To do so, we propose a model architecture capable of analyzing both types of activation maps by combining different deep learning networks. Specifically, one of the inputs is the ROI time series activation map as described above, constructed by computing the correlation matrix between all pairs of ROI, and the second is the fMRI $\times$ ROI activation map. The pooling technique used in our model is a concatenation of the two feature vectors, which is then used as input to four fully-connected layers before the network outputs its prediction. The resulting classification system is a multimodal model, an automated disease classification system that uses two types of activation maps to predict whether the given patient is healthy or has autism. With both input modalities, the resulting diagnosis system is both more accurate and offers a more complete understanding of the functional data, and provides a powerful aid to physicians during the diagnostic process.

The main contributions of our method are highlighted as follows:

1. We propose an end-to-end deep neural network-based multimodal architecture that incorporates features from two different types of modalities. Our proposed architecture incorporates all connectomic information from the functional imaging data, which allows for a more comprehensive and holistic functional image analysis.
2. By incorporating both types of activation maps from the functional data, the overall performance of the classifier is improved and thus creates a more powerful diagnostic tool to assist doctors. Moreover, we also provide 'visual explanations' of the regions in fMRI images that our model utilizes to make diagnosis predictions. We believe this visualization offers transparency on the model and is crucial in providing effective assistance to the diagnostic process.

The remainder of this paper is organized as follows: in Section 2, we present the dataset and imaging modalities that were analyzed in our study, and our methods for analysis, including the preprocessing pipeline and network architectures; in Section 3, we discuss the details behind the training and testing of our constructed models; in Section 4, we present the results and performance metrics of each model and discuss them with respect to other publications in the field; and we present our conclusions and future work in Section 5.

2. Methods and Data

2.1. Data

In this study, we focus on the analysis of functional magnetic resonance imaging, or fMRI scans. The purpose of these images is to track changes in blood oxygen level-dependent (BOLD) signal in the brain across a period of time. Functional images are thus four-dimensional, where the dimensions (H, W, D, T) represent the height, width, depth, and time dimensions of the image volume, respectively [3]. fMRI scans can also be represented as regions of interest (ROI) mean time series data [17,18], which is constructed from the fMRI scan after preprocessing, and can be considered of as an abridged or summarized version of the complete multidimensional fMRI image volume. The ROI time series data is constructed by first segmenting the original fMRI scan functionally homogeneous regions (ROI), and then taking the average BOLD signal from each area. These ROIs are typically segmented using a functional parcellation brain atlas [19]; different atlases "segment" the full brain scan into different ROIs. For the purposes of our research, we chose to use the Automated Anatomical Labeling (AAL) atlas. After the regions have been specified, the BOLD signal intensities of each voxel are averaged across all voxels enclosed in the region, to return one intensity value for each time frame. The result is a T-dimensional vector for every ROI, where T represents the number of seconds for which the signal was measured. Thus, for each subject, one ROI mean time series volume is a 2D matrix with dimensions (N, T), where N represents the number of ROIs [8].

However, the BOLD signal measured by fMRI images represents changes in the blood oxygenation of brain tissue, and are not equivalent to neural activity [20]. Thus, it is not appropriate to directly use the fMRI scan of BOLD signals nor the ROI time series data as input for analysis. Instead, correlations between the time series data must be computed, either between voxels and ROIs or only pairs of ROIs—these correlations serve as the two different features used in our model. The resulting output from this step is a correlation matrix or activation map, which indicates points in the scan where there is neural activity.

This study was conducted on the ABIDE dataset [21], a multi-site open-access MRI study containing anonymized patient neuroimaging data. Data from the first phase of the study (ABIDE-I) was used in our analysis, which consisted of fMRI images and regions of interest (ROI) time series signals from both control and disease groups. The original ABIDE-I dataset consists of 1112 subjects; in this study, 77 subjects were removed from consideration due to low quality or missing scans. This yielded a total of 1035 subjects, with 505 individuals diagnosed with ASD and 530 typical controls, from 17 sites.

2.2. Preprocessing

Prior to classification, neuroimaging and connectomic data must be appropriately preprocessed in order to allow efficient and precise analysis. Preprocessing can be divided into two steps, as outlined in the following sections: (1) preparation and quality assessment of neuro-images and extraction of time series data and (2) feature preprocessing.

2.2.1. Preprocessing of Neuro-images

As previously mentioned (see Section 2.1), the dataset used in this study consists of images collected from 17 different sites [21]. The standard preprocessing steps were taken to prepare the neuroimages for analysis using the Configurable Pipeline for the Analysis of Connectomes (CPAC) toolbox [10], which compiles preprocessing tools from multiple state-of-the-art neuroimaging analysis libraries, such as AFNI, FSL, ANTs, etc. Namely, the preprocessing frameworks in this pipeline include slice timing correction, motion correction, global mean intensity normalization and standardization of functional data to MNI space ($3 \times 3 \times 3$ mm resolution). We used data extracted with global signal regression and band-pass filtering (0.01–10Hz) in our analysis. After preprocessing was complete with the CPAC pipeline, ROI time series data was then extracted from the resulting fMRI images using the Automated Anatomical Labeling (AAL) functional parcellation brain atlas, which consists of $N = 116$ labeled regions [19].

2.2.2. Feature Preprocessing

As previously described in Section 3.1, connectomic data consists of the fMRI image scan, as well as the ROI time series data. While most state-of-the-art neuroimaging analysis studies focus on only one form of functional data, we computed both ROI connectivity matrices, i.e., ROI $\times$ ROI activation maps, and full-brain connectivity fingerprints, i.e., fMRI voxels $\times$ ROI activation maps, using the fMRI scan and ROI signal intensities.

Activation map of fMRI and ROI. The connectivity fingerprints between the functional images and mean time series data were computed by calculating correlation coefficients between every pair of voxels from the fMRI scan and ROI from the time series data [9]. We first restructured the 4D fMRI scan into a 2D matrix, such that each row of the matrix corresponds to one voxel, and each column is one intensity value at a given time T. The reshaped matrix would have thus have dimensions $(H \times W \times D, T)$. We then compute a correlation matrix between the voxel intensities and the ROI time series data; the resulting matrix will be of dimensions $(H \times W \times D, N)$, where N is the number of ROI.

Activation map of only ROI. The ROI functional connectivity maps were constructed by computing a correlation matrix for each subject, where each cell of the matrix contains the correlation coefficient between a pair of regions, i.e., the level of co-activation in the signals between any two given regions. Since the resulting correlation matrix is symmetrical along its diagonal, we removed the values in the lower triangle to delete the duplicates, and also deleted the main diagonal of the matrix, which represents the correlations of each region with itself. The remaining matrix values were then reshaped into a vector of features to use as input into the model. The number of features in the final vector is given by $\frac{1}{2}((N-1)N)$, where N is the total number of regions [8]. Since the AAL brain atlas was used to extract the ROI time series data ($N = 116$), the resulting vector consisted of 6670 features. The entire feature extraction and connectivity matrix construction workflow is illustrated in Figure 1.

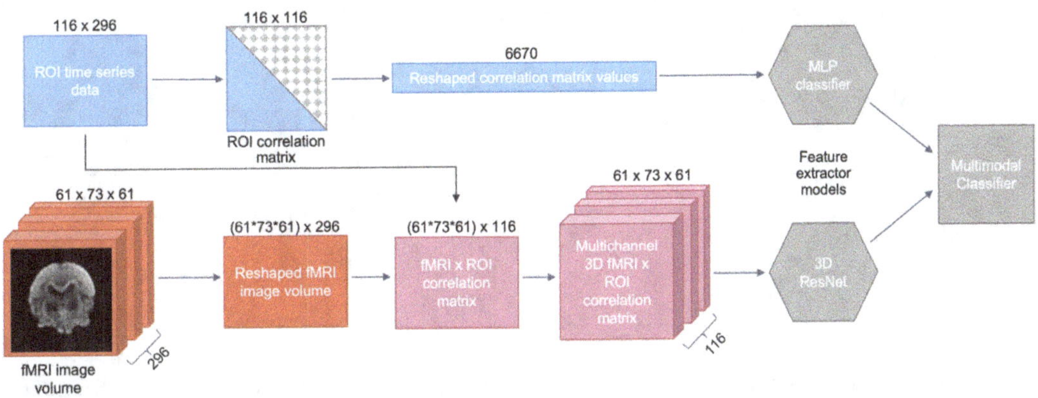

Figure 1. Preprocessing workflow. Construction of correlation matrices, or activation maps (terms are used interchangeably) between fMRI voxels $\times$ ROI time series and between pairs of ROI time series alone. Numbers on edges of the objects indicate matrix dimensions at the current step, e.g., the dimensions of the fMRI scan and ROI time series data are ($H = 61, W = 73, D = 61, T = 296$) and ($N = 116, T = 296$), respectively. For more detail on ResNet and MLP network architectures, refer to Figure 2.

2.3. Network Architectures

In this neuroimaging classification problem, the input to the model is an fMRI $\times$ ROI connectivity fingerprint and a vector of ROI correlation coefficients, and the goal is to diagnose the subject as either positive (with autism) or negative (healthy) based on both inputs. The proposed multimodal model extracts representations for both the fMRI scan and the ROI input, pools the feature vectors using simple vector concatenation, and arrives at a diagnosis using the combined features, which are propagated through four fully-connected layers before being classified into one of two classes.

We extracted features from fMRI $\times$ ROI correlation matrices using a modified 18-layer Residual Network (ResNet-18) [22]. All 2-dimensional convolution layers were replaced by their 3-dimensional equivalents in order to process the multichannel 3D correlation matrices. The correlation matrices were all uniformly of the dimensions $(61, 73, 61, 116)$, corresponding to (H, W, D, T) respectively. During training, the data is reshaped to be $(116, 61, 73, 61)$ so that the ROI dimension is used as the number of input channels into the first convolutional layer of the ResNet-18 network. Max-pooling is performed following the input convolutional layer over a $1 \times 3 \times 3$ pixel window, with a stride of $(1, 2, 2)$. The stride attribute determines how far the window or filter is moved in each dimension after every computation; e.g., with a stride of 2, the filter moves 2 pixels in the specified dimension. The matrix is then passed through a stack of convolutional blocks (Res-blocks), each with multiple convolutional layers, where we pass filters across the image to convolve over the height, width, and depth dimensions. The filters have very small receptive fields: $3 \times 3 \times 3$ (which is the smallest size to capture the notion of left/right, up/down, center). In the first two convolutional blocks, we also use $1 \times 3 \times 3$ or convolution filters. The convolution stride varies between 1 and 2 pixels depending on the dimension. Following the convolutional blocks, average pooling is performed over a $32 \times 3 \times 2$ window, and the resulting output is a 512-D vector. The vector is then passed through a fully connected layer before returning the final model output.

ROI $\times$ ROI connectivity map features were extracted using a multilayer perceptron (MLP) classifier, which was a simple fully-connected network. The MLP consisted of three hidden layers, each with 100 nodes. As stated above, the ROI correlation matrices were reshaped into 6670-D vectors, where each element represents a pairwise correlation coefficient between the averageBOLD signal of two ROIs.

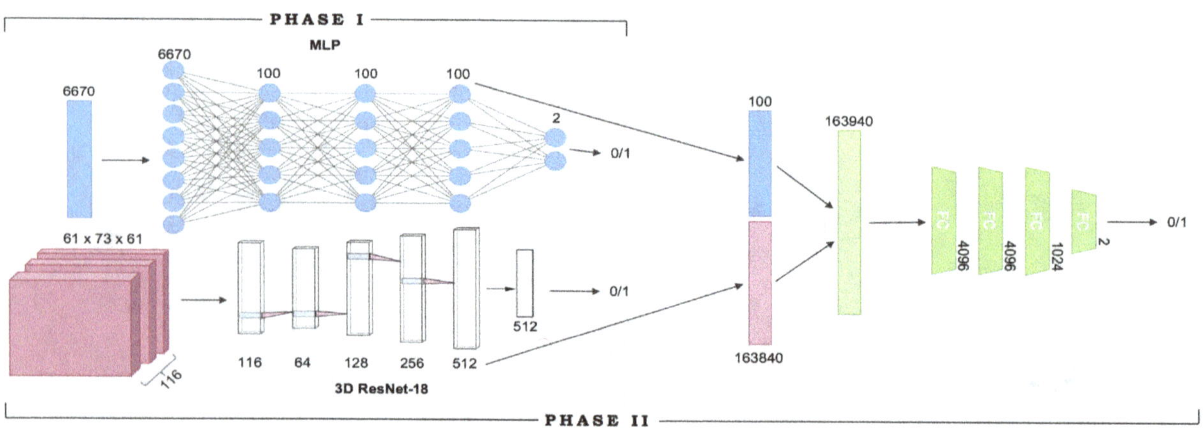

Figure 2. Multimodal network architectures and training phases. Visualization of the structure of the complete deep multimodal network. Numbers denote nodes or input channels in the labeled layer; FC implies fully connected layers. Phase I of training refers to the training of Resnet-18 and MLP for feature extraction; Phase II refers to the end-to-end training of the entire multimodal model after removing output layers from the feature extractors (as shown in the figure, the last 2-node layer of the MLP and the 512-channel layer of the ResNet are bypassed during Phase II of training.)

3. Experimental Details

Training occurred in two separate phases due to the nature of the model architecture, as described in Section 4.2. In Phase I, the feature extractors were separately trained as independent networks. Namely, the MLP was trained on ROI activation maps, and ResNet-18 was trained on fMRI $\times$ ROI activation maps. Upon completion of training for both networks, Phase II of training began. Both MLP and ResNet-18 models were truncated to remove their output layers to be used as feature extractors, and then combined with the four fully-connected layers to form the end-to-end model. The resulting multimodal network, built from the pretrained MLP and ResNet-18 models (the learned network weights of both models were saved and loaded into the multimodal network), was trained from scratch in Phase II, initialized with the learned weights from Phase I. After training is complete, we report performance metrics of classification accuracy, precision, recall, and F1 score for each feature extractor model, as well as the final end-to-end multimodal model. The full network architecture and the two training phases are visualized in Figure 2.

3.1. Training Details

Prior to training, the neuroimaging datasets was randomly split into the training and testing sets. 900 subjects were used to train the model, and the remaining 135 subjects were used to evaluate the trained model. The same training and testing sets were used in both phases of training, i.e., to train both the feature extractor models and the overall combined multimodal network to avoid polluting the test set with training data, or vice versa.

The ResNet-18 network used in this work is detailed in Table 1. We used a rectified linear unit (ReLU) activation function [23] after each layer and Softmax cross-entropy loss to train the network using minibatch stochastic gradient descent. We used a batch size = 8 and momentum = 0.9 to train both the feature extractor models and the end-to-end multimodal model. Both the feature extractor models were trained from scratch. To train the 3D CNN feature extractor, we used a learning rate of 1×10^{-2} for 30 epochs and dropped the learning rate after every 6 epochs by a factor of 1×10^{-1}; with the MLP, we used a learning rate of 1×10^{-2} across 50 epochs and dropped the learning rate by a factor of 1×10^{-1} after every 5 epochs. In the second phase of training for the end-to-end model, the feature extractor layers were initialized using the MLP and ResNet's weights learned during Phase I of training; the entire network was then trained end to end with a learning rate of 1×10^{-5} for 30 epochs. The learning rate was dropped after every 8 epochs for this network with a factor of 1×10^{-1}. All models were constructed using Pytorch [24] and were trained on a single Nvidia P6000 GPU. The end-to-end training process of both feature extractors and the complete multimodal model took roughly two hours.

Table 1. ResNet-18 architecture. Network architecture for 3D ResNet-18 model used for corr (fMRI, ROI) feature extraction. Building blocks are shown in brackets, with the numbers of blocks stacked.

Layer Name	3D ResNet-18	Output Size
conv1	$5 \times 5 \times 5$, 64, stride(2,2,2)	$32 \times 38 \times 32 \times 64$
Max Pool	$1 \times 3 \times 3$ max pool, stride(1,2,2)	$32 \times 19 \times 16 \times 64$
Res-block 1	$\begin{bmatrix} 1 \times 3 \times 3, 64, \text{stride}(1,1,1) \\ 1 \times 3 \times 3, 64, \text{stride}(1,1,1) \end{bmatrix} \times 2$	$32 \times 19 \times 16 \times 64$
Res-block 2	$\begin{bmatrix} 1 \times 3 \times 3, 128, \text{stride}(1,2,2) \\ 1 \times 3 \times 3, 128, \text{stride}(1,1,1) \end{bmatrix} \times 2$	$32 \times 10 \times 8 \times 128$
Res-block 3	$\begin{bmatrix} 3 \times 3 \times 3, 256, \text{stride}(1,2,2) \\ 3 \times 3 \times 3, 256, \text{stride}(1,1,1) \end{bmatrix} \times 2$	$32 \times 5 \times 4 \times 256$
Res-block 4	$\begin{bmatrix} 3 \times 3 \times 3, 512, \text{stride}(1,2,2) \\ 3 \times 3 \times 3, 512, \text{stride}(1,1,1) \end{bmatrix} \times 2$	$32 \times 3 \times 2 \times 512$
Average Pool	$32 \times 3 \times 2$ average pool	$1 \times 1 \times 1 \times 512$
Fully connected	512×2 fully connected layer	2

We present details of the ResNet-18 network architecture in Table 1 above.

4. Results

Due to the absence of any standardized benchmarks or training-testing set splits, it is difficult to compare against other published works in this field. Previous papers also do not evaluate networks using the same metrics, and thus do not all report precision, recall and F1 scores, and thus cannot be directly compared with our results. The following studies use different architectures and do not specify the data used for training and testing, and are meant to serve only as a reference to the present paper.

Previous studies on functional imaging analysis used only one type of correlation matrix or activation map as input. Khosla et. al. [9] analyzed the fMRI voxel and ROI time series activation map, and achieved 73% accuracy with their ensemble model. Guo et. al. [16] conducted studies on the ROI time series activation map, and achieved 81% accuracy using a fully-connected DNN network.

Heinsfeld et. al. [8], also only used the ROI time series activation map, and report classification accuracies ranging from 52% to 70% using DNNs. They also studied the same data using support vector machines and random forests, which achieved 62% and 58% accuracy, respectively.

When trained on a random subset of 90% of the total ABIDE-I dataset and evaluated on the remaining patients, our proposed multimodal model is able to achieve an accuracy of 74% and an F1-score of 0.805. More importantly, we are able to reach a very high recall of 95%, which is crucial for a computer-assisted diagnosis system—when physicians diagnose patients for disease, a false negative can have extremely adverse consequences.

4.1. Ablation Results

We compare the performance of the feature extractor models and the combined multimodal model in Table 2. The ResNet-18 network, trained on fMRI × ROI activation maps, achieved a classification accuracy of 73.1%; the MLP classifier, trained on ROI × ROI activation maps, achieved a classification accuracy of 70.8%. When the feature vectors from both networks are pooled and used in the combined multimodal model, the resulting network has a higher classification accuracy of 74%, as well as a very high recall of 95% and an F1 score of 0.805, indicating that integrating both types of input in the model improves the overall network performance and be able to more accurately predict the correct diagnosis.

Table 2. Results and performance metrics. Classification accuracy, precision, recall, and F1 scores for both feature extractor networks and final end-to-end multimodal model.

Training Phase	Input	Model	Accuracy	Precision	Recall	F1 Score
Phase I	corr(fMRI, ROI)	ResNet-18	0.731	0.726	0.849	0.783
	corr(ROI, ROI)	MLP	0.708	**0.737**	0.759	0.749
Phase II	**Both** corr	Multimodal	**0.740**	0.699	**0.949**	**0.805**

4.2. Explanation of Model Predictions

Many medical imaging analysis techniques, especially those involving complex deep learning models, are difficult to interpret—it is difficult to decipher the inner workings of the networks or understand how they arrive at their predictions. To make our multimodal model more transparent, we visualized the regions of the fMRI images where the network focused on during the prediction process, as shown in Figure 3. Using gradient-weighted class activation mapping (Grad-CAM) as proposed by Selvaraju et. al. [25], we computed the activation gradients on the fMRI and ROI correlation matrices that were computed during the feature preprocessing stage of our study. We then overlaid these gradient-maps (heatmaps) on the original ABIDE fMRI scans to provide a clearer visual on which areas of the scan the model focuses on during the training and learning process. Through this visualization process, we were able to construct 'visual explanations' for the decisions made by our model by highlighting the important regions in the functional image for predicting the diagnosis. In doing so, we can clearly see the areas of the brain the model focuses on to identify differences between healthy control subjects and patients with autism. Moreover, this visualization will also aid doctors and physicians in the diagnostic process for ASD by assisting them in pinpointing the regions most likely to contain neural anomalies.

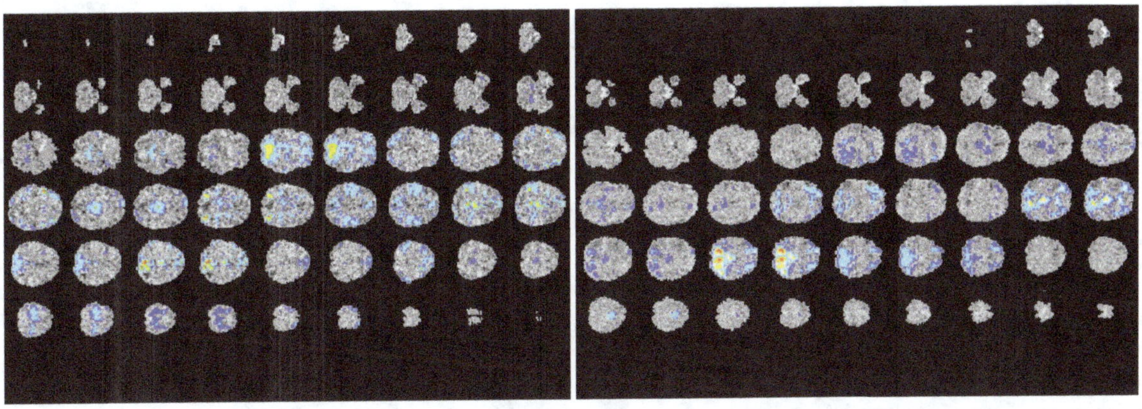

Figure 3. Explanations of model predictions. Cross-sections of fMRI scans indicating the regions that the network focused on when making predictions. Left: scans from a patient with autism; right: scans from a healthy individual with normal development. These images depict the regions the model used to predict the diagnosis of the scan, offering transparency on the model's decision-making process. The visualizations were produced using techniques proposed by Selvaraju et al. [25].

5. Conclusions

In this paper, we proposed a deep multimodal learning model for neuroimaging classification on the ABIDE dataset. Two types of functional imaging data, namely the activation maps calculated between fMRI image voxels $\times$ ROI time series and between only ROI time series, were used as input to two separate classifiers, a 3D ResNet-18 network and a multilayer perceptron classifier. The resulting feature vectors from these networks were pooled and used as input into several fully-connected layers to make the final prediction either control (healthy) or diseased (with autism). By proposing a model architecture that incorporates both types of activation maps, we use all the information provided by the functional data and demonstrate that the new model is capable of more accurate performance and thus makes for a better diagnosis system to assist doctors and medical practitioners.

However, at this point in time, the prediction accuracy of the multimodal model has only reached 74%, due to the limited amount of training data. This leads to the overfitting of our model.In the future, we plan to expand the training dataset by data augmentation and collecting more images to train our models in an effort to achieve higher accuracy. We hope that with further optimization and testing, we can eliminate any overfitting and reduce the amount of time needed for training. Moreover, we will be able to expand our analysis to other neuroimaging datasets, and demonstrate the generalizability of our methods by applying our automated system to diagnose more neurological diseases in addition to autism. With more testing and a larger quantity of data, we also hope to perform separate analysis on the visualizations of the model predictions, and to study the trends in which regions our model focuses on when making a diagnosis.

Author Contributions: M.T. conceptualized the research problem, collected and analyzed the data, and drafted the manuscript. A.S. supervised M.T., assisted development and edited the manuscript. All the authors have read and approved this version of the manuscript. Conceptualization, M.T. and A.S.; methodology, M.T.; validation, M.T., P.K.; visualization, P.K.; formal analysis, M.T.; investigation, M.T.; resources, A.S.; data curation, M.T., H.C.; writing–original draft preparation, M.T.; writing–review and editing, M.T., H.C., P.K., A.S.; visualization, P.K.; supervision, A.S.; project administration, M.T., A.S. All authors have read and agreed to the published version of the manuscript.

Abbreviations

The following abbreviations are used in this manuscript:

MDPI	Multidisciplinary Digital Publishing Institute

DOAJ	Directory of open access journals
ABIDE	Autism Brain Imaging Data Exchange
CNN	convolutional neural network
Grad-CAM	gradient-weighted class activation mapping
ROI	regions of interest

References

1. Sparks, B.; Friedman, S.; Shaw, D.; Aylward, E.H.; Echelard, D.; Artru, A.; Maravilla, K.; Giedd, J.; Munson, J.; Dawson, G.; et al. Brain structural abnormalities in young children with autism spectrum disorder. *Neurology* **2002**, *59*, 184–192. [CrossRef] [PubMed]
2. Huerta, M.; Lord, C. Diagnostic evaluation of autism spectrum disorders. *Pediatr. Clin. N. Am.* **2012**, *59*, 103. [CrossRef] [PubMed]
3. Glover, G.H. Overview of functional magnetic resonance imaging. *Neurosurg. Clin.* **2011**, *22*, 133–139. [CrossRef] [PubMed]
4. Biswal, B.; Zerrin Yetkin, F.; Haughton, V.M.; Hyde, J.S. Functional connectivity in the motor cortex of resting human brain using echo-planar MRI. *Magn. Reson. Med.* **1995**, *34*, 537–541. [CrossRef] [PubMed]
5. Zhou, Y.; He, X.; Huang, L.; Liu, L.; Zhu, F.; Cui, S.; Shao, L. Collaborative Learning of Semi-Supervised Segmentation and Classification for Medical Images. In Proceedings of the IEEE Conference on Computer Vision and Pattern Recognition, Long Beach, CA, USA, 15–20 June 2019; pp. 2079–2088.
6. Friman, O.; Cedefamn, J.; Lundberg, P.; Borga, M.; Knutsson, H. Detection of neural activity in functional MRI using canonical correlation analysis. *Magn. Reson. Med.* **2001**, *45*, 323–330. [CrossRef]
7. Nielsen, J.A.; Zielinski, B.A.; Fletcher, P.T.; Alexander, A.L.; Lange, N.; Bigler, E.D.; Lainhart, J.E.; Anderson, J.S. Multisite functional connectivity MRI classification of autism: ABIDE results. *Front. Hum. Neurosci.* **2013**, *7*, 599. [CrossRef] [PubMed]
8. Heinsfeld, A.S.; Franco, A.R.; Craddock, R.C.; Buchweitz, A.; Meneguzzi, F. Identification of autism spectrum disorder using deep learning and the ABIDE dataset. *Neuroimage Clin.* **2018**, *17*, 16–23. [CrossRef] [PubMed]
9. Khosla, M.; Jamison, K.; Kuceyeski, A.; Sabuncu, M.R. 3D convolutional neural networks for classification of functional connectomes. In *Deep Learning in Medical Image Analysis and Multimodal Learning for Clinical Decision Support*; Springer: Berlin/Heidelberg, Germany, 2018; pp. 137–145.
10. Craddock, C.; Benhajali, Y.; Chu, C.; Chouinard, F.; Evans, A.; Jakab, A.; Khundrakpam, B.S.; Lewis, J.D.; Li, Q.; Milham, M.; et al. The Neuro Bureau Preprocessing Initiative: Open sharing of preprocessed neuroimaging data and derivatives. *Front. Neuroinf.* **2013**, *7*. [CrossRef]
11. Xu, Y.; Mo, T.; Feng, Q.; Zhong, P.; Lai, M.; Eric, I.; Chang, C. Deep learning of feature representation with multiple instance learning for medical image analysis. In Proceedings of the 2014 IEEE International Conference on Acoustics, Speech and Signal Processing (ICASSP), Florence, Italy, 4–9 May 2014; pp. 1626–1630.
12. Ayyachamy, S.; Alex, V.; Khened, M.; Krishnamurthi, G. Medical image retrieval using Resnet-18. In Proceedings of the Medical Imaging 2019: Imaging Informatics for Healthcare, Research, and Applications. International Society for Optics and Photonics, San Diego, CA, USA, 16–21 February 2019; Volume 10954, p. 1095410.
13. Zhang, Z.; Yang, L.; Zheng, Y. Translating and segmenting multimodal medical volumes with cycle-and shape-consistency generative adversarial network. In Proceedings of the IEEE Conference on Computer Vision and Pattern Recognition, Salt Lake City, UT, USA, 16–20 June 2018; pp. 9242–9251.
14. Fukui, A.; Park, D.H.; Yang, D.; Rohrbach, A.; Darrell, T.; Rohrbach, M. Multimodal compact bilinear pooling for visual question answering and visual grounding. *arXiv* **2016**, arXiv:1606.01847.
15. Gao, Y.; Beijbom, O.; Zhang, N.; Darrell, T. Compact bilinear pooling. In Proceedings of the IEEE Conference on Computer Vision and Pattern Recognition, Las Vegas, NV, USA, 26 June–1 July 2016; pp. 317–326.
16. Guo, X.; Dominick, K.C.; Minai, A.A.; Li, H.; Erickson, C.A.; Lu, L.J. Diagnosing autism spectrum disorder from brain resting-state functional connectivity patterns using a deep neural network with a novel feature selection method. *Front. Neurosci.* **2017**, *11*, 460. [CrossRef] [PubMed]
17. Logothetis, N.K. What we can do and what we cannot do with fMRI. *Nature* **2008**, *453*, 869. [CrossRef] [PubMed]

18. Arthurs, O.J.; Boniface, S. How well do we understand the neural origins of the fMRI BOLD signal? *Trends Neurosci.* **2002**, *25*, 27–31. [CrossRef]
19. Wang, J.; Wang, L.; Zang, Y.; Yang, H.; Tang, H.; Gong, Q.; Chen, Z.; Zhu, C.; He, Y. Parcellation-dependent small-world brain functional networks: A resting-state fMRI study. *Hum. Brain Mapp.* **2009**, *30*, 1511–1523. [CrossRef] [PubMed]
20. Smith, S.M. Overview of fMRI analysis. *Br. J. Radiol.* **2004**, *77*, S167–S175. [CrossRef] [PubMed]
21. Di Martino, A.; Yan, C.G.; Li, Q.; Denio, E.; Castellanos, F.X.; Alaerts, K.; Anderson, J.S.; Assaf, M.; Bookheimer, S.Y.; Dapretto, M.; et al. The autism brain imaging data exchange: Towards a large-scale evaluation of the intrinsic brain architecture in autism. *Mol. Psychiatry* **2014**, *19*, 659. [CrossRef] [PubMed]
22. He, K.; Zhang, X.; Ren, S.; Sun, J. Deep residual learning for image recognition. In Proceedings of the IEEE Conference on Computer Vision and Pattern Recognition, Las Vegas, NV, USA, 26 June–1 July 2016; pp. 770–778.
23. Nair, V.; Hinton, G.E. Rectified linear units improve restricted boltzmann machines. In Proceedings of the 27th International Conference on Machine Learning (ICML-10), Haifa, Israel, 21–24 June 2010; pp. 807–814.
24. Ketkar, N., Introduction to PyTorch. In *Deep Learning with Python, a Hands-on Introduction*, Apress ed.; Apress: New York, NY, USA, 2017; pp. 195–208. [CrossRef]
25. Selvaraju, R.R.; Cogswell, M.; Das, A.; Vedantam, R.; Parikh, D.; Batra, D. Grad-cam: Visual explanations from deep networks via gradient-based localization. In Proceedings of the IEEE International Conference on Computer Vision, Venice, Italy, 22–29 October 2017; pp. 618–626.

6

Comparative Study of First Order Optimizers for Image Classification using Convolutional Neural Networks on Histopathology Images

Ibrahem Kandel [1,*], Mauro Castelli [1] and Aleš Popovič [2]

[1] Nova Information Management School (NOVA IMS), Campus de Campolide, Universidade Nova de Lisboa, 1070-312 Lisboa, Portugal; mcastelli@novaims.unl.pt

[2] School of Economics and Business, University of Ljubljana, Kardeljeva Ploščad 17, 1000 Ljubljana, Slovenia; ales.popovic@ef.uni-lj.si

* Correspondence: d20181143@novaims.unl.pt

Abstract: The classification of histopathology images requires an experienced physician with years of experience to classify the histopathology images accurately. In this study, an algorithm was developed to assist physicians in classifying histopathology images; the algorithm receives the histopathology image as an input and produces the percentage of cancer presence. The primary classifier used in this algorithm is the convolutional neural network, which is a state-of-the-art classifier used in image classification as it can classify images without relying on the manual selection of features from each image. The main aim of this research is to improve the robustness of the classifier used by comparing six different first-order stochastic gradient-based optimizers to select the best for this particular dataset. The dataset used to train the classifier is the PatchCamelyon public dataset, which consists of 220,025 images to train the classifier; the dataset is composed of 60% positive images and 40% negative images, and 57,458 images to test its performance. The classifier was trained on 80% of the images and validated on the rest of 20% of the images; then, it was tested on the test set. The optimizers were evaluated based on their AUC of the ROC curve. The results show that the adaptative based optimizers achieved the highest results except for AdaGrad that achieved the lowest results.

Keywords: image classification; convolutional neural networks; deep learning; medical images; transfer learning; optimizers

---

1. Introduction

To evaluate whether tissue is cancerous, a sample is taken from the suspicious area and then evaluated, under an optical microscope, by the pathologist. This procedure is very time-consuming and extremely complicated [1], and therefore, it requires an expert pathologist with years of experience. Depending on the particular task, even an expert pathologist could make errors. This complicated procedure often demands a second opinion or even assistance, which is where artificial intelligence assumes a role. Artificial intelligence (AI) can provide significant help, whether through a lot it is automation or to furnish the pathologist with a second opinion. AI can be defined as using a computer to generate a prediction of each image by training a deep neural network model. The training process consists of feeding the system labeled pathology images, after which the algorithm seeks; first, to map a function between the input label and the prediction and second, measures the error and tries to minimize it. The state-of-the-art algorithm used in the image classification is the convolutional neural network.

In the context of image classification, deep learning may be defined as a computer program is said to learn from experience E, like pathology images, concerning some task T, like image classification that differentiates between cancerous and non-cancerous images, and is capable of recognizing the relevant image without being explicitly programmed to do so, and using a performance measure like the AUC of the ROC curve. The algorithm's performance on the image classifier, as measured by the AUC, improves by adding more images. Practically speaking, machine learning is the task of recognizing patterns from training images and applying these patterns to identify an image with an unknown label.

The convolutional neural network (CNN) has been used as an image classification algorithm for nearly two decades [2]. The real power of CNN was rediscovered in the context of the ImageNet competition, where millions of images, with thousands of labels, were classified with 85% accuracy; at that time, CNN resumed its former role as one of the most important algorithms for image classification [3]. CNN has been applied in different image classification domains, such as agriculture [4–6] and traffic detection [7,8]. With the rapid improvements in GPU cards and the increasing size of datasets, many influential and robust architectures, like AlexNet [9], VGG16 [10], VGG19 [10], ResNet50 [11], and InceptionV3 [12], were introduced. Transfer learning is a deep learning technique, which allows the knowledge acquired during training on previous models to be applied to new tasks. Transfer learning has many advantages. It saves time by starting from the end point of the most recent training, instead of training the new model from scratch; it extends the knowledge it acquired from previous models; transfer learning is particularly useful when the size of the new training dataset is small. Transfer learning has made significant contributions to the fields of computer vision, audio classification, and natural language processing.

The difference between the predicted label and the correct label is called the cost function; the whole point of the algorithm is to minimize this cost function. As the algorithm most commonly used to minimize the cost function, backpropagation is an iterative algorithm, where each of its iterations consists of two passes: A forward pass throughout the entire network, where the inputs are propagated from the input layer to the output layer. At this point, the cost function is be calculated to measure the performance of the network; then there is the backward pass, where the weights are backpropagated from the output to the input of the network. The optimizers are used to minimize this cost function.

This work evaluates different first-degree optimizers used to classify pathology images as cancerous or non-cancerous. Each optimizer is evaluated based on its performance and convergence time. Four CNN architectures will be used to compare the performance of each optimizer to those of the others.

2. Related Works

Many works compared the performance of different optimizers in the context of different neural network architectures; the reported approaches differ in relation to the network architecture, datasets, and the optimizers under study.

In a study by Dogo et al. [13], the authors evaluated the performance of seven optimizers on three image datasets: Natural Images dataset, Cats and Dogs dataset, and Fashion MNIST dataset. The authors evaluated the performance of each optimizer based on accuracy achieved and the convergence time, where convergence consists of reaching the minimum of the function. To determine the performance quality of each optimizer, the authors proposed a simple CNN architecture, with three convolutional layers, and one dense layer with 64 neurons. For the Cats and Dogs dataset, the Nadam optimizer achieved the best performance, and the Adadelta optimizer produced the most mediocre performance; the RMSProp represents the shortest convergence time, and the Nadam optimizer achieved the longest convergence. For the Fashion dataset, the Adam optimizer achieved the highest degree of accuracy, and the Adadelta optimizer displayed the lowest accuracy; the Adamax optimizer achieved the shortest convergence time, and the Adadelta optimizer had the longest convergence time was the Adadelta optimizer. For the Natural dataset, the Nadam optimizer was the best performer, and the Adagrad optimizer exhibited the most inferior accuracy; the SGD algorithm achieved the shortest convergence time, and the Adadelta algorithm had the longest convergence time. The authors concluded that the Nadam optimizer was the best of all tested optimizer, due to its combined mastery of the momentum and the adaptive gradient estimation.

The authors Prilianti et al. [14] compared the performance of seven optimizers on the digital plant dataset. To evaluate each optimizer, the authors used three CNN architectures; the first was a shallow network with only one convolutional layer and without any dense layers; the second CNN architecture used was the LeNet architecture, which was introduced by Lecun et al., [15]; and the third CNN architecture was the AlexNet [9]. The authors evaluated the performance of each optimizer on each CNN architecture, based on the mean square error (MSE). The Adam optimizer achieved the lowest MSE for the shallow net architecture, as well as the LeNet architecture, while the Adadelta achieved the lowest MSE on the AlexNet architecture. The authors concluded that Adam optimizer achieved the best performance.

Jangid and Srivastava [16] assessed the performance of three optimizers on handwritten Devanagari characters. The optimizers tested were Adam, Adamax, and RMSProp. To evaluate each optimizer, the authors introduced a CNN architecture with three convolutional layers and one dense layer with 1000 neurons. For this architecture, RMSProp achieved the best accuracy. Swastika et al. [17] evaluated three optimizers to classify vehicle types: Adam, Adadelta, and SGD. The authors used three CNN architectures to evaluate each optimizer: a shallow network, LeNet, and MiniVGGNet. The optimizers were evaluated based on their accuracy, which meant that the Adadelta optimizer was the best for the Mini VGGNet architecture.

This study uses four CNN architectures to perform a comparative evaluation of six first-degree stochastic gradient descent optimizers: the optimizers tested are Nesterov gradient descent, Adagrad, Adam, Adamax, Nadam, and RMSProp; and the CNN architectures tested are VGG16, InceptionV3, DenseNet, and ResNet50. The optimizers are evaluated based on their AUC of the ROC curve and their convergence time. All the optimizers' default hyperparameters were kept constant throughout the experiment, except the learning rate, which was set to three values 0.001, 0.0001, and 0.0001. Fine-tuning was applied to each network to adjust its weight to the new dataset.

3. Methodology

3.1. Dataset

The public available PatchCamelyon dataset [18,19] was used in this study. The images represent sentinel axillary lymph nodes to investigate the spread of breast cancer. The dataset was sampled from two hospitals in the Netherlands, experienced pathologists from the Netherlands annotated the dataset labels. The dataset was acquired from the Kaggle platform [20]. The dataset consists of 220,025 images to train the classifier; the dataset is composed of 60% positive images and 40% negative images, and it includes 57,458 unlabeled images to test the classifier performance. All images have dimensions of 96 × 96 pixels. Eighty percent of the dataset is used to train the classifier, which is subsequently evaluated with the other 20% of the dataset images; the classifier is also tested on the online set of 57,458 images, and the results are uploaded to the Kaggle platform to detect the model performance. A sample of images is presented in Figure 1.

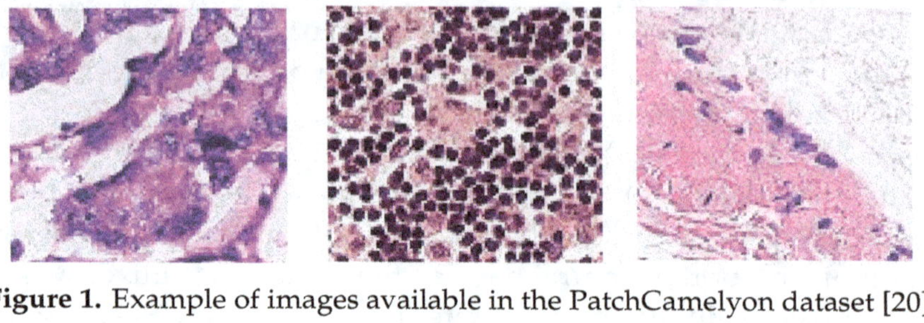

Figure 1. Example of images available in the PatchCamelyon dataset [20].

3.2. *Convolutional Neural Networks*

CNN is the most used algorithm in image classification, where it is understood to be a deep learning algorithm that serves as a feed-forward neural network with more than one hidden layer. The CNN for image classification was introduced by Fukushima [2] to mimic the biological visual cortex of the brain. CNN combines sophisticated features obtained from the higher layers of the network with the generic features obtained from the lower layers of the network. The most critical layer of CNN is the convolution layer, which is responsible for capturing the temporal and spatial information of each image; the convolutional layer must conduct the convolution operation, which is a mathematical operation performed between the input and the filter to produce the feature map. Equation (1) shows the convolution operation,

$$O[u,v] = F[m,n] * I[u,v] = \sum_m \sum_n F[m,n] \cdot I[u+m, v+n] \tag{1}$$

where $F[m,n]$ is the convolution filter, $I[u,v]$ is the input image and $O[u,v]$ is the output feature map.

A filter is convolved over the input image to produce a feature map. Another CNN layer is the activation function, which is used to present non-linearity because usually, the image classification task is highly non-linear. To reduce overfitting and to reduce the spatial footprint of each filter, two main techniques can be used to extract the essential pixels and removing the noise. The first involves using a stride value larger than 1, which reduces the output of each filter. The second technique is called pooling, where a pooling layer usually follows the activation layer. Pooling layers can strengthen network spatial invariance [21]. The two main types of pooling layers are the maximum pooling layer and the average pooling layer.

Then, fully connected layers follow, usually defined at the end of the network, which takes the output of the feature extraction layers. The primary purpose of the dense layer is to consider all the features extracted from the previous layers and employ these features to classify the output. The dense layers are followed by an activation function, which usually consists of a rectified linear unit (ReLU) layer; finally, at the end of the network, a softmax or sigmoid function is used to output the target probability.

3.3. *Optimizers*

The model learns (trains) on a given dataset by comparing the actual label of the input (available in the training set) to the predicted label, thereby, minimizing the cost function. Hypothetically, if the cost function is zero, the model has learned the dataset correctly. However, an optimization algorithm is needed to achieve the minimum of a cost function. The next section discusses different optimization algorithms, introduced in the literature, to minimize the cost function.

3.3.1. Vanilla Gradient Descent Optimizers

Gradient descent is the primary class of optimizers capable of finding the minimum value of the cost function. The literature has introduced three versions of gradient descent.

Batch Gradient Descent

The first optimization algorithm was the batch gradient descent optimization algorithm (BGD), which updates the network weights after scanning the whole training dataset; in the case of images, convergence takes much time, as there may be millions of weights to optimize and the whole dataset needs to be reevaluated at every step (i.e., epoch). For convex loss function, it is guaranteed that the BGD will converge to the global minimum, while it converges to a local minimum for non-convex functions. The weights are updated based on Equation (2):

$$w_{t+1} = w_t - \eta \frac{\partial C}{\partial w_t} \tag{2}$$

$$\frac{\partial C}{\partial w_t} = \nabla_w C(w_t) \tag{3}$$

where Equation (3) is the gradients update equation, and η is the learning rate hyperparameter. w_t are the weights at step t, $C(.)$ is the cost function and $\nabla_w C(w_t)$ is the gradient of weight parameters w_t.

Stochastic Gradient Descent

To overcome the shortcomings of BGD, stochastic gradient descent (SGD) was introduced. SGD allows to update the network weights per each training image, that is why SGD is sometimes called online training. However, such updates engender massive fluctuation in the loss function, due to the high variance between different images, which can create much noise in the training phase:

$$w_{t+1} = w_t - \eta \frac{\partial C}{\partial w_t} \tag{4}$$

$$\frac{\partial C}{\partial w_t} = \nabla_w C\left(w_t; x^{(i)}; y^{(i)}\right) \tag{5}$$

The weights are updated based on Equation (4), where Equation (5) is the gradient update equation, and η is the learning rate hyperparameter. w_t are the weights at step t, $C(.)$ is the cost function, and $\nabla_w C(w_t)$ is the gradient of weight parameters w_t for image x and its corresponding label y.

Mini-Batch Gradient Descent

Mini-batch gradient descent was introduced to overcome the shortcomings of the previous two algorithms, because it allows for the weights to be updated per batch, and not per image. As such, mini-batch gradient descent may be regarded as a particular case of SGD, where the number of samples is more than one. In the literature and it follows, in this paper, the mini-batch is referred to as stochastic gradient descent (SGD):

$$w_{t+1} = w_t - \eta \frac{\partial C}{\partial w_t} \tag{6}$$

$$\frac{\partial C}{\partial w_t} = \nabla_w C\left(w_t; x^{(i:i+n)}; y^{(i:i+n)}\right) \tag{7}$$

The weights are updated based on Equation (6), and Equation (7) is the gradient update equation. η is the learning rate hyperparameter, w_t are the weights at step t, n is the number of data points, $C(.)$ is the cost function and $\nabla_w C(w_t)$ is the gradient of weight parameters w_t for image x and its corresponding label y.

3.3.2. Momentum-Based Gradient Descent Optimizers

The main drawback of using mini-batch SGD is the presence of oscillations during the updating of the weights. These oscillations usually result in a long time to reach convergence. Momentum, also known as moving average gradients, was introduced, in order to overcome this issue and to fix the gradients' direction.

Momentum Gradient Descent

Understanding the right direction for the gradient avoids oscillations in the wrong directions, and knowing the right direction relies on using the previous position for guidance. Considering the previous position, the updating rule adds a fraction of the previous update, which gives the optimizer the momentum needed to continue moving in the right direction. The weights are updated based on Equation (10),

$$V_t = \lambda V_{t-1} + \eta \frac{\partial C}{\partial w_t} \tag{8}$$

$$\frac{\partial C}{\partial w_t} = \nabla_w \, C\left(w_t; x^{(i:i+n)}; y^{(i:i+n)}\right) \tag{9}$$

$$w_{t+1} = w_t - V_t \tag{10}$$

where V is the velocity, and it is initialized to 0. λ is used to select the amount of information needed from the previous update. η is the learning rate hyperparameter, w_t are the weights at step t, n is the number of data points, $C(.)$ is the cost function, and $\nabla_w \, C(w_t)$ is the gradient of weight parameters w_t for image x and its corresponding label y.

Nesterov Momentum Gradient Descent

If the momentum is sufficiently high, close to the minimum, the optimizer may overshoot the minimum. The previous optimization algorithms take the current and the previous gradients into account for updating the weights. However, to make the optimization algorithm more robust, we must take the future gradients into account as well, to approximate the gradients' direction. The weights are updated based on Equation (13),

$$V_t = \lambda V_{t-1} + \eta \frac{\partial C}{\partial w_t} \tag{11}$$

$$\frac{\partial C}{\partial w_t} = \nabla_w \, C\left(w_t - \lambda V_{t-1}; x^{(i:i+n)}; y^{(i:i+n)}\right) \tag{12}$$

$$w_{t+1} = w_t - V_t \tag{13}$$

where V is the velocity, and it is initialized to 0, λ is used to select the amount of information needed from the previous update. While, η is the learning rate hyperparameter, w_t are the weights at step t, n is the number of data points, $C(.)$ is the cost function, and $\nabla_w \, C(w_t)$ is the gradient of weight parameters w_t for image x and its corresponding label y. $(w_t - \lambda V_{t-1})$ is the look-ahead position that is capable of approximating the next gradient position, thereby allowing it to slow down if it threatens to overshoot the minimum.

3.3.3. Adaptive Gradient Descent Optimizers

All the optimization mentioned above has a fixed learning rate, while, in practice, deep learning algorithms are non-convex problems. That may be a problem, as we may face a sparse weight matrix, where we require different updates for different weights, especially for infrequent weights, where significant updates are needed to reach to avoid oscillating.

AdaGrad Optimizer

To scale the learning rate for each weight, the AdaGrad optimization algorithm [22] was introduced to establish different updates for different weights. The learning rate is tuned automatically, by dividing the learning rate by the sum of squares of all previous gradients. The weights are updated based on Equation (14),

$$w_t^i = w_{t-1}^i - \frac{\eta}{\sqrt{\sum_{\mathcal{T}=1}^{t}\left(\nabla_w C\left(w_{\mathcal{T}}^i\right)\right)^2 + \epsilon}} \cdot \nabla_w C\left(w_t^i\right) \tag{14}$$

where η is the learning rate hyperparameter, w_t are the weights at step t, $C(.)$ is the cost function, and $\nabla_w \, C(w_t)$ is the gradient of weight parameters w_t for image x and its corresponding label y. The sum of squares $\sqrt{\sum_{\mathcal{T}=1}^{t}\left(\nabla_w C\left(w_{\mathcal{T}}^i\right)\right)^2}$ is used to scale the learning rate; it gives a high learning rate for the least frequent gradients and a low learning rate for the more frequent gradients.

RMSProp Optimizer

The main drawback of AdaGrad is that the learning rate decreases monotonically because every added term is positive. After many epochs, the learning rate is so small that it stops updating the weights. RMSProp was introduced to address the problem of the monotonically decreasing learning rate [23]. The weights are updated based on Equation (17),

$$G = \nabla_w C(w_t) \tag{15}$$

$$E\left[G^2\right]_t = \lambda\, E\left[G^2\right]_{t-1} + (1-\lambda)G_t^2 \tag{16}$$

$$w_t^i = w_{t-1}^i - \frac{\eta}{\sqrt{E[G^2]_t + \epsilon}} \cdot \nabla_w C\left(w_t^i\right) \tag{17}$$

where η is the learning rate hyperparameter, w_t are the weights at step t, $C(.)$ is the cost function, and $\nabla_w\, C(w_t)$ is the gradient of weight parameters w_t for image x and its corresponding label y. λ is used to select the amount of information needed from the previous update. $E\left[G^2\right]_t$ is the running average of the squared gradients, which has been used to avoid the monotonically decreasing gradients of the AdaGrad optimizer.

Adam Optimizer

The Adam optimization [24] algorithm was introduced to combine the benefits of Nesterov momentum, AdaGrad, and RMSProp algorithms. The weights are updated based on Equation (18):

$$w_t^i = w_{t-1}^i - \frac{\eta}{\sqrt{\hat{v}_t} + \epsilon} \cdot \hat{m}_t \tag{18}$$

where:

$$\hat{m}_t = \frac{m_t}{1-\beta_1^t} \tag{19}$$

$$\hat{v}_t = \frac{v_t}{1-\beta_2^t} \tag{20}$$

$$m_t = \beta_1 m_{t-1} + (1-\beta_1)G \tag{21}$$

$$v_t = \beta_2 v_{t-1} + (1-\beta_2)[G]^2 \tag{22}$$

$$G = \nabla_w C(w_t) \tag{23}$$

where η is the learning rate hyperparameter, w_t are the weights at step t, $C(.)$ is the cost function, and $\nabla_w\, C(w_t)$ is the gradient of weight parameters w_t for image x and its corresponding label y, β_i is used to select the amount of information needed from the previous update, where $\beta_i \in [0, 1]$, m_t is the running average of the gradients, also known as the first moment, v_t is the running average of the squared gradients, and known as the second moment. If the first and second moments get initialized at zero, they are biased toward it, to solve this zero-biased problem, these moments are bias-corrected by dividing them by their respective β.

Adamax Optimizer

Adamax [24] is the update of the Adam algorithm, where the uncentered variance tends to ∞. The weights are updated based on Equation (24):

$$w_t^i = w_{t-1}^i - \frac{\eta}{v_t + \epsilon} \cdot \hat{m}_t \tag{24}$$

where:

$$\hat{m}_t = \frac{m_t}{1-\beta_1^t} \tag{25}$$

$$v_t = \max(\beta_2 \cdot v_{t-1}, |G_t|) \tag{26}$$

$$m_t = \beta_1 m_{t-1} + (1-\beta_1)G \tag{27}$$

$$G = \nabla_w C(w_t) \tag{28}$$

where η is the learning rate hyperparameter, w_t are the weights at step t, $C(.)$ is the cost function, and $\nabla_w C(w_t)$ is the gradient of weight parameters w_t for image x and its corresponding label y. β_i is used to select the amount of information needed from the previous update, where $\beta_i \in [0,1]$. m_t is the first moment, v_t is the second moment.

Nadam Optimizer

Nadam [25] is an extension of the Adam algorithm by combining it with Nesterov momentum gradient descent. The weights are updated based on Equation (29):

$$w_t^i = w_{t-1}^i - \frac{\eta}{\sqrt{v_t + \epsilon}} \cdot \widetilde{m}_t \tag{29}$$

where:

$$\widetilde{m}_t = \beta_1^{t+1} \hat{m}_t + \left(1 - \beta_1^t\right) \hat{g}_t \tag{30}$$

$$\hat{m}_t = \frac{m_t}{1 - \prod_{i=1}^{t} \beta_1^i} \tag{31}$$

$$\hat{g}_t = \frac{g_t}{1 - \prod_{i=1}^{t} \beta_1^i} \tag{32}$$

where η is the learning rate hyperparameter, and w_t are the weights at step t. While, β_i is used to select the amount of information needed from the previous update, where $\beta_i \in [0,1]$, m_t is the first moment.

Fine-Tuning

According to [26,27] transfer learning can be formalized as follows: by having a domain D, where $D = \{X, P(X)\}$, in which X is the feature space and $P(X)$ is the marginal probability distribution and task $\mathcal{T} = \{Y, f(.)\}$, where Y is the label space and $f(.)$ is the predictive function which models $P(y|x)$ for $y \in Y$ and $x \in X$. By having a source domain D_s and learning task $\mathcal{T}_S$ and a target domain D_T and learning task $\mathcal{T}_T$, by using weights from D_S and $\mathcal{T}_S$, learning the target predictive function $f(.)$ in $\mathcal{T}_T$ can be improved a lot, where $D_S \neq D_T$, $\mathcal{T}_S \neq \mathcal{T}_T$, or both. Fine-tuning is very important in the classification of medical images, because the neural network usually needs many images to be trained. However, in the medical field, for many reasons, labeled medical images are scarce. Instead of initializing the weights from scratch, ImageNet weights can be used. In this paper, the networks were trained on ImageNet dataset and all the networks blocks were fine-tuned using the PatchCamelyon dataset [18,19].

3.3.4. VGG16 Network

VGG16 [10] was introduced in 2014 by the researchers at Oxford's Visual Geometry Group. It was one of the top algorithms involved in the ImageNet classification challenge, and it had an 8.1% error rate. VGG16 consists of five convolution blocks, where the first block contains two convolution layers, stacked together with 64 filters. The second block consists of two stacked convolution layers with 128 filters, where the second convolution block is separated from the first block by a max pool layer. The third block consists of three convolution layers, stacked together with 256 filters and separated from the second block by another max pool layer. The fourth and fifth layers have the same architecture, but instead, have 512 filters. The convolution filter used throughout this network is of size 3×3 and stride of 1. Then, a flatten layer is added between the convolution blocks and the dense layers, converting the 3D vector into a 1D vector. The last block consists of three dense layers, each of which has 4096 neurons, to classify each image. The last layer is a softmax layer, which is used to ensure that the probability summation of the output is one. ReLU was used as an activation layer throughout the network. This network was trained on the ImageNet dataset for three weeks on four GPUs to detect the ImageNet classification task. A summary of VGG16 network is presented in Table 1.

Table 1. Number of layers and parameters of the CNNs used in this study.

Networks	Number of Layers	Number of Parameters
VGG16	16	14,714,688
InceptionV3	48	21,802,784
ResNet50	50	23,587,712
DenseNet121	121	7,037,504

3.3.5. InceptionV3 Network

The authors Szegedy et al. [28] introduced a novel architecture, called Inception, to participate in the ImageNet competition in 2015; Inception had an accuracy rate of 92.2%. The architecture consists of 48 layers and total parameters of 22,000,000. This architecture has a concatenated layer of convolutions, stacked in parallel to decrease the size of the architecture while maintaining its complexity. InceptionV3 network architecture is shown in Figure 2. A summary of InceptionV3 network is presented in Table 1.

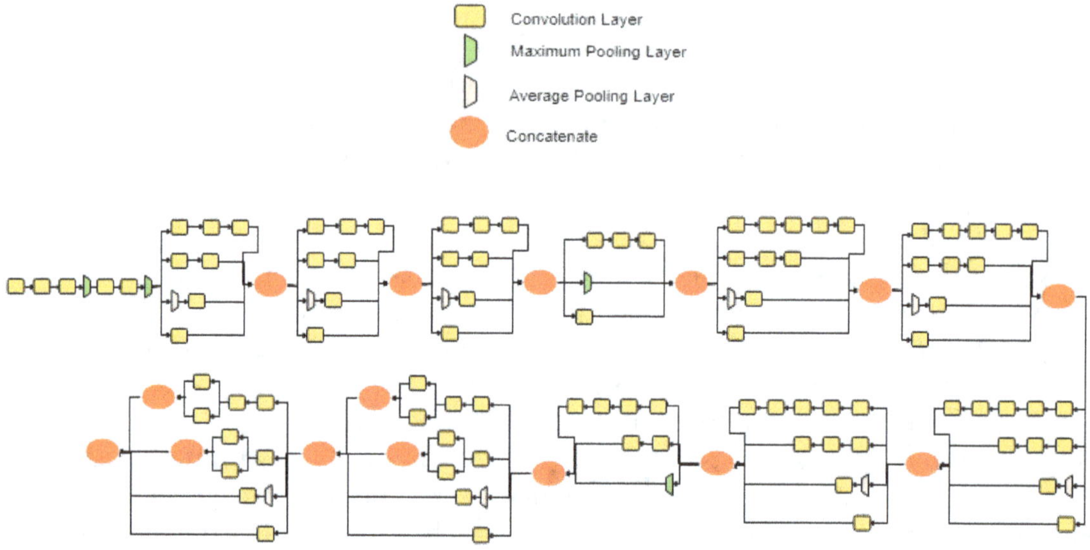

Figure 2. InceptionV3 network architecture.

3.3.6. ResNet Network

The authors, He et al. [11], investigated the effect of increasing the depth of the convolutional neural network and its impact on network performance. The authors noticed that increasing the depth of the network decreases the generalizability of the network, which means that the test error of the network is higher than a shallow network. This may be due to the vanishing gradients, where the weights are not updated in deep layers. Therefore, He et al. [11] introduced a novel architecture called ResNet, where Res signifies the application of a residual connection between the convolutional layers, which is then passed to the ReLU activation layer. One of the main benefits of adding the residual connection is that the weights learned from the previous layers can be carried to the next layers during the backpropagation step. ResNet won the ImageNet competition in 2015 with Top-5 accuracy of 94.29%. It has a total of 23,587,712 parameters, and its ImageNet weights are available in the Keras package. A summary of ResNet network is presented in Table 1.

3.3.7. DenseNet Network

DenseNet network [29] was inspired by the residual connection of the ResNet architecture. All the layers are connected to all their subsequent layers, meaning that a residual connection is established between all the layers. Merging will be used instead of adding to combine the layers. DenseNet has many variants depends on the number of layers; some of the variants are DenseNet 121, DenseNet169, and DenseNet201. In this paper, we opted for the DenseNet121 network. A summary of DenseNet network is presented in Table 1.

3.4. Overcoming Overfitting

Overfitting generally consists of memorization of the training dataset and usually leads to poor performance on the test dataset. This means that the performance on the training set can be excellent, but the performance on the test set is quite poor. The loss of the generalizability of the network may be due to many issues, such as the capacity of the network or the nature of the training dataset itself. Many measures have been introduced in the literature to overcome overfitting. Below are some techniques that were used in this research to overcome overfitting.

3.4.1. Dropout

A regularization layer introduced by [30] can be applied to any layer in the network. During network training, some neurons are disabled with a pre-defined dropout-rate probability P. This can be understood as a sort of bagging for neural networks.

3.4.2. Image Augmentation

Increasing the size of the training set improves the performance of the network. For image datasets, many duplicates can be created with simple changes to the original dataset, including rotation, flipping, zooming, and cropping. These transformations make the network more robust in defending against overfitting, and it enhances network performance as well. In our case, the original images are flipped, rotated, zoomed, and shifted. The rotation range used was 180°; and the images were randomly flipped horizontally and vertically; the shifting range used was 25%; and the zoom range used was 40%.

3.4.3. Early Stopping

Early stopping is a precautionary measure used to prevent the network from overfitting, which may be defined as stopping the training phase of the network when the performance on the validation set stops improving for a pre-defined number of epochs. This pre-defined number usually ranges from 10–50 epochs. In our case, the number of epochs is 10.

3.5. Evaluation Metrics

To assess the quality of the trained CNN, many measures have been developed. For classification tasks, a confusion matrix is constructed to assess the model quality; it categorizes the model predictions, according to whether they match the correct label of the image. It has four central values:

TP: True positive (A positive example, classified as a positive example)
TN: True negative (A negative example, classified as a negative example)
FP: False positive (A negative example, but classified as a positive example)
FN: False-negative (A positive example, but classified as a negative example)

To visualize the model performance, the ROC curve was introduced to examine the trade-off between sensitivity and specificity visually. The main idea of the ROC curve is to plot the specificity of the algorithms, which is the percentage of the correctly classified negatives against the sensitivity, which is the percentage of the correctly classified positives of the algorithm [31]. The ROC curve has a diagonal line, which represents a random guess model. It means that the model cannot differentiate between true positives and false positives; this diagonal line can be considered as the baseline where models can be judged. The best model has a curve that passes through the top left corner for "100% Sensitivity" and has a 0% false-positive rate. To measure the quality of the model using the ROC curve, a statistic known as AUC or "Area under the ROC curve," is used; this treats the ROC diagram as a two-dimensional square and measures the area under the curve. AUC has a minimum value of 0.5 and a maximum value of 1, where 0.5 represents a model with no predictive power, and 1 represents a model with 100% predictive power. According to Vuk [32], the AUC is calculated by Equation (33):

$$\mathrm{AUC} = \int_0^1 \frac{\mathrm{TP}}{\mathrm{P}}\, \mathrm{d}\frac{\mathrm{FP}}{\mathrm{N}} = \frac{1}{\mathrm{PN}} \int_0^{\mathrm{N}} \mathrm{TP}\, \mathrm{dFP} \tag{33}$$

where $\mathrm{TP} + \mathrm{FN} = \mathrm{P}$ and $\mathrm{TN} + \mathrm{FP} = \mathrm{N}$.

4. Results

The following section details the results obtained from training the four network architectures using the six selected optimizers with three learning rates, namely, 1×10^{-3}, 1×10^{-4}, and 1×10^{-5}. Many experiments have been conducted on this dataset, to determine the behavior of each optimizer with each network architecture to determine the best combination. The performance of each optimizer with the VGG16 architecture is presented in Table 2, with the InceptionV3 architecture in Table 3, with the ResNet architecture in Table 4, and with the DenseNet architecture in Table 5. To test the performance of each configuration, two types of evaluation were used; the first consists of splitting the training dataset into 80%/20% to train and validate the dataset. After training, the model is used to predict the class of the images in the test set, and the result is submitted to the Kaggle platform to assess the performance of each model. The AUC of the ROC curve measured the performance. The optimizers are ranked based on their test AUC that was acquired from the Kaggle platform.

In all the experiments, the default settings of each optimizer were chosen, except the learning rate, and image augmentation used for rotating, flipping, and cropping all the images. The size of the images was kept constant at 96 × 96; a batch size of 64 images was used, and early stopping was applied with the number of epochs equal to 10.

4.1. VGG16 Architecture Result

Table 2 shows the results for the VGG16 architecture, which shows that the highest AUC was achieved by Adam optimizer, which also took the shortest time to achieve convergence. At the same time, the lowest test AUC was achieved by RMSProp and Adamax optimizers that did not converge at all. For the highest learning rate (1×10^{-3}) the highest AUC achieved was by the Adam optimizer, and the lowest AUC achieved was by the RMSProp and Adamax optimizers. For the medium learning rate (1×10^{-4}) the highest AUC achieved was by NAG optimizer, and the lowest AUC achieved was by both AdaGrad and Adam optimizers. For the lowest learning rate (1×10^{-5} The AdaGrad optimizer achieved), the highest AUC achieved by the Adam optimizer and the lowest AUC. Overall, the medium learning rate achieved the best results, followed by the lowest learning rate. Adam optimizer was the most stable optimizer with high results and low variance between different learning rates.

Table 2. Results obtained with the VGG16 architecture. Where LR stands for learning rate; NAG represents Nesterov momentum; AdaGrad represents the adaptive gradient optimizer; RMSProp represents the root mean square propagation optimizer; Adam represents adaptive moment estimation optimizer; AdaMax represents maximum adaptive moment estimation optimizer; and Nadam represents Nesterov and Adam optimizer.

Optimizers	LR = 10^{-3}	LR = 10^{-4}	LR = 10^{-5}
NAG	89.45%	94.64%	94.25%
AdaGrad	88.50%	87.40%	88.07%
RMSProp	50.00%	94.33%	93.45%
Adam	90.88%	90.39%	95.01%
Adamax	50.00%	94.02%	94.20%
Nadam	85.00%	91.14%	94.33%

4.2. *InceptionV3 Architecture Result*

Table 3 shows the results for the InceptionV3 architecture, which shows that the highest AUC was achieved by the RMSProp optimizer, which also took the shortest time to achieve convergence. At the same time, the lowest test AUC was achieved by AdaGrad optimizer, which also took the longest time to convergence. For the highest learning rate (1×10^{-3}), the AdaGrad optimizer achieved the highest AUC, while, the Adam optimizer achieved the lowest AUC. For the medium learning rate (1×10^{-4}) the highest AUC achieved was by the RMSProp optimizer, and the lowest AUC achieved was by the AdaGrad optimizer. For the lowest learning rate (1×10^{-5} The AdaGrad optimizer achieved), the highest AUC achieved by the AdaMax optimizer and the lowest AUC. Overall, the medium learning rate achieved the best results, followed by the lowest learning rate. Adamax optimizer was the most stable optimizer with high results and low variance between different learning rates.

Table 3. Results obtained with the InceptionV3 architecture. Where LR stands for learning rate; NAG represents Nesterov momentum; AdaGrad represents the adaptive gradient optimizer; RMSProp represents the root mean square propagation optimizer; Adam represents adaptive moment estimation optimizer; AdaMax represents maximum adaptive moment estimation optimizer; and Nadam represents Nesterov and Adam optimizer.

Optimizers	LR = 10^{-3}	LR = 10^{-4}	LR = 10^{-5}
NAG	93.18%	93.25%	90.81%
AdaGrad	93.64%	90.46%	86.32%
RMSProp	91.41%	94.91%	92.65%
Adam	90.44%	92.53%	93.22%
Adamax	93.44%	93.11%	93.95%
Nadam	91.97%	91.33%	92.46%

4.3. *ResNet Architecture Result*

Table 4 shows the results for the ResNet architecture, which shows that the best AUC was achieved by the Nadam optimizer, while the AdaGrad optimizer achieved the lowest AUC. For the highest learning rate (1×10^{-3}) the highest AUC achieved was by the AdaGrad optimizer, and the lowest AUC achieved was by the RMSProp optimizer. For the medium learning rate (1×10^{-4}) the highest AUC achieved was by the NAG optimizer, and the lowest AUC achieved was by the AdaGrad optimizer. For the lowest learning rate (1×10^{-5} The AdaGrad optimizer achieved), the highest AUC achieved by the Nadam optimizer and the lowest AUC. Overall, the medium learning rate achieved the best results, followed by the lowest learning rate. Adamax optimizer was the most stable optimizer with high results and low variance between different learning rates.

Table 4. Results obtained with the ResNet architecture. Where LR stands for learning rate; NAG represents Nesterov momentum; AdaGrad represents the adaptive gradient optimizer; RMSProp represents the root mean square propagation optimizer; Adam represents adaptive moment estimation optimizer; AdaMax represents maximum adaptive moment estimation optimizer; and Nadam represents Nesterov and Adam optimizer.

Optimizers	LR = 10^{-3}	LR = 10^{-4}	LR = 10^{-5}
NAG	90.07%	93.84%	89.00%
AdaGrad	93.04%	89.11%	83.46%
RMSProp	89.56%	89.62%	93.04%
Adam	90.24%	90.24%	93.84%
Adamax	90.24%	92.24%	93.70%
Nadam	91.91%	89.36%	93.85%

4.4. *DenseNet Architecture Result*

Table 5 shows the results for the DenseNet architecture, where the best AUC was achieved by Adamax optimizer, while the Adam optimizer achieved the lowest AUC. For the highest learning rate (1×10^{-3}) the highest AUC achieved was by the AdaGrad optimizer, and the lowest AUC achieved was by the Adam optimizer. For the medium learning rate (1×10^{-4}) the highest AUC achieved was by Adamax optimizer, and the lowest AUC achieved was by the Adam optimizer. For the lowest learning rate (1×10^{-5} The AdaGrad optimizer achieved), the highest AUC was achieved by the RMSProp optimizer and the lowest AUC. Overall, the medium learning rate achieved the best results, followed by the lowest learning rate. Adamax optimizer was the most stable optimizer with high results and low variance between different learning rates.

Table 5. Results obtained with the DenseNet architecture. Where LR represents learning rate; NAG represents Nesterov momentum; AdaGrad represents the adaptive gradient optimizer; RMSProp represents the root mean square propagation optimizer; Adam represents adaptive moment estimation optimizer; AdaMax represents maximum adaptive moment estimation optimizer; and Nadam represents Nesterov and Adam optimizer.

Optimizers	LR = 10^{-3}	LR = 10^{-4}	LR = 10^{-5}
NAG	93.08%	94.31%	91.64%
AdaGrad	93.89%	93.57%	87.70%
RMSProp	88.19%	93.98%	94.61%
Adam	84.18%	89.69%	94.43%
Adamax	90.62%	95.12%	93.91%
Nadam	86.77%	94.21%	93.77%

Overall, in terms of performance across all four networks, the highest results were achieved by the adaptive learning optimizers, like Adam, Adamax, Nadam, and RMSProp. However, these optimizers needed a lower learning rate to be able to converge, while the high learning rate did not achieve good results. One exception was the AdaGrad optimizer that did not achieve high results with a low learning rate; on the contrary, it needed a high learning rate to be able to converge to an acceptable result. From our results and the results obtained by Prilianti et al. [14], it is apparent that every combination of network and optimizer will produce a unique combination. However, the general behavior of each optimizer can be noted, which can be concluded from the results. Overall, NAG optimizer did achieve high results overall the four architectures and overall the three learning rates used with the medium learning rate $\left(1 \times 10^{-4}\right)$ achieved the best results. The AdaGrad optimizer did not achieve high results compared to other optimizers used, especially when trained using low learning rates. RMSProp optimizer did achieve high results with a low learning rate but was unstable with high learning rates. Adam optimizer needed a low learning rate to be able to converge to high results. While, the AdaMax optimizer behaved similarly to the Adam optimizer, except for a high learning rate with the VGG16, where it did not converge at all, one reason may be the shallow depth of the VGG16 network. Nadam optimizer did achieve high results with both the medium learning rate and the low learning rate.

5. Discussion

Taking into account the results achieved from the experimental campaign, it is possible to draw some interesting observations of the behavior of the CNNs and optimizers considered in this paper. By focusing on the choice of the optimizer and its relation with the learning rate, the experimental results confirm that the choice of the learning rate may result in an unstable behavior of the training process. This is particularly evident, for some of the considered networks and optimizers, when considering the smallest learning rate used in the experiments. As one can see, when $LR = 10^{-3}$, the training process of VGG16 with both RMSProp and Adamax optimizer result in a poor performance of the model. As explained in the previous sections, this can be motivated by the fact that the weights of the network change abruptly from one epoch to the next. Moving to lower LR values allows the convergence of the training process in all the configurations that were investigated. Overall, the results match the theoretical expectation: A lower LR value allows for a smoother convergence, but it requires more time with respect to a greater LR value.

Another interesting observation relates to the importance of the hyperparameters. While this is a topic of fundamental importance in the area of deep learning, it is particularly evident from the results of the experimental phase. In particular, all the considered architecture produced a comparable performance when the best configuration of the learning rate and optimizer (that is different for each type of architecture) was considered. In other words, it seems that the choice of the hyperparameters not only plays an essential role in determining the performance of the model, but the CNNs under exam are indistinguishable in terms of performance. We believe that this is an interesting observation that should further stress the importance of the tuning of the hyperparameters.

Focusing on the optimizers, AdaGrad produces the best performance with $LR = 10^{-3}$ and, under this aspect, it behaves differently with respect to the other optimizers under analysis. Conversely, Adam, Adamax, and Nadam obtained the best performance on the considered CNNs when $LR = 10^{-5}$ (except Adamax on the DenseNet architecture, where the best performance is obtained with $LR = 10^{-4}$).

Globally, the best result on the considered dataset was achieved by Adamax optimizer and DenseNet network. Anyway, the differences in terms of performance among the best configurations of each network, are not statistically significant. Overall, every optimizer behaved differently according to the particular architecture. For instance, for the deep architectures like ResNet, AdaGrad outperformed Adam and Adamax. For the shallow architectures like VGG16, AdaMax and NAG had the same performance. Given a specific network, each optimizer requires a different amount of time for converging (i.e., concluding ten epochs). In particular, RMSProp was the fastest optimizer, whereas training a CNN with AdaGrad resulted in the slowest training process. This result is coherent with respect to the one discussed proposed by Dogo et al. [13], in which the authors investigated the effect of different optimizers in terms of required time to reach. More in detail, training the VGG16 architecture requires a minimum of 90 min (RMSProp optimizer and learning rate of 10^{-3}) and a maximum of nine hours (AdaGrad optimizer and learning rate of 10^{-5}). InceptionV3 requires approximately one hour more than VGG16; in this case, the use of RMSProp (with a learning rate of 10^{-3}) resulted in the fastest training process (approximately 150 min), while the use of AdaGrad (with a learning rate of 10^{-5}) required approximately 10 h to finish. An identical pattern was observed for ResNet and DenseNet, that are requiring approximately two hours more than VGG16 for concluding the training process.

Finally, it is important to compare the results achieved with transfer learning against the ones obtained with CNNs that were specifically built for classifying the images of the PatchCamelyon dataset. The winner of the Kaggle competition obtained an AUC of 1, while the second-best performing network obtained an AUC of 0.98. On the other hand, the best performing network obtained with transfer learning (DenseNet architecture, with Adamax optimizer, and a learning rate of 10^{-4}) was able to obtain an AUC of 0.95. This result confirms the suitability of transfer learning for the task at hand. More in detail, we believe that, by considering deeper architectures and more epochs, it could be possible to improve the results of this study, thus equaling the performance achieved by the winner of the Kaggle competition. On the other hand, we highlight a fundamental difference between the best performance reported in the present study and the best performance of the Kaggle competition: The former was obtained using an existing network (used for addressing different computer vision tasks) and by fine-tuning it, while the latter was achieved by designing an ad hoc CNN, a time-consuming task that requires some expertise.

6. Conclusions

CNN represents an analysis of images created using current computation techniques. This is mostly due to their ability to obtain a performance that is similar to, or better than, the one achieved by human beings. Nevertheless, similarly to other deep learning models, training a CNN is a task that usually requires a vast amount of images. This is an essential limitation in all the domains, like the medical one, in which data are scarce and difficult to obtain. In such a situation, transfer learning may provide a viable option. The idea of transfer learning is to use a model trained over thousands of observations (i.e., images in this study) to provide an initial architecture and set of weights for addressing a similar problem over a different domain. Motivated by the success of transfer learning in the analysis of medical images, and for further studying this promising research area, this paper compared the performance optimizers used in popular CNNs for the classification of histopathology images. In particular, four network architectures were used in the evaluation process. These networks were trained on the ImageNet dataset, which consists of millions of images, and their weights were fine-tuned to suit the considered histopathology images dataset. The results obtained from the experimental phase, in which different combinations of network, optimizer, and learning rate were considered, corroborated the initial hypothesis on the importance of the optimizer and the learning rate. While the choice of CNN is essential, it is clear that by fixing the value of the learning rate, the results obtained using different optimizers could be significantly different. On the other hand, once a particular optimizer is selected, the choice of the learning rate plays an essential role in determining the final performance of CNNs.

Interestingly, for each of the different CNNs under exam, it is possible to notice that the best performing configuration of optimizer and learning rate produces an AUC that is approximately 94%. This result strengthens the importance of selecting the hyperparameters of the network, and, in a future investigation, we will extend this work to include additional hyperparameters and datasets aiming at providing formal guidelines for medical experts that want to use CNN models to support their daily work.

Author Contributions: Conceptualization, I.K. and M.C.; methodology, I.K.; software, I.K.; validation, I.K., M.C.; formal analysis, I.K.; investigation, I.K., M.C.; resources, M.C.; data curation, I.K.; writing—original draft preparation, I.K.; writing—review and editing, I.K. and M.C; visualization, I.K.; supervision, M.C. and A.P.; project administration, M.C. and A.P.; funding acquisition, M.C. and A.P. All authors have read and agreed to the published version of the manuscript.

References

1. Jukić, D.M.; Drogowski, L.M.; Martina, J.; Parwani, A.V. Clinical examination and validation of primary diagnosis in anatomic pathology using whole slide digital images. *Arch. Pathol. Lab. Med.* **2011**, *135*, 372–378. [CrossRef] [PubMed]
2. Fukushima, K. Neocognitron: A self-organizing neural network model for a mechanism of pattern recognition unaffected by shift in position. *Biol. Cybern.* **1980**, *36*, 193–202. [CrossRef] [PubMed]
3. Tajbakhsh, N.; Shin, J.Y.; Gurudu, S.R.; Hurst, R.T.; Kendall, C.B.; Gotway, M.B.; Liang, J. Convolutional

Neural Networks for Medical Image Analysis: Full Training or Fine Tuning? *IEEE Trans. Med Imaging* **2016**, *35*, 1299–1312. [CrossRef] [PubMed]

4. Fuentes, A.; Yoon, S.; Kim, S.C.; Park, D.S. A Robust Deep-Learning-Based Detector for Real-Time Tomato Plant Diseases and Pests Recognition. *Sensors* **2017**, *17*, 2022. [CrossRef] [PubMed]
5. Mohanty, S.P.; Hughes, D.P.; Salathé, M. Using Deep Learning for Image-Based Plant Disease Detection. *Front. Plant Sci.* **2016**, *7*, 1419. [CrossRef] [PubMed]
6. Singh, A.K.; Ganapathysubramanian, B.; Sarkar, S.; Singh, A. Deep Learning for Plant Stress Phenotyping: Trends and Future Perspectives. *Trends Plant Sci.* **2018**, *23*, 883–898. [CrossRef] [PubMed]
7. John, V.; Yoneda, K.; Qi, B.; Liu, Z.; Mita, S. Traffic light recognition in varying illumination using deep learning and saliency map. In *17th International IEEE Conference on Intelligent Transportation Systems (ITSC)*; Institute of Electrical and Electronics Engineers (IEEE): Piscataway, NJ, USA, 2014; pp. 2286–2291. [CrossRef]
8. Tae-Hyun, H.; In-Hak, J.; Seong-Ik, C. *Detection of Traffic Lights for Vision-Based Car Navigation System BT-Advances in Image and Video Technology*; Springer: Berlin/Heidelberg, Germany, 2006; pp. 682–691.
9. Krizhevsky, A.; Sutskever, I.; Hinton, G.E. ImageNet Classification with Deep Convolutional Neural Networks. *Neural Inf. Process. Syst.* **2012**, *25*. [CrossRef]
10. Simonyan, K.; Zisserman, A. Very Deep Convolutional Networks for Large-Scale Image Recognition. *arXiv* **2014**, arXiv:1409.1556.
11. He, K.; Zhang, X.; Ren, S.; Sun, J. Deep Residual Learning for Image Recognition. In *2016 IEEE Conference on Computer Vision and Pattern Recognition (CVPR)*; Institute of Electrical and Electronics Engineers (IEEE): Piscataway, NJ, USA, 2016; pp. 770–778. [CrossRef]
12. Szegedy, C.; Vanhoucke, V.; Ioffe, S.; Shlens, J.; Wojna, Z. Rethinking the Inception Architecture for Computer Vision. In *IEEE Conference on Computer Vision and Pattern Recognition (CVPR)*; Institute of Electrical and Electronics Engineers (IEEE): Piscataway, NJ, USA, 2016; pp. 2818–2826. [CrossRef]
13. Dogo, E.M.; Afolabi, O.J.; Nwulu, N.I.; Twala, B.; Aigbavboa, C.O. Aigbavboa, A Comparative Analysis of Gradient Descent-Based Optimization Algorithms on Convolutional Neural Networks. In Proceedings of the 2018 International Conference on Computational Techniques, Electronics and Mechanical Systems (CTEMS), Belgaum, India, 21–22 December 2018.
14. Prilianti, K.R.; Brotosudarmo, T.H.P.; Anam, S.; Suryanto, A. *Performance Comparison of the Convolutional Neural Network Optimizer for Photosynthetic Pigments Prediction on Plant Digital Image*; AIP Publishing: University Park, MA, USA, 2019.
15. LeCun, Y.; Bottou, L.; Bengio, Y.; Haffner, P. Gradient-based learning applied to document recognition. In Proceedings of the IEEE; IEEE: Piscataway, NJ, USA, 1998; Volume 86, pp. 2278–2324. [CrossRef]
16. Jangid, M.; Srivastava, S. Deep ConvNet with different stochastic optimizations for handwritten devanagari character. In Proceedings of the IC4S 2017, Patong Phuket, Thailand, 11–12 October 2017; Volume 1, pp. 51–60.
17. Swastika, W.; Ariyanto, M.F.; Setiawan, H.; Irawan, P.L.T. Appropriate CNN Architecture and Optimizer for Vehicle Type Classification System on the Toll Road. *J. Phys. Conf. Ser.* **2019**, *1196*, 012044. [CrossRef]
18. Bejnordi, B.E.; Veta, M.; Van Diest, P.J.; Van Ginneken, B.; Karssemeijer, N.; Litjens, G.; Van Der Laak, J.A.W.M.; The CAMELYON16 Consortium; Hermsen, M.; Manson, Q.F.; et al. Diagnostic Assessment of Deep Learning Algorithms for Detection of Lymph Node Metastases in Women With Breast Cancer. *JAMA* **2017**, *318*, 2199–2210. [CrossRef] [PubMed]
19. Veeling, B.S.; Linmans, J.; Winkens, J.; Cohen, T.; Welling, M. *Rotation Equivariant CNNs for Digital Pathology BT-Medical Image Computing and Computer Assisted Intervention–MICCAI 2018*; Springer: Berlin/Heidelberg, Germany, 2018; pp. 210–218.
20. Kaggle. PatchCamelyon. Available online: https://www.kaggle.com/c/histopathologic-cancer-detection/data (accessed on 1 September 2020).
21. Scherer, D.; Müller, A.; Behnke, S. Evaluation of Pooling Operations in Convolutional Architectures for Object Recognition. *Computer Vision* **2010**, *6354*, 92–101.
22. Duchi, J.C.; Hazan, E.; Singer, Y. Adaptive Subgradient Methods for Online Learning and Stochastic Optimization. *J. Mach. Learn. Res.* **2011**, *12*, 2121–2159.
23. Hinton, G.; Srivastava, N.; Swersky, K. Neural Networks for Machine Learning, Lecture 6a Overview of Mini-Batch Gradient Descent. Available online: http://www.cs.toronto.edu/-hinton/coursera/lecture6/lec6.pdf (accessed on 24 August 2020).

24. Kingma, D.; Ba, J. Adam: A Method for Stochastic Optimization. Available online: https://arxiv.org/abs/1412.6980 (accessed on 22 August 2020).
25. Dozat, T. Incorporating Nesterov Momentum into Adam. In Proceedings of the 4th International Conference on Learning Representations, Workshop Track, San Juan, Puerto Rico, 2–4 May 2016.
26. SPan, S.J.; Yang, Q. A Survey on Transfer Learning. *IEEE Trans. Knowl. Data Eng.* **2009**, *22*, 1345–1359. [CrossRef]
27. Xie, M.; Jean, N.; Burke, M.; Lobell, D.; Ermon, S. Transfer learning from deep features for remote sensing and poverty mapping. In Proceedings of the 30th AAAI Conference on Artificial Intelligence, AAAI 2016, Phoenix, AZ, USA, 12–17 February 2016; pp. 3929–3935.
28. Szegedy, C.; Liu, W.; Jia, Y.; Sermanet, P.; Reed, S.; Anguelov, D.; Erhan, D.; Vanhoucke, V.; Rabinovich, A. Going deeper with convolutions. In Proceedings of the 2015 IEEE Conference on Computer Vision and Pattern Recognition (CVPR), Boston, MA, USA, 7–12 June 2015; pp. 1–9. [CrossRef]
29. Huang, G.; Liu, Z.; Van Der Maaten, L.; Weinberger, K.Q. Densely Connected Convolutional Networks. In Proceedings of the 2017 IEEE Conference on Computer Vision and Pattern Recognition (CVPR), Honolulu, HI, USA, 21–26 July 2017; pp. 2261–2269. [CrossRef]
30. Srivastava, N.; Hinton, G.; Krizhevsky, A.; Sutskever, I.; Salakhutdinov, R. Dropout: A Simple Way to Prevent Neural Networks from Overfitting. *J. Mach. Learn. Res.* **2014**, *15*, 1929–1958.
31. Fawcett, T. ROC Graphs: Notes and Practical Considerations for Data Mining Researchers. Available online: https://www.hpl.hp.com/techreports/2003/HPL-2003-4.pdf (accessed on 27 August 2020).
32. Vuk, M. ROC Curve, Lift Chart and Calibration Plot. *Comput. Sci.* **2006**, *3*, 89–108.

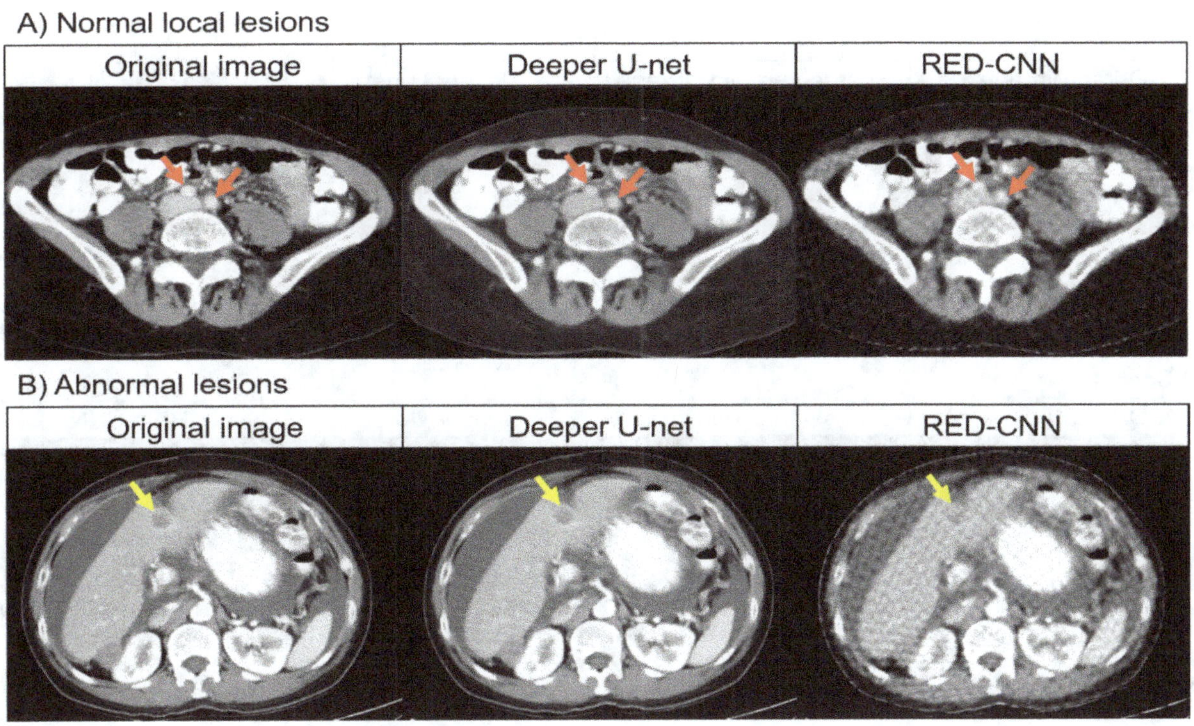

Figure 2. Representative images of the original CT and denoised CT obtained using deeper U-net and RED-CNN. Note: (**A**) Visual scores of common iliac artery (red arrow): 5 points for deeper U-net, 2 points for RED-CNN for reader 1; 4 points for deeper U-net, 2 points for RED-CNN for reader 2. (**B**) Visual scores of liver metastasis (yellow arrow): 3 points for deeper U-net, 2 points for RED-CNN for reader 1; 4 points for deeper U-net, 2 points for RED-CNN for reader 2. Abbreviation: RED-CNN, Residual Encoder-Decoder Convolutional Neural Network.

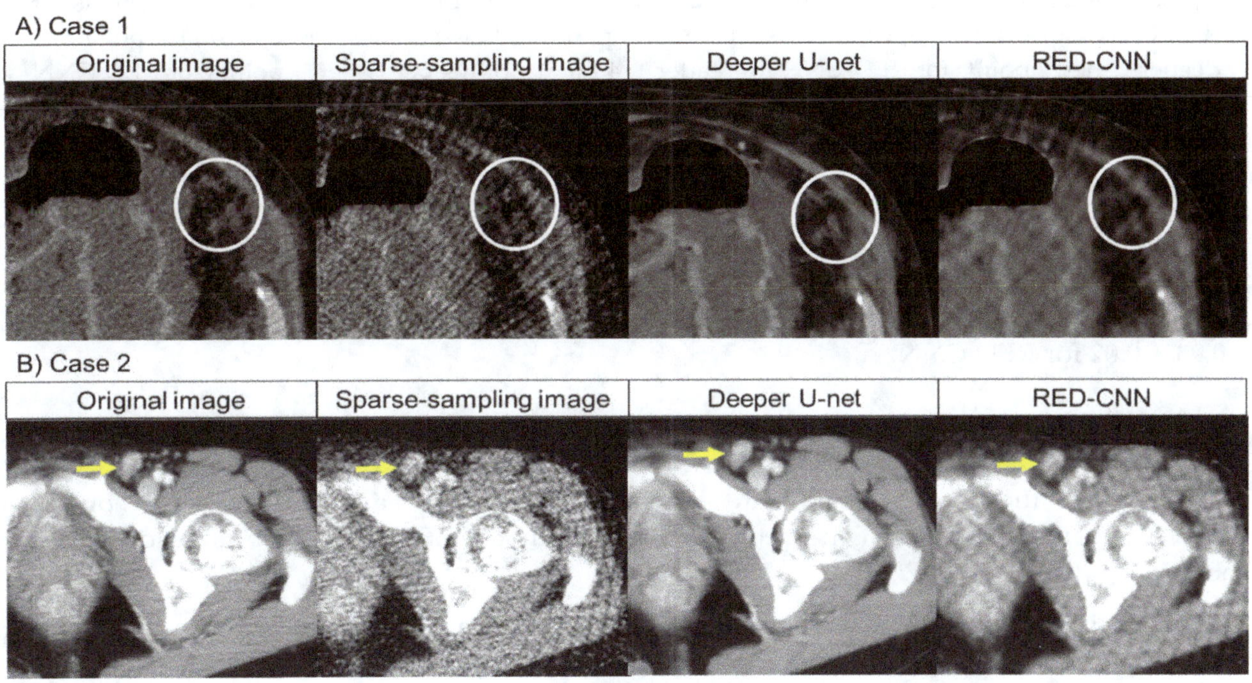

Figure 3. *Cont.*

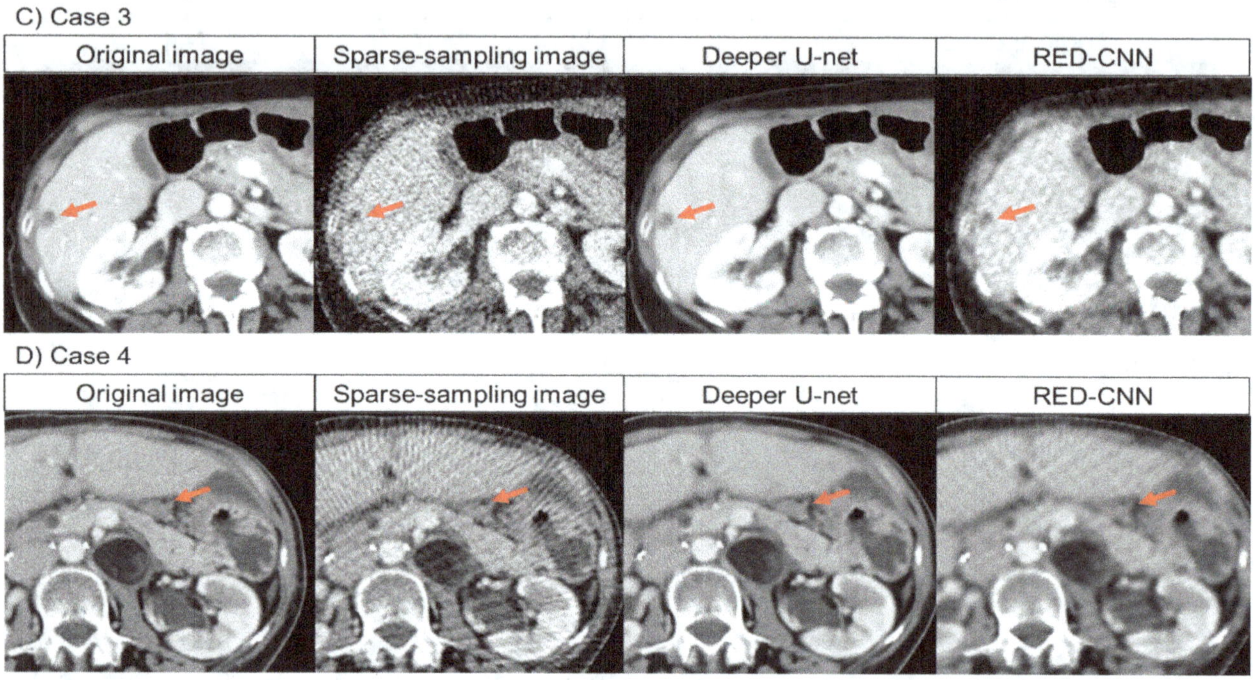

Figure 3. Representative images of the original CT, sparse-sampling CT before denoising, and denoised CT obtained using deeper U-net and RED-CNN. Note: (**A**) Case 1: Visual scores of peritoneal dissemination (white circle): 4 points for deeper U-net, 1 points for RED-CNN for reader 1; 4 points for deeper U-net, 1 points for RED-CNN for reader 2. (**B**) Case 2: Visual scores of lymph node metastasis (yellow arrow): 5 points for deeper U-net, 2 points for RED-CNN for reader 1; 4 points for deeper U-net, 2 points for RED-CNN for reader 2. (**C**) Case 3: Visual scores of liver metastasis (red arrow): 4 points for deeper U-net, 2 points for RED-CNN for reader 1; 4 points for deeper U-net, 2 points for RED-CNN for reader 2. (**D**) Case 4: Visual scores of peritoneal dissemination (red arrow): 4 points for deeper U-net, 2 points for RED-CNN for reader 1; 4 points for deeper U-net, 1 points for RED-CNN for reader 2.

3.1. *Quantitative Image Analysis*

We evaluate the PSNR and SSIM on the 4667 CT images from 50 test cases. The number of samples for calculating PSNR and SSIM was 4667. The PSNR and SSIM were 29.2 ± 1.49 and 0.75 ± 0.04 for the sparse-sampling images before denoising, 48.5 ± 2.69 and 0.99 ± 0.01 for deeper U-net, and 37.3 ± 1.97 and 0.93 ± 0.02 for RED-CNN.

3.2. *Qualitative Image Analysis*

The results of the visual evaluation are shown in Figures 4 and 5 and Tables 5 and 6. For all items of the visual evaluation, deeper U-net scored better than that of RED-CNN for both readers as shown in Table 7.

Streak artifacts tended to be stronger on images at the upper abdomen level, especially where the lung and abdominal organs were visualized on the same image.

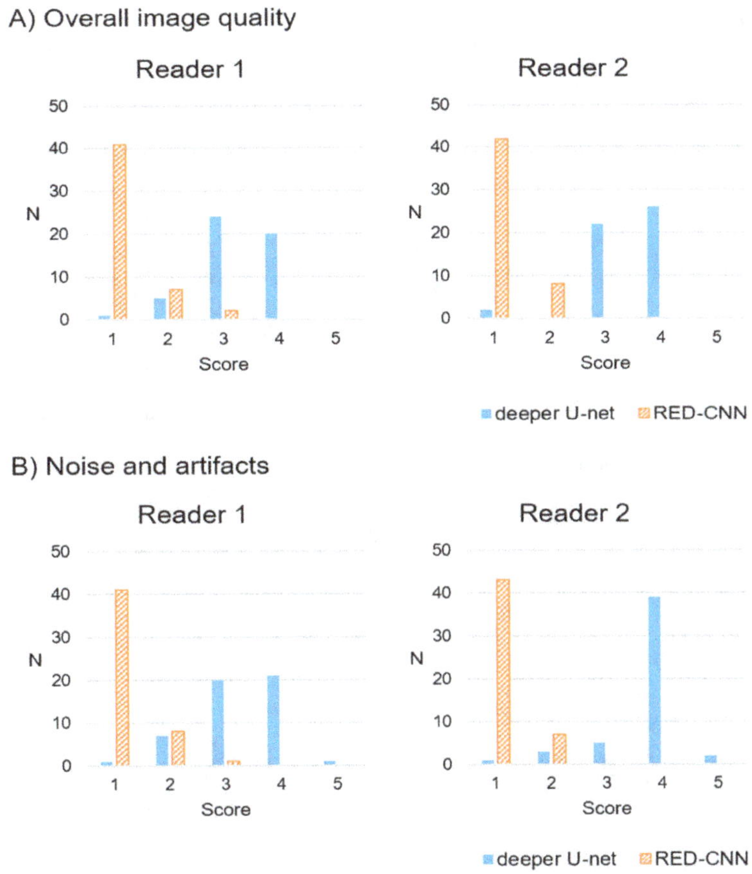

Figure 4. Visual evaluation of entire CT image quality by the two readers using different deep learning algorithms.

Table 5. Visual evaluation of entire CT image quality by the two readers using different deep learning algorithms.

(A) Overall Image Quality					
	Reader 1			Reader 2	
score	Deeper U-net	RED-CNN	score	Deeper U-net	RED-CNN
1	1	41	1	2	42
2	5	7	2	0	8
3	24	2	3	22	0
4	20	0	4	26	0
5	0	0	5	0	0
(B) Noise and Artifacts					
	Reader 1			Reader 2	
score	Deeper U-net	RED-CNN	score	Deeper U-net	RED-CNN
1	1	41	1	1	43
2	7	8	2	3	7
3	20	1	3	5	0
4	21	0	4	39	0
5	1	0	5	2	0

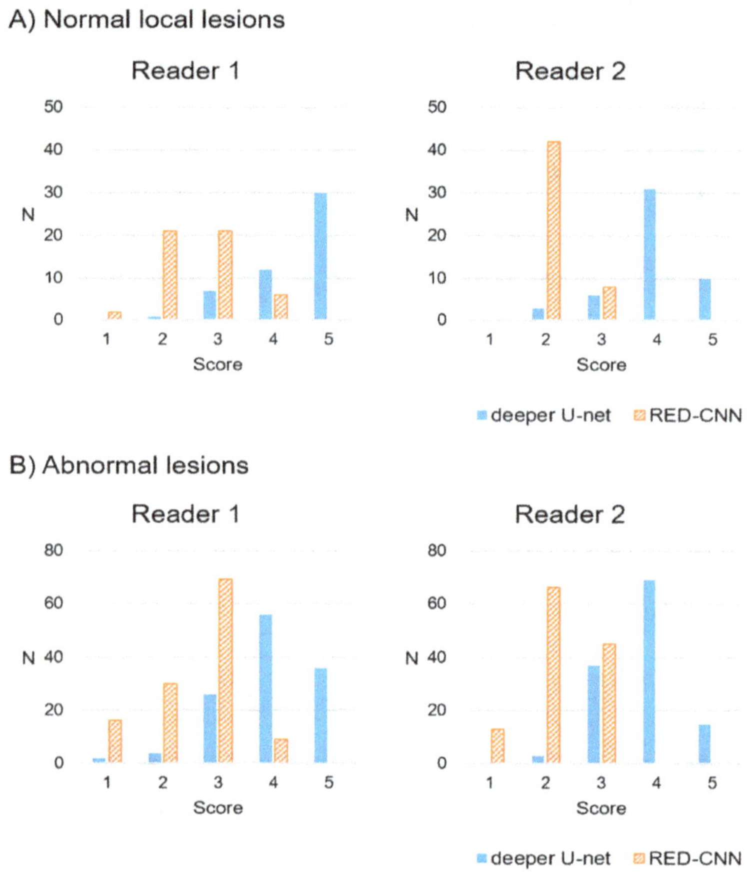

Figure 5. Visual evaluation of normal local lesions and abnormal lesions by the two readers using different deep learning algorithms.

Table 6. Visual evaluation of normal local lesions and abnormal lesions by the two readers using different deep learning algorithms.

(A) Normal Local Lesions					
	Reader 1			Reader 2	
score	Deeper U-net	RED-CNN	score	Deeper U-net	RED-CNN
1	0	2	1	0	0
2	1	21	2	3	42
3	7	21	3	6	8
4	12	6	4	31	0
5	30	0	5	10	0
(B) Abnormal Lesions					
	Reader 1			Reader 2	
score	Deeper U-net	RED-CNN	score	Deeper U-net	RED-CNN
1	2	16	1	13	0
2	6	30	2	66	5
3	26	69	3	44	35
4	56	9	4	0	68
5	34	0	5	0	15

Table 7. Results of visual evaluations by the two readers using different deep learning algorithms.

		Deeper U-net	RED-CNN	*p*
Entire CT image quality				
(A) Overall image quality	Reader 1	median, 3; IQR, 3 to 4	median, 1; IQR, 1 to 1	<0.0001
	Reader 2	median, 4; IQR, 3 to 4	median, 1; IQR, 1 to 1	<0.0001
(B) Noise and artifacts	Reader 1	median, 3; IQR, 3 to 4	median, 1; IQR, 1 to 1	<0.0001
	Reader 2	median, 4; IQR, 4 to 4	median, 1; IQR, 1 to 1	<0.0001
Normal local lesions	Reader 1	median, 5; IQR, 4 to 5	median, 3; IQR, 2 to 3	<0.0001
	Reader 2	median, 4; IQR, 4 to 4	median, 2; IQR, 2 to 2	<0.0001
Abnormal lesions	Reader 1	median, 4; IQR, 3 to 5	median, 3; IQR, 2 to 3	<0.0001
	Reader 2	median, 4; IQR, 3 to 4	median, 2; IQR, 2 to 3	<0.0001

Abbreviation: IQR, interquartile range; RED-CNN, Residual Encoder-Decoder Convolutional Neural Network.

The detectability of abnormal lesions with deeper U-net was significantly better than that with RED-CNN: 95.2% (118/124) vs. 62.9% (78/124) ($p < 0.0001$) for reader 1 and 97.6% (121/124) vs. 36.3% (45/124) ($p < 0.0001$) for reader 2. The number of FN with deeper U-net were six and three for readers 1 and 2, respectively. All these abnormal lesions were non-measurable peritoneal dissemination, which were identified as slight subtle soft-tissue infiltration and reticulonodular lesions on the original CT image. The representative images of the FN case are shown in Figure 6.

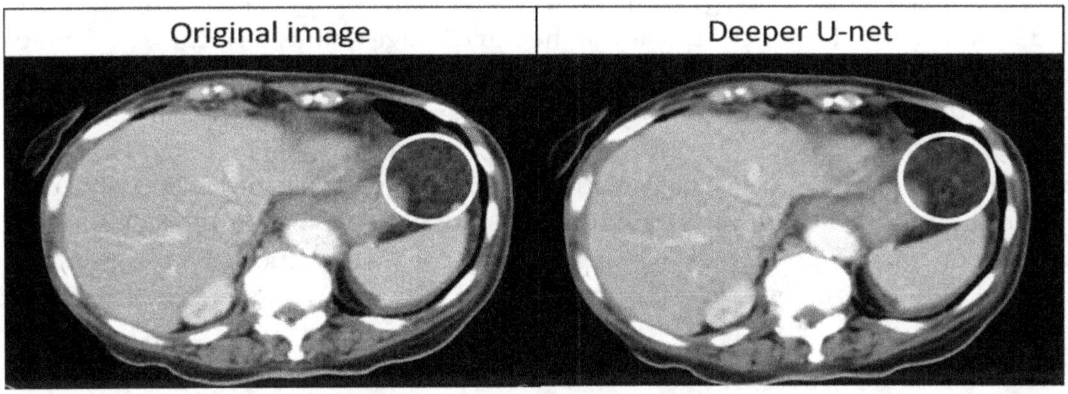

Figure 6. A representative undiagnosable lesion on denoised CT image with deeper U-net. Note: The circle shows non-measurable peritoneal dissemination. With deeper U-net, the score was 1 point for reader 1 and 2 points for reader 2.

4. Discussion

In the current study, we compared the quantitative and qualitative image quality of sparse-sampling CT denoised with deeper U-net and RED-CNN. RED-CNN was compared with our deeper U-net because of its similar network structure [7]. For quantitative analysis, mean scores of PSNR and SSIM of CT image quality with deeper U-net were better than those with RED-CNN. For all of the visual evaluation items, the scores of CT image quality with deeper U-net were significantly better than those of RED-CNN. In addition, the detectability of ovarian cancer metastasis was more than 95% in deeper U-net.

A few studies on deep learning-based reconstruction have shown that it improved image quality and reduced noise and artifacts better than hybrid IR and MBIR [8,16,28]. Nakamura et al. reported that deep learning reconstruction could reduce noise and artifacts more than hybrid IR could and that it may improve the detection of low-contrast lesions when evaluating hypovascular hepatic metastases [16]. While their study did not evaluate low-dose CT, the deep learning model is also considered an effective method with the potential to use lower-dose CT techniques such as sparse sampling with clinically acceptable results [5]. Our results showed that denoising with deeper U-net could be used to detect ovarian cancer metastasis.

To the best of our knowledge, this was the first study that evaluated the detectability of cancer metastasis, including peritoneal dissemination, liver metastasis, and lymph node metastasis on deep learning-based reconstructed CT images. The usefulness of sparse-sampling CT with deep learning has been previously reported [6,7,9,10], but image evaluation was limited to quantitative measures in most of these studies. While Nakai et al. reported on quantitative and qualitative assessments of the efficacy of deep learning on chest CT images [6], our study evaluated the usefulness of sparse-sampling CT denoised with deep learning techniques from the clinical viewpoint. We have proven that deeper U-net has an excellent ability to improve image quality and detectability of metastasis, and it could prove effective in clinical practice.

The performance difference between deeper U-net and RED-CNN was significant when assessing sparse-sampling CT images. A strong streak artifact around bony structures affected the image quality of sparse-sampling CT [29]. Therefore, to improve the image quality of sparse-sampling CT, an ideal deep learning model should reduce streak artifact associated with anatomical structures. RED-CNN used an image patch (size 55×55 pixels) for its training, therefore the algorithm had difficulty discerning between a streak artifact and anatomical structures. As a result, reducing the streak artifact related to anatomical structure may be limited in RED-CNN. In contrast, since deeper U-net used the entire CT image (size 512×512 pixels) for training, deeper U-net could be optimized to reduce streak artifact related to anatomical structures. This difference between the two deep learning models may lead to performance differences shown in the current study.

Since score 5 was defined as image quality and visualization equivalent to original CT (Tables 1–3), the denoised CT images of deeper U-net was not the same image quality as original CT images from the viewpoint of score. However, the visual scores and detectability of deeper U-net were sufficiently high.

Although patients with peritoneal dissemination are diagnosed as advanced stage, complete debulking surgery can be expected to improve the prognosis in epithelial malignant ovarian tumor [30]. In addition, there are some histological types with a favorable prognosis due to successful chemotherapy, such as yolk sac tumor [31]. Thus, the reduction of CT-radiation exposure is essential for patients with ovarian cancer. With our proposed method, theoretically, the CT radiation exposure can be reduced to one-tenth of that of the original CT. The reduction of radiation exposure may reduce the incidence of radiation-induced cancer. Furthermore, while we evaluated about only the detection of metastasis of malignant ovarian tumors in the current study, we speculate that the proposed method may be applied to other diseases.

While our results show that deeper U-net proved useful in detecting cancer metastasis, there were several drawbacks in the model. First, fine anatomical structures were obscured due to excessive denoising. This effect might be minimized by blending images of FBP and deep learning-based reconstruction, such as hybrid IR and MBIR, by adjusting radiation exposure (rate of sparse sampling) and blending rate. Secondly, the strong streak artifacts around the prosthesis and the upper abdomen compromised diagnostic ability near these anatomical lesions. Furthermore, streak artifacts tended to be stronger on images at the upper abdomen level, especially where the lung and abdominal organs were visualized on the same image. This effect may have resulted from the relatively small number of training data images that included both lung and abdominal organs compared to images that included only abdominal organs. Since ovarian cancer primarily metastasizes to the peritoneal liver surface and the liver, improving the image quality in these areas is considered a future research area. Increasing the number of training data images with cross-sections displaying both the lung and abdominal organs may help improve image quality and reduce streak artifacts in deep learning models, including deeper U-net.

Our study had several limitations. First, we used images from only one public database. The application of our deep learning model should be further evaluated in other databases. Second, sparse-sampling images cannot be obtained from real CT scanners at the current time. Our simulated subsampled images may differ from the images on real scanners. In future, we need to evaluate the performance of our deeper U-net using real CT acquisitions. Third, images obtained with the deep learning model of GAN tended to be more "natural" than those obtained with conventional deep learning model. However, the noise reduction of GAN is weaker than that of a conventional deep learning model [17]. There was a concern that the radiologist's ability to detect metastasis might decline if the noise reduction was insufficient. Therefore, GAN was not used in the current study. Finally, because of our study design, we did not evaluate false positives, true negatives, and specificity in the current study. Therefore, it is necessary to conduct radiologists' observer studies in which false positives and true negatives are evaluated.

5. Conclusions

Sparse-sampling CT with deep learning reconstruction could prove useful in detecting metastasis of malignant ovarian tumors and might contribute to reducing CT radiation exposure. With our proposed method, theoretically, the CT radiation exposure can be reduced to one-tenth of that of the original CT, while keeping the detectability of ovarian cancer metastasis more than 95%. It may reduce the incidence of radiation-induced cancer.

Author Contributions: Conceptualization, M.N. (Mizuho Nishio); methodology, M.N. (Mizuho Nishio); software, M.N. (Mizuho Nishio); validation, M.N. (Mizuho Nishio), Y.U. (Yasuyo Urase); formal analysis, Y.U. (Yasuyo Urase), M.N. (Mizuho Nishio); investigation, Y.U. (Yasuyo Urase), M.N. (Mizuho Nishio), Y.U. (Yoshiko Ueno), A.K.K.; resources, M.N. (Mizuho Nishio); data curation, M.N. (Mizuho Nishio); writing—original draft preparation, Y.U. (Yasuyo Urase); writing—review and editing, Y.U. (Yasuyo Urase), M.N. (Mizuho Nishio), Y.U. (Yoshiko Ueno), A.K.K., K.S., T.K., T.M. (Takaki Maeda), M.N. (Munenobu Nogami), M.H., T.M. (Takamichi Murakami); visualization, Y.U. (Yasuyo Urase), and M.N. (Mizuho Nishio); supervision, T.M. (Takamichi Murakami); project administration, M.N. (Mizuho Nishio); funding acquisition, M.N. (Mizuho Nishio). All authors have read and agreed to the published version of the manuscript.

Acknowledgments: The authors would like to thank Izumi Imaoka from department of Radiology, Kobe Minimally invasive Cancer Center for her suggestion about defining metastatic lesions of ovarian cancer.

Appendix A. Network Structure of Deeper U-Net

The network structure of our deeper U-net is slightly modified from original deeper U-net [6]. The differences between the two networks were as follows:

1. The numbers of maxpooling and upsampling were 9 in our deeper U-net.
2. The numbers of feature maps in the first convolution layer of our U-net was 104. After the maxpooling layer, the number of feature maps in the convolution layer was doubled. However, if the numbers of feature maps were 832, the number of feature maps was not increased even after the maxpooling layer.
3. Rectified Linear Unit (ReLU) was used, instead of Leaky ReLU.
4. Probability of Dropout was changed. 0.2% was used in our deeper U-net.

Appendix B. Detail Procedure of Qualitative Evaluation by Radiologists

The detail procedure of qualitative evaluation was as follows. Two board-certified radiologists (17 and 10 years of experience, respectively) independently performed the visual evaluation as readers. The patient IDs of TCGA-OV in 50 test cases were sorted in alphabetical and numerical order, and the two radiologists interpreted the CT images in this order. All the 50 sets of denoised CT images with deeper U-net were evaluated first, then followed by those with RED-CNN. Image quality evaluation of the entire CT and the local normal lesions were performed by comparing the original image and the denoised image on 3D Slicer (version 4.10.2, https://www.slicer.org/) [24], and then the abnormal lesions were evaluated. Two other board-certified radiologists (6 and 14 years of experience, respectively) determined the abnormal lesions on the original image by consensus, and recorded the locations of the abnormal lesions on a file. In evaluating the abnormal lesions, the two readers referred to the file for the locations of abnormal lesions. At the time of interpretation, the two readers were informed of patient's age, and blind to all other clinical data. The image quality differed greatly between the two models, therefore the readers could easily determine the deep learning model with which the given CT images were denoised. Therefore, the interpretation order of the denoised images with deeper U-net and RED-CNN was not randomized. It was presumed that bias in evaluation of denoised CT images was inevitable even if interpretation order of deeper U-net and RED-CNN was randomized or the evaluations of CT images denoised with the two models were performed separately at long interval.

References

1. Ferlay, J.; Colombet, M.; Soerjomataram, I.; Mathers, C.; Parkin, D.M.; Piñeros, M.; Znaor, A.; Bray, F. Estimating the global cancer incidence and mortality in 2018: GLOBOCAN sources and methods. *Int. J. Cancer* **2019**, *144*, 1941–1953. [CrossRef]
2. Heints, A.; Odicino, F.; Maisonneuve, P.; Qiomm, M.A.; Benedet, J.L.; Creasman, W.T.; Ngan, H.Y.S.; Pecorelli, S.; Beller, U. Carcinoma of the ovary. *Int. J. Gynecol. Obstet.* **2006**, *95*, s161–s192. [CrossRef]
3. Webb, P.M.; Jordan, S.J. Epidemiology of epithelial ovarian cancer. *Best Pract. Res. Clin. Obstet. Gynaecol.* **2017**, *41*, 3–14. [CrossRef]
4. Shao, Y.-H.; Tsai, K.; Kim, S.; Wu, Y.-J.; Demissie, K. Exposure to Tomographic Scans and Cancer Risks. *JNCI Cancer Spectr.* **2019**, *4*, pkz072. [CrossRef] [PubMed]
5. Willemink, M.J.; Noël, P.B. The evolution of image reconstruction for CT—From filtered back projection to artificial intelligence. *Eur. Radiol.* **2019**, *29*, 2185–2195. [CrossRef] [PubMed]
6. Nakai, H.; Nishio, M.; Yamashita, R.; Ono, A.; Nakao, K.K.; Fujimoto, K.; Togashi, K. Quantitative and Qualitative Evaluation of Convolutional Neural Networks with a Deeper U-Net for Sparse-View Computed Tomography Reconstruction. *Acad. Radiol.* **2019**, *27*, 563–574. [CrossRef] [PubMed]
7. Chen, H.; Zhang, Y.; Kalra, M.K.; Lin, F.; Chen, Y.; Liao, P.; Member, S.; Wang, G. Low-Dose CT with a Residual Encoder-Decoder Convolutional Neural Network (RED-CNN). *IEEE Trans. Med. Imaging* **2017**, *36*, 2524–2534. [CrossRef]
8. Tatsugami, F.; Higaki, T.; Nakamura, Y.; Yu, Z.; Zhou, J.; Lu, Y.; Fujioka, C.; Kitagawa, T.; Kihara, Y.; Iida, M.; et al. Deep learning–based image restoration algorithm for coronary CT angiography. *Eur. Radiol.* **2019**, *29*, 5322–5329. [CrossRef]
9. Jin, K.H.; McCann, M.T.; Froustey, E.; Unser, M. Deep Convolutional Neural Network for Inverse Problems in Imaging. *IEEE Trans. Image Process.* **2017**, *26*, 4509–4522. [CrossRef]
10. Han, Y.; Ye, J.C. Framing U-Net via Deep Convolutional Framelets: Application to Sparse-View CT. *IEEE Trans. Med. Imaging* **2018**, *37*, 1418–1429. [CrossRef]
11. Nishio, M.; Nagashima, C.; Hirabayashi, S.; Ohnishi, A.; Sasaki, K.; Sagawa, T.; Hamada, M.; Yamashita, T. Convolutional auto-encoders for image denoising of ultra-low-dose CT. *Heliyon* **2017**, *3*, e00393. [CrossRef]
12. Kang, E.; Koo, H.J.; Yang, D.H.; Seo, J.B.; Ye, J.C. Cycle-consistent adversarial denoising network for multiphase coronary CT angiography. *Med. Phys.* **2019**, *46*, 550–562. [CrossRef]
13. Wolterink, J.M.; Leiner, T.; Viergever, M.A.; Išgum, I. Generative adversarial networks for noise reduction in low-dose CT. *IEEE Trans. Med. Imaging* **2017**, *36*, 2536–2545. [CrossRef] [PubMed]
14. Kang, E.; Min, J.; Ye, J.C. A deep convolutional neural network using directional wavelets for low-dose X-ray CT reconstruction. *Med. Phys.* **2017**, *44*, e360–e375. [CrossRef]
15. Mookiah, M.R.K.; Subburaj, K.; Mei, K.; Kopp, F.K.; Kaesmacher, J.; Jungmann, P.M.; Foehr, P.; Noel, P.B.; Kirschke, J.S.; Baum, T. Multidetector Computed Tomography Imaging: Effect of Sparse Sampling and Iterative Reconstruction on Trabecular Bone Microstructure. *J. Comput. Assist. Tomogr.* **2018**, *42*, 441–447. [CrossRef] [PubMed]
16. Nakamura, Y.; Higaki, T.; Tatsugami, F.; Zhou, J.; Yu, Z.; Akino, N.; Ito, Y.; Iida, M.; Awai, K. Deep Learning–based CT Image Reconstruction: Initial Evaluation Targeting Hypovascular Hepatic Metastases. *Radiol. Artif. Intell.* **2019**, *1*, e180011. [CrossRef]
17. Blau, Y.; Michaeli, T.; Israel, T. The Perception-Distortion Tradeoff Yochai. *Proc. IEEE Conf. Comput. Vis. Pattern Recognit.* **2018**, 6228–6237. [CrossRef]

18. Clark, K.; Vendt, B.; Smith, K.; Freymann, J.; Kirby, J.; Koppel, P.; Moore, S.; Phillips, S.; Maffitt, D.; Pringle, M.; et al. The cancer imaging archive (TCIA): Maintaining and operating a public information repository. *J. Digit. Imaging* **2013**, *26*, 1045–1057. [CrossRef]
19. TCGA-OV. Available online: http://doi.org/10.7937/K9/TCIA.2016.NDO1MDFQ (accessed on 20 December 2019).
20. TCGA Attribution. Available online: http://cancergenome.nih.gov/ (accessed on 20 December 2019).
21. Van Aarle, W.; Palenstijn, W.J.; Cant, J.; Janssens, E.; Bleichrodt, F.; Dabravolski, A.; De Beenhouwer, J.; Joost Batenburg, K.; Sijbers, J. Fast and flexible X-ray tomography using the ASTRA toolbox. *Opt. Express* **2016**, *24*, 25129. [CrossRef]
22. Van Aarle, W.; Palenstijn, W.J.; De Beenhouwer, J.; Altantzis, T.; Bals, S.; Batenburg, K.J.; Sijbers, J. The ASTRA Toolbox: A platform for advanced algorithm development in electron tomography. *Ultramicroscopy* **2015**, *157*, 35–47. [CrossRef]
23. Wang, Z.; Bovik, C.; Sheikh, H.R.; Simoncelli, E.P. Image Quality Assessment: From Error Visibility to Structural Similarity. *IEEE Trans. Image Process.* **2004**, *13*, 600–612. [CrossRef] [PubMed]
24. Fedorov, A.; Beichel, R.; Kalpathy-Cramer, J.; Finet, J.; Fillion-Robin, J.-C.; Pujol, S.; Jennings, D.; Bauer, C.; Sonka, M.; Fennessy, F. 3D Slicer as an Image Computing Platform for the Quantitative Imaging Network. *Magn. Reson. Imaging* **2012**, *30*, 1323–1341. [CrossRef]
25. Nougaret, S.; Addley, H.C.; Colombo, P.E.; Fujii, S.; Al Sharif, S.S.; Tirumani, S.H.; Jardon, K.; Sala, E.; Reinhold, C. Ovarian carcinomatosis: How the radiologist can help plan the surgical approach. *Radiographics* **2012**, *32*, 1775–1800. [CrossRef] [PubMed]
26. Eisenhauer, E.A.; Therasse, P.; Bogaerts, J.; Schwartz, L.H.; Sargent, D.; Ford, R.; Dancey, J.; Arbuck, S.; Gwyther, S.; Mooney, M.; et al. New response evaluation criteria in solid tumours: Revised RECIST guideline (version 1.1). *Eur. J. Cancer* **2009**, *45*, 228–247. [CrossRef] [PubMed]
27. Mutch, D.G.; Prat, J. 2014 FIGO staging for ovarian, fallopian tube and peritoneal cancer. *Gynecol. Oncol.* **2014**, *133*, 401–404. [CrossRef]
28. Akagi, M.; Nakamura, Y.; Higaki, T.; Narita, K.; Honda, Y.; Zhou, J.; Yu, Z.; Akino, N.; Awai, K. Deep learning reconstruction improves image quality of abdominal ultra-high-resolution CT. *Eur. Radiol.* **2019**, *29*, 6163–6171. [CrossRef]
29. Jin, S.O.; Kim, J.G.; Lee, S.Y.; Kwon, O.K. Bone-induced streak artifact suppression in sparse-view CT image reconstruction. *Biomed. Eng. Online* **2012**, *11*, 1–13. [CrossRef]
30. Du Bois, A.; Reuss, A.; Pujade-Lauraine, E.; Harter, P.; Ray-Coquard, I.; Pfisterer, J. Role of surgical outcome as prognostic factor in advanced epithelial ovarian cancer: A combined exploratory analysis of 3 prospectively randomized phase 3 multicenter trials: By the arbeitsgemeinschaft gynaekologische onkologie studiengruppe ovarialkarzin. *Cancer* **2009**, *115*, 1234–1244. [CrossRef]
31. Faure Conter, C.; Xia, C.; Gershenson, D.; Hurteau, J.; Covens, A.; Pashankar, F.; Krailo, M.; Billmire, D.; Patte, C.; Fresneau, B.; et al. Ovarian yolk sac tumors; does age matter? *Int. J. Gynecol. Cancer* **2018**, *28*, 77–84. [CrossRef]

8

Detection of HER2 from Haematoxylin-Eosin Slides through a Cascade of Deep Learning Classifiers via Multi-Instance Learning

David La Barbera [1], António Polónia [2,3], Kevin Roitero [1], Eduardo Conde-Sousa [3,4] and Vincenzo Della Mea [1,*]

1 Department of Mathematics, Computer Science and Physics, University of Udine, 33100 Udine, Italy; labarbera.david@spes.uniud.it (D.L.B.); roitero.kevin@spes.uniud.it (K.R.)

2 Department of Pathology, Ipatimup Diagnostics, Institute of Molecular Pathology and Immunology, University of Porto, 4169-007 Porto, Portugal; apolonia@ipatimup.pt

3 i3S—Instituto de Investigação e Inovação em Saúde, Universidade do Porto, 4169-007 Porto, Portugal; econdesousa@gmail.com

4 INEB—Instituto de Engenharia Biomédica, Universidade do Porto, 4169-007 Porto, Portugal

* Correspondence: vincenzo.dellamea@uniud.it

Abstract: Breast cancer is the most frequently diagnosed cancer in woman. The correct identification of the HER2 receptor is a matter of major importance when dealing with breast cancer: an over-expression of HER2 is associated with aggressive clinical behaviour; moreover, HER2 targeted therapy results in a significant improvement in the overall survival rate. In this work, we employ a pipeline based on a cascade of deep neural network classifiers and multi-instance learning to detect the presence of HER2 from Haematoxylin–Eosin slides, which partly mimics the pathologist's behaviour by first recognizing cancer and then evaluating HER2. Our results show that the proposed system presents a good overall effectiveness. Furthermore, the system design is prone to further improvements that can be easily deployed in order to increase the effectiveness score.

Keywords: digital pathology; whole slide image processing; multiple instance learning; convolutional neural networks; deep learning classification; HER2

---

1. Introduction

Breast cancer is the most frequently diagnosed cancer in women. As shown by Siegel et al. [1], breast cancer in 2020 is expected to account for 30% of female cancer in United States. The diagnosis of breast cancer, including its morphological subtypes, is that was carried out by a pathologist by examining a microscope histologic slide obtained from a breast biopsy or from a surgical sample. The slide is stained with a two-colors staining, called Haematoxylin-Eosin (HE), which enables the recognition of morphological features of the cancer. Haematoxylin-Eosin (HE) is universally used for histologic diagnosis. In addition to that, further sections are prepared and stained with immunohistochemical techniques (IHC) to evidentiate the expression of specific proteins. In the case of breast cancer, routine examination includes oestrogen and progesterone receptors, MIB2, and HER2. Visually, HE-stained slides show blue (for nuclei) and pink (for cytoplasm), while IHC slides are brown where the investigated protein is expressed, and counterstained in blue by means of haematoxylin.

According to current guidelines of the College of American Pathologists for HER2 testing in breast cancer [2], Human Epidermal growth factor Receptor 2 (HER2) quantification must be routinely tested, in invasive breast cancer, recurrences, and metastases. HER2 is a trans-membrane protein receptor with tyrosine kinase activity; studies have shown that HER2 is amplified and/or over-expressed in about 25% of breast cancer cases [3]. The over-expression and/or amplification of the HER2 receptor have been associated with aggressive clinical behaviour; nevertheless, the accurate assessment of the HER2 receptor has proven to be essential for identifying breast cancer patients who will benefit from HER2-targeted therapy [4]. It has been demonstrated by many clinical trials that the HER2-targeted therapy (both when administrated during and/or after chemotherapy) results in a significant improvement in both disease-free and overall survival in patients who have shown either an amplification or over-expression of the HER2 receptor [4]. Consequently, the correct identification of the HER2 receptor lead to select patients who are expected to benefit from the targeted therapy; this makes HER2 a helpful marker for the therapy decision making process.

Many researchers tried to develop IHC techniques that are able to identify HER2 with a sufficient precision and therefore be able to help the pathologist with the characterization of breast cancer [5–13]. The current approach to HER2 testing consists in cutting an additional section for the IHC evaluation of the positivity, negativity, or uncertain status of HER2 expression. In uncertain cases, a further examination has to be done based on In-Situ Hybridization, increasing costs and time. This, in addition to the HE stained slide, which is always prepared because needed for morphological diagnosis of cancer and of its subtypes. In the context of digital pathology, there is an increasing interest in developing Deep Learning (DL) techniques that can support the decision making process of the pathologist, especially when dealing with cancer related topics [10]. The practical use of deep learning in the context of breast cancer diseases is mainly due the performance achieved by deep learning algorithms over the last decade in the field of image recognition [14–16].

The recent HEROHE challenge proposed a peculiar research question: is it possible to identify HER2 from Hematoxylin–Eosin images of invasive breast cancer? In case of success, this would allow obtaining HER2 status without the corresponding IHC image, thus reducing time and costs. In fact, it is known that HER2 positivity is associated with aggressiveness of the tumour, which, in turn, is associated with certain morphological features, such as high histological grade. Thus, the idea is to exploit such morphological features as a proxy for HER2 status. For this, the Challenge organizers provided a set of 400 digitized haematoxylin-eosin slides accompanied by their HER2 status, and subsequently 150 slides for testing.

The objective of our study is the same behind the HEROHE challenge: to find a method to recognize the therapeutically useful HER2 status from the morphological aspects of the breast cancer only, as recognisable in the HE slides that are already used for diagnosis.

More in detail, our approach is based on deep learning algorithms employed in the setting of image recognition and Multiple Instance Learning (MIL) [17–21].

Digitized microscope slides, normally called digital slides or Whole Slide Images (WSI), correspond to huge scanned images that are difficult to process with standard Machine Learning (ML) or Deep Learning (DL) approaches due to hardware limitations [22]. A technique that is used to overcome such limitations is represented by MIL [23,24]. Opposed to the classical ML and DL classification setting where the learning algorithm receives in input a set of individually labelled instances, in MIL the learning algorithm receives a set of labelled instances (in our case, each instance is a WSI), each of these containing many unlabelled instances (in our case, the WSI is divided into tiles). Subsequently, the final class for the instance (i.e., the WSI) is decided upon the predicted classes of the unlabelled instances (i.e., the tiles). For example, in the simplest case, the main instance may be labelled as negative if all its unlabelled instances in it are labelled as negative negative [25].

We now detail some work related to the work of this paper.

MIL has been proven to be effective in the setting of image recognition and, in particular, in the context of cancer detection: Campanella et al. [26] used MIL to tackle the problem of prostate cancer detection, basal cell carcinoma, and breast cancer metastases to axillary lymph nodes. Their approach resulted in areas under the ROC curve (AUC) above 0.98 for the cancer types considered in the study.

MIL has also been used in the setting of breast cancer image detection. P J et al. [27] conducted experiments on a public dataset of biopsy images of benign and malignant breast cancers; according to their findings, MIL provides better results than state-of-the-art approaches in the setting of the detection of breast cancer in images. A more relevant work to our setting is the study conducted by Couture et al. [28], which investigated a method to predict cancer subtypes from histologic images. Couture et al. used MIL to model the problem and account for intra-cancer variations in cancer subtypes, improving the correct classification of cancer subtypes with reference to the state of the art approaches, and providing also insights about cancer heterogeneity.

Other researchers tried to detect HER2 from HER2 stained digital slides, using ML or not ML methods [29–34]; we do not detail their methodology, since they are out of scope for this work.

Thus, our specific contribution is a pipeline based on a cascade of deep neural network classifiers and multi-instance learning, which partly mimics the pathologist' behaviour by first recognizing cancer and then evaluating HER2, and able to currently provide state-of-the-art performance for the novel problem of detecting HER2 from Haematoxylin–Eosin slides.

2. Materials and Methods

2.1. Dataset and Materials

In our study, we used the dataset made available from the Instituto de Investigação and Inovação em Saúde and Instituto de Engenharia de Sistemas e Computadores, Tecnologia e Ciência from Porto University in Porto, Portugal, who together organized the HEROHE Grand Challenge for ECDP2020 (see https://ecdp2020.grand-challenge.org). The classification of this dataset used the latest American Society of Clinical Oncology/College of American Pathologists (ASCO/CAP) classification of breast cancer (Focused Update 2018) [2]. The HEROHE training dataset is composed of 144 positive slides (i.e., WSI of cases which are labelled as HER2 positive) and 216 negative slides (i.e., WSI of cases that are labelled as HER2 negative). Figure 1 shows an example of positive and negative slides present in the dataset.

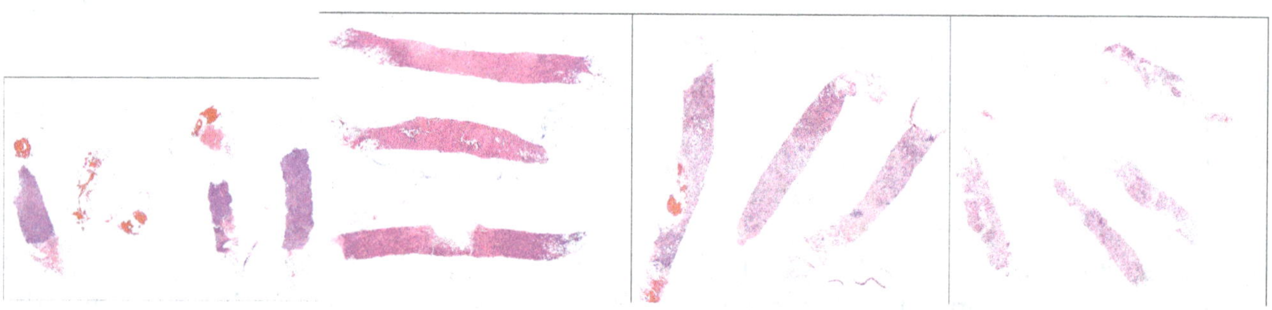

A B C D

Figure 1. Example of tiles from the HEROHE dataset. The left-most two slides (**A**,**B**) have been labelled as positive for HER2; The right-most two slides (**C**,**D**) have been labelled as negative.

After implementing the proposed solution (as detailed in the next section), we tested it on the HEROHE Grand Challenge test set that is composed of 60 positive and 90 negative slides. The training, validation, and testing phase has been carried out using either a Titan XP GPU or using the Google Cloud Platform. The proposed solution has been implemented on the fast.ai Framework. Due to the nature of the data used in this study, we cannot publicly release the images used to train our algorithms. However, we release all of the code used to conduct the experiments as well as the trained models (Supplementary Materials).

2.2. Our Approach: A Cascade of Deep Learning Classifiers

The idea behind this work is to build a system that mimics the actions a pathologist performs when detecting the presence of the HER2 receptor. The actions include to divide each slide into tiles under the "divide et impera" principle, filter the tiles in order to keep only the most informative ones for the purpose of HER2 detection (i.e., only the tiles containing cancer), check for the presence of

HER2 into the individual tiles, and finally aggregate the tile information at the slide level to perform the decision whether the whole slide expresses or not the HER2 receptor.

To this aim, we developed a multi-stage pipeline as graphically represented in Figure 2. We considered a multi-stage system because this architectural design allowed us to try different techniques (or different variants of a single technique) for each stage, and then deploy to the final version of the system using only the most effective combination of stages. Furthermore, a multi-stage pipeline is the ideal scenario to test different approaches and compare single techniques at different levels of the pipeline. The pipeline we implemented is composed, as follows: the first stage extracts the tiles (Section 2.2.1), second stage considers either all tiles (Section 2.2.2), or a subset of them (Section 2.2.3), third stage details the main classifier architecture (Section 2.2.4), fourth stage formalize the features considered (Section 2.2.5), and fifth stage consider the post-training aggregation by means of either majority voting (Section 2.2.6) or a Tabular learner (Section 2.2.7). In the following sections, we discuss the role of each stage in detail.

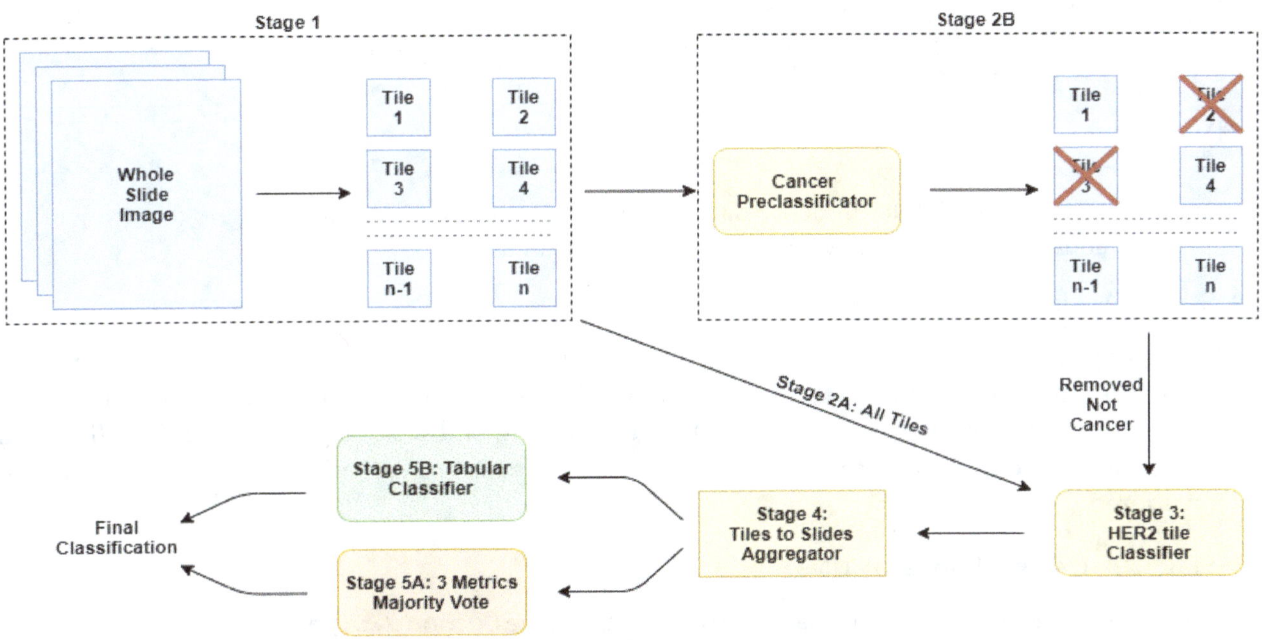

Figure 2. Graphical overview of the multi-stage deep learning pipeline.

2.2.1. Stage 1: The Tiles Extractor

The first stage of our pipeline is devoted to extract the tiles from every WSI present in the dataset. We consider each tile to be an instance necessary? (using the DL nomenclature) of our problem formulation. Slides provided by the HEROHE challenge were scanned at 40× magnification (which corresponds to a pixel size of 0.25 μm/pixel), with a 3DHistech Pannoramic 1000 scanner, and stored in their proprietary format. For the present work, slides were subsampled to 20× magnification (which has proven to reduce the computational complexity, but not decrease the overall accuracy with reference to the 40× magnification [26]) and converted to TIFF format. Therefore, the pixel size of the used slides corresponds to 0.50 μm/pixel.

After such process, each slide is then decomposed into squares (i.e., the tiles) of 512 × 512 pixels, with no stride. Figure 3 shows an example of the decomposition of two slides into tiles. Note that the slides in the dataset might have different dimensions, thus each of them is decomposed in a variable number of tiles.

Subsequently, in order to increase the overall accuracy model and preserve salient features [35], we dropped the tiles that have an average grey-scale value (i.e., the pixel value that represents the brightness of the pixel; the lower the value, the darker the pixel) greater than 0.8. This allows to discard background slides, including those presenting very small amounts of tissue.

After this stage, we considered two different approaches: the former consists in passing forward to the next stage all of the tiles; the latter in considering only an informative subset of tiles. Such approaches are detailed respectively in Sections 2.2.2 and 2.2.3.

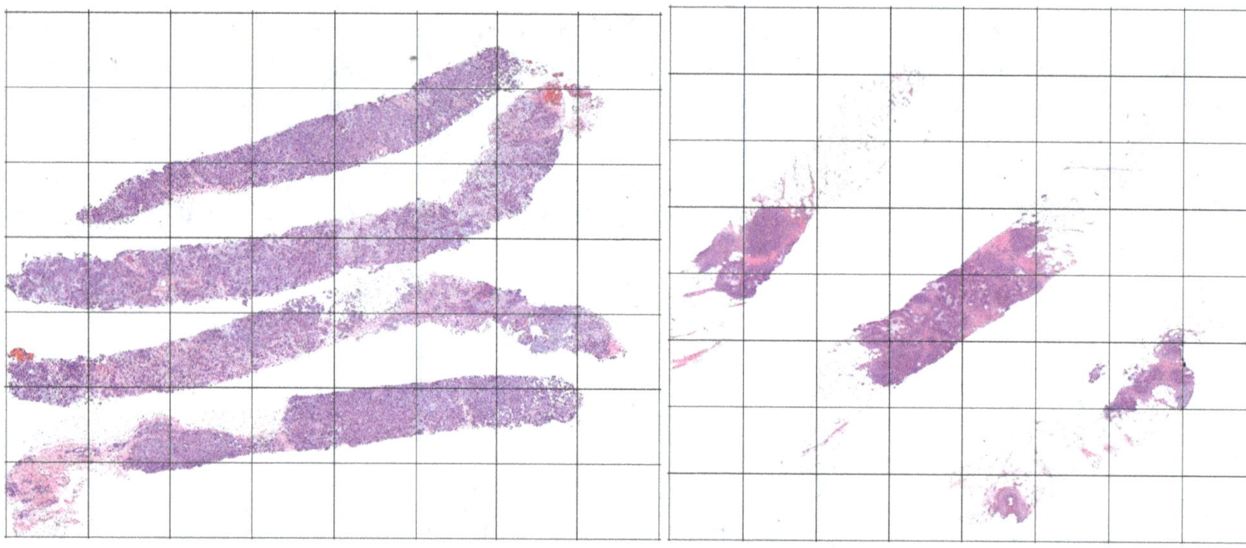

Figure 3. An example of slides from our dataset in which we applied a rectangular grid (shown with the continuous black lines) to show the division of a slide in tiles.

2.2.2. Stage 2A: Using All the Tiles

This stage simply consists in keeping all the tiles, without discarding any, and forwarding them without any modification to the next stage. The rationale behind this stage is that by maintaining all of the tiles we do not discard any potentially useful information, and we delegate to (the classifier of) the next stages the task to discern between relevant and not relevant information (i.e., noise) for all of the tiles considered.

2.2.3. Stage 2B: Using a Subset of Tiles

This stage takes in input all of the tiles from Stage 1 (see Section 2.2.1) and filters them, under the rationale that a subset of tiles is more informative for the model than the whole set of (potentially noisy) tiles. Moreover, this process simulates the real case scenario; in fact, when looking for the presence of HER2 in slides, the pathologist focus the search only in the part of slides (similar to our tiles) containing cancer, and more specifically in the tiles containing invasive cancer. One additional reason is that HER2 might also be expressed outside the cancer tissue, in normal ducts, or as extracellular accumulation, or also as staining artifacts. While we might expect that DL is able to cope with these situations too, we did not want to expose the network to spurious data, or at least to reduce the amount of noise. We perform a pre-classification task, with the purpose of discerning between the tiles that contain cancer and those that do not, in order to filter the input tiles. To this aim, we developed a model based on a Convolutional Neural Network (CNN), relying on the model detailed by Della Mea and Pilutti [36], which is based on the `densenet-201` architecture [37–39] pretrained on the `ImageNet` dataset [40]. However, the HEROHE data set did not include annotations for identifying cancer areas inside the slides, which may as well contain normal tissue or tissue representing other not tumoral diseases. Thus, although not optimal, we had to exploit a different set of training images. For this aim, we fine-tuned the model on 400 images from the BACH Challenge Part A (see https://iciar2018-challenge.grand-challenge.org/) [41] dataset. These images are 2048 × 1536; by means of SlideJ [42] we extracted tiles of 512 × 512 size, with a stride of 256, obtaining 35 tiles per image. Thus, we trained for three epochs to fine-tune the last layer, plus three epochs for the whole network. We applied the default fast.ai data augmentation transforms, including random mixtures of flips, rotations, moderate zoom (up to 1.1 ×), warping, luminosity, and contrast variations. We collapsed the original labels (i.e., "normal", "benign", "in situ carcinoma", and "invasive carcinoma", 100 images for each class, corresponding to 3500 tiles) into two binary categories, as follows: we mapped the original labels "normal" and "benign" into the label "no cancer", and the labels "in situ carcinoma" and "invasive carcinoma" into the label "cancer". Note that we also consider tiles that contain in-situ cancer because, at high resolution, it would be impossible to distinguish them from the ones with invasive cancer.

After the training phase, we fed all of the tiles considered in this work to the fine-tuned classifier, and we removed the tiles classified as not containing cancer. Overall, we fed the model with 90.068 test tiles, and we removed 29.429 tiles (32.68%), maintaining 60.639 (67.32%). On average, we removed the 29.27% of tiles from each slide; more in detail, on average, we removed 32.02% of tiles from negative slides and 25.16% from positive slides. Figure 4 shows an example of the classification outcome in term of slides.

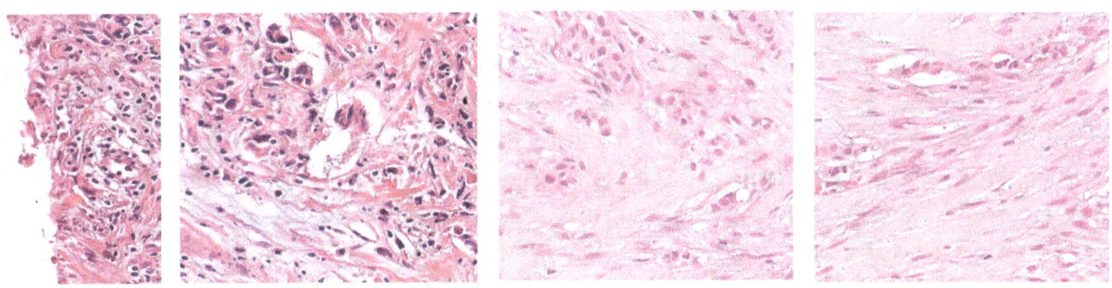

A B C D

Figure 4. Tiles identified by the cancer classifier as: positive (first two tiles, tile (**A**) is a true positive, tile (**B**) is a false positive), and negative (last two tiles, tile (**C**) is a true negative, tile (**D**) is a false negative).

2.2.4. Stage 3: The Main Classifier

After the second stage, we trained the main classifier, either with all tiles (from stage 2A) or with the subset of tiles labelled as containing cancer (from stage 2B). Our main architecture is as follows. We trained a classifier based on the `ResNet152` architecture [43], a well-known architecture for image recognition [43–46] based on the concept of residual learning [43]. Figure 5 provides a schema of the model architecture and the block for residual learning. We fed the classifier each tile with the associated HER2 status. We did not expect to obtain high accuracy, because in a positive slide HER2 is not expressed everywhere; on the other side, in a negative slide, we expect HER2 not to be expressed, although it is known that it could also be present in normal tissue, which is one reason why we wanted to discard not cancer tiles. We trained the classifier using the HEROHE training set for three epochs while using precision as loss function. For data augmentation, we applied the same transforms as the first classifier. Learning rate has been set according the One-cycle policy developed by L.Smith [47].

Figure 6 shows an example of the classification outcome in terms of tiles.

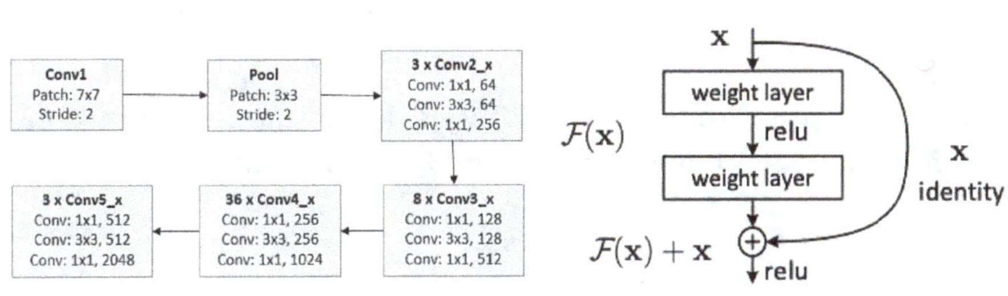

Figure 5. The basic architecture of Resnet152 (**left**, from [48]), and the building block for the residual learning (**right**, from [43]).

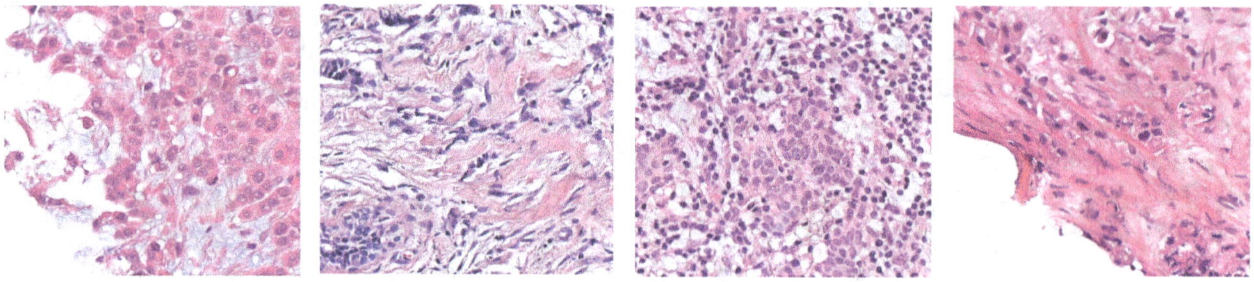

A B C D

Figure 6. Tiles identified by the HER2 classifier as positive (first two tiles, tile (**A**) is a true positive, tile (**B**) is a false positive), and negative (last two tiles, tile (**C**) is a true negative, and tile (**D**) is a false negative).

2.2.5. Stage 4: Computing the Features

The classifier detailed in the previous stage returns as output, for each test instance, the probability that the test instance belongs to a given class, for all of the classes. In our setting, the classifier returns a probability value in the $[0,1]$ range that denotes the probability of each tile in be positive for the HER2 receptor. Those are the probabilities we will consider in this section. After training our main classifier to determine for each tile its probability of containing the HER2 receptor, we aggregated the results at the tile level to determine the overall classification outcome, which correspond to assess whether the whole slide contains or not the HER2 receptor. To this aim, we used two strategies detailed in the following, which take advantage of the features described in this section.

Suppose that we have $\mathcal{S}$ slides, and that each slide is divided into $\mathcal{T}$ tiles. We denote with p_i^j is the probability of the i-th tile (belonging to the j-th slide) to be tested positive for HER2.

Subsequently, in the first case we compute the binary positivity $P_1(s_i)$ of the slide s_i by considering the simple arithmetic average of the probabilities p_i^j for all of the tiles; formally:

$$P_1(s_i) = \begin{cases} 1 & \text{if } \frac{1}{\mathcal{T}} \sum_{i=1}^{\mathcal{T}} p_i^j \geq 0.5, \\ 0 & \text{otherwise.} \end{cases}$$

In the second case, we compute the binary positivity $P_2(s_i)$ of the slide s_i by considering the simple arithmetic average of the probabilities p_i^j for tiles having probability $p_i^j \geq 0.5$.; formally:

$$P_2(s_i) = \begin{cases} 1 & \text{if } \frac{1}{\mathcal{T}} \sum_{i=1}^{\mathcal{T}} p_i^j \cdot G(p_i^j) \geq 0.66, \\ 0 & \text{otherwise,} \end{cases}$$

where

$$G(p_i^j) = \begin{cases} 1 & \text{if } p_i^j \geq 0.5, \\ 0 & \text{otherwise.} \end{cases}$$

In the third case, we compute the binary positivity $P_3(s_i)$ of the slide s_i by considering the slide positive if at least the 35% of its tiles have a probability $p_i^j \geq 0.5$; formally:

$$P_3(s_i) = \begin{cases} 1 & \text{if } \frac{1}{\mathcal{T}} \sum_{i=1}^{\mathcal{T}} G(p_i^j) \geq 0.35, \\ 0 & \text{otherwise.} \end{cases}$$

Apart from the three positivity indices $P_1(s_i)$, $P_2(s_i)$, and $P_3(s_i)$ of each slide, we consider, as additional set of features, the frequency of the probabilities p_i^j for each slide, for each interval $[h, h+0.1)$, $h \in \{0.5, 0.6, 0.7, 0.8, 0.9\}$; formally,

$$F_h(s_i) = \frac{1}{\mathcal{T}} \sum_{i=1}^{\mathcal{T}} C(p_i^j, h),$$

where

$$C(p_i^j, h) = \begin{cases} 1 & \text{if } p_i^j \in [h, h+0.1), \\ 0 & \text{otherwise.} \end{cases}$$

After computing the positivity indices $P_1(s_i)$, $P_2(s_i)$, and $P_3(s_i)$, and the set of features $F_h(s_i)$, $h \in \{0.5, 0.6, 0.7, 0.8, 0.9\}$, we aggregate such indices to compute the overall positivity of the i-th slide. To do so, we adopt two strategies, detailed in the following.

2.2.6. Stage 5A: Post-Trainer Aggregation Using Majority Vote

The first strategy we adopt to compute the overall positivity of each slide is to simply compute the majority vote of the $P_1(s_i)$, $P_2(s_i)$, and $P_3(s_i)$ indices. In this way, we assume that all of the features are equally informative for the final decision.

2.2.7. Stage 5B: Post-Trainer Aggregation Using a Tabular Learner

The second strategy we adopt to the overall positivity of each slide consists in train a classifier to learn the best weights for the indices. More in detail, in this phase, we use the $P_1(s_i)$ probabilities not binarized, denoted as $P_1^*(s_i)$ (i.e., $\frac{1}{\mathcal{T}} \sum_{i=1}^{\mathcal{T}} p_i^j$), as well as the set of features $F_h(s_i), h \in \{0.5, 0.6, 0.7, 0.8, 0.9\}$ to build the feature matrix detailed in Table 1. Following this approach, we delegate to the algorithm the task of learning how to combine the features in the best possible way. We trained the Tabular learning while using an architecture with three layers composed by respectively 500, 250, and 125 fully connected layers, and we used accuracy as loss function. We did some experiments to include all the $P_1(s_i)$, $P_2(s_i)$, and $P_3(s_i)$ indices in the feature matrix, but we found that the additional indices did not provide a significant increase in the effectiveness scores.

Table 1. Training matrix for the Tabular Learner. $P_1^*(s_i)$ represents the non binarized $P_1(s_i)$ probability. $P(s_i)$ represents the true positivity for the i-th tile (used only for the training phase).

	P_1^*	$F_{0.5}$	$F_{0.6}$	$F_{0.7}$	$F_{0.8}$	$F_{0.9}$	P
s_1	$P_1^*(s_1)$	$F_{0.5}(s_1)$	$F_{0.6}(s_1)$	$F_{0.7}(s_1)$	$F_{0.8}(s_1)$	$F_{0.9}(s_1)$	$P(s_1)$
s_2	$P_1^*(s_2)$	$F_{0.5}(s_2)$	$F_{0.6}(s_2)$	$F_{0.7}(s_2)$	$F_{0.8}(s_2)$	$F_{0.9}(s_2)$	$P(s_2)$
$\vdots$	$\vdots$	$\vdots$	$\vdots$	$\vdots$	$\vdots$	$\vdots$	$\vdots$
s_i	$P_1^*(s_i)$	$F_{0.5}(s_i)$	$F_{0.6}(s_i)$	$F_{0.7}(s_i)$	$F_{0.8}(s_i)$	$F_{0.9}(s_i)$	$P(s_i)$
$\vdots$	$\vdots$	$\vdots$	$\vdots$	$\vdots$	$\vdots$	$\vdots$	$\vdots$
$s_{\mathcal{S}}$	$P_1^*(s_{\mathcal{S}})$	$F_{0.5}(s_{\mathcal{S}})$	$F_{0.6}(s_{\mathcal{S}})$	$F_{0.7}(s_{\mathcal{S}})$	$F_{0.8}(s_{\mathcal{S}})$	$F_{0.9}(s_{\mathcal{S}})$	$P(s_{\mathcal{S}})$

3. Results

Table 2 reports the effectiveness of our approach measured on the HEROHE Grand Challenge test set. To the best of our knowledge, there are no other published results (up to current date) that investigate our same problem or use the same test data as we do. For this reason, Table 2 reports the effectiveness scores of our method and the leaderboard of the HEROHE challenge only. Note that the leaderboard has been chosen by the organising committee of the HEROE challenge on the basis of the F1 score alone.

Table 2. Evaluation metrics for our two approaches and the leaderboard of the HEROHE challenge. In bold we highlight the best result obtained for each evaluation metric.

	All Tiles		Subset of Tiles		Best
	Majority Vote	Tabular Classifier	Majority Vote	Tabular Classifier	HEROHE
Accuracy	0.687	0.673	0.667	**0.707**	-
Precision	0.570	0.560	0.580	**0.603**	0.5682
Recall	**0.883**	0.864	0.783	0.797	0.8333
F1-Score	**0.693**	0.680	0.667	0.687	0.6757

As we can see from the table, if we consider the variants of our approach separately, it is always the case that our system outperforms the leaderboard of the HEROHE challenge, even though different metrics are maximized by different algorithms. The only variant that outperforms the leaderboard of the HEROHE challenge on all the considered metrics is the "All Tiles–Majority Vote" variant.

Turning to compare the different approaches that we propose, we see that it is not always the case that employing the Tabular classifier lead to obtain higher effectiveness scores; more in detail, we see that for precision oriented metrics (i.e., Accuracy and Precision) consider a subset of tiles lead to higher effectiveness scores, and for the metrics affected by recall (i.e., Recall and F1) when considering all of the tiles lead to higher effectiveness scores.

Investigating the most effective approach for each metric separately, we see that our approach leads to obtain an accuracy score of about 0.7 and a precision score of about 0.6, suggesting that our model is able to correctly identify positives in the majority of positive cases. We also see that our model finds almost all positive cases in our dataset (recall of 0.88). When considering the metric used to rank systems in the HEROHE challenge, we see that our model has an F1 score of about 0.7, indicating a good overall balance between precision and recall.

4. Discussion and Conclusions

By looking at the results, we can draw different remarks. First, we see that recall (and F1 as result) is maximized when all the tiles are kept in the dataset; this an expected outcome. It is natural that by keeping all of the tiles (i.e., by keeping more data) we obtain a higher recall score. Nevertheless, this behaviour suggests that, when considering the effectiveness metrics all together, it is not straightforward to choose whether to remove or not a subset of tiles, as some tiles might be more informative than others for some metrics, but not for all of them. Finally, this behaviour can be caused not only by the fact that we keep more data, but also by complex interactions between the classification algorithm and some particular feature of the tile. We plan to address this matter in future work. When considering that our problem is a high recall problem, we can say that the best variant of our approach is the "All Tiles–Majority Vote" one. In other terms, considering our setting we want to find all of the patients that actually are positive for HER2, and we can accept a lower precision if the effort to conduct a clinical test to detect HER2 is not significant, which we believe is a more than reasonable assumption to make: we are willing to spend a little more in clinical testing but be able to save more lives. Summarising the remarks drawn from the results section, we can state that our results indicate that our multi-stage pipeline is indeed effective in detecting HER2. Furthermore, the results indicate that our approach is not over- nor under-dimensioned, given that both the filtering of tiles and the post classifier aggregation done with learners boost the results for some evaluation metric. Finally, we remark that a multi-stage pipeline has the advantage of being easily maintainable, and the accuracy of the single levels can be increased independently.

In this paper, we tackled the problem of classification of the HER2 status on HE slides of invasive breast cancer. Our approach based on a cascade of deep learning classifiers and multi instance learning shows good effectiveness scores for different evaluation metrics. We show that pre-filtering tiles lead to remove potentially noisy tiles and overall leads to an improvement of some effectiveness metrics. We also found that combining different predictors by means of a Tabular classifier is more effective than doing that by the means of a majority voting scores for precision oriented metrics, indicating that, indeed, different predictors need to be weighted and provide signals of different importance for the overall task. However, the overall effectiveness if far from being usable in clinical practice a substitution of the traditional IHC- and ISH-based testing. While this could be due to the intrinsic independency of the information provided by morphology and by HER2 expression, it is also surely conditioned by the relatively low number of slides used for training. In fact, while the overall number of images is high, they correspond to the about 400 cases provided by the Challenge, which are likely too few for Multiple Instance Learning. While no direct comparison is possible about HER2 detection, in other MIL-based related works on digital slides, larger data sets have been used with better results than ours. In particular, in [26] a dataset of about 44,000 slides has been used; although not directly comparable, they reached an AUC of 0.99. In the work of Couture et al. [28] the dataset is closer in size (571 slides) to ours, but also measures of effectiveness, while higher, are not too dissimilar (e.g., 0.80 accuracy for estrogen receptor status, which is a similar but not identical problem as HER2 status). Overall, we think that our work is an important step towards the development of a supervised approach that can serve the purpose of helping medical experts in the delicate task of selecting the appropriate treatment when dealing with clinical cases of breast cancer. For future work, we plan to develop the presented pipeline in order to increase the effectiveness metrics by increasing the impact and the effectiveness of the different stages of the pipeline. One way is to include further case details in the last stage of the pipeline, e.g., the other IHC results, patient data, etc. The other relatively easy enhancement will come from training the cancer classifier on slides acquired with the same setup as the other classifier. In fact, as is the cancer classifier is sub-optimal. In this way, we can provide even more information to the medical experts with the aim of providing a more sound and robust tool that can be practically used in the clinical decision making process.

Author Contributions: (In alphabetical order within each category) Conceptualization, V.D.M., D.L.B., and K.R.; methodology, V.D.M., D.L.B., and K.R.; validation, V.D.M., D.L.B., and K.R.; formal analysis, D.L.B.; investigation, V.D.M., and D.L.B.; resources, V.D.M., A.P. and E.C.-S.; data curation, D.L.B., A.P. and E.C.-S.; writing—original draft preparation, V.D.M., D.L.B., and K.R.; writing—review and editing, V.D.M., D.L.B., K.R., A.P. and E.C.-S.; visualization, D.L.B.; supervision, V.D.M. and K.R.; project administration, V.D.M., A.P. and E.C.-S.; funding acquisition, V.D.M. and A.P. All authors have read and agreed to the published version of the manuscript.

Acknowledgments: The digital slides of breast cancer tissue samples stained with HE were digitized at IPATIMUP Diagnostics, University of Porto, Portugal. We thank Nvidia for providing the GPU used to train the models, and Google for providing the grant consisting in Google Cloud credits used to carry out the experiments detailed in this paper.

Abbreviations

The following abbreviations are used in this manuscript:

CNN	Convolutional Neural Network
DL	Deep Learning
HER2	Human Epidermal growth factor Receptor 2
MIL	Multiple Instance Learning
ML	Machine Learning
WSI	Whole Slide Image

References

1. Siegel, R.L.; Miller, K.D.; Jemal, A. Cancer statistics, 2020. *CA A Cancer J. Clin.* **2020**, *70*, 7–30. [CrossRef] [PubMed]
2. Wolff, A.C.; Hammond, M.E.H.; Allison, K.H.; Harvey, B.E.; Mangu, P.B.; Bartlett, J.M.S.; Bilous, M.; Ellis, I.O.; Fitzgibbons, P.; Hanna, W.; et al. Human Epidermal Growth Factor Receptor 2 Testing in Breast Cancer:

American Society of Clinical Oncology/College of American Pathologists Clinical Practice Guideline Focused Update. *Arch. Pathol. Lab. Med.* **2018**, *142*, 1364–1382. [CrossRef] [PubMed]
3. Dean-Colomb, W.; Esteva, F.J. Her2-positive breast cancer: Herceptin and beyond. *Eur. J. Cancer* **2008**, *44*, 2806–2812. [CrossRef] [PubMed]
4. Nahta, R.; Esteva, F.J. HER-2-Targeted Therapy. *Clin. Cancer Res.* **2003**, *9*, 5078–5084.
5. Gutierrez, C.; Schiff, R. HER2: Biology, detection, and clinical implications. *Arch. Pathol. Lab. Med.* **2011**, *135*, 55–62.
6. Al-Khafaji, Q.; Harris, M.; Tombelli, S.; Laschi, S.; Turner, A.; Mascini, M.; Marrazza, G. An electrochemical immunoassay for HER2 detection. *Electroanalysis* **2012**, *24*, 735–742. [CrossRef]
7. Riethdorf, S.; Müller, V.; Zhang, L.; Rau, T.; Loibl, S.; Komor, M.; Roller, M.; Huober, J.; Fehm, T.; Schrader, I. Detection and HER2 expression of circulating tumor cells: Prospective monitoring in breast cancer patients treated in the neoadjuvant GeparQuattro trial. *Clin. Cancer Res.* **2010**, *16*, 2634–2645. [CrossRef]
8. Gevensleben, H.; Garcia-Murillas, I.; Graeser, M.K.; Schiavon, G.; Osin, P.; Parton, M.; Smith, I.E.; Ashworth, A.; Turner, N.C. Noninvasive detection of HER2 amplification with plasma DNA digital PCR. *Clin. Cancer Res.* **2013**, *19*, 3276–3284. [CrossRef]
9. Gohring, J.T.; Dale, P.S.; Fan, X. Detection of HER2 breast cancer biomarker using the opto-fluidic ring resonator biosensor. *Sens. Actuators B Chem.* **2010**, *146*, 226–230. [CrossRef]
10. Vandenberghe, M.E.; Scott, M.L.; Scorer, P.W.; Söderberg, M.; Balcerzak, D.; Barker, C. Relevance of deep learning to facilitate the diagnosis of HER2 status in breast cancer. *Sci. Rep.* **2017**, *7*, 45938. [CrossRef]
11. Yaziji, H.; Goldstein, L.C.; Barry, T.S.; Werling, R.; Hwang, H.; Ellis, G.K.; Gralow, J.R.; Livingston, R.B.; Gown, A.M. HER-2 testing in breast cancer using parallel tissue-based methods. *JAMA* **2004**, *291*, 1972–1977. [CrossRef] [PubMed]
12. Basavanhally, A.N.; Ganesan, S.; Agner, S.; Monaco, J.P.; Feldman, M.D.; Tomaszewski, J.E.; Bhanot, G.; Madabhushi, A. Computerized image-based detection and grading of lymphocytic infiltration in HER2+ breast cancer histopathology. *IEEE Trans. Biomed. Eng.* **2009**, *57*, 642–653. [CrossRef] [PubMed]
13. Cruz-Roa, A.; Gilmore, H.; Basavanhally, A.; Feldman, M.; Ganesan, S.; Shih, N.N.; Tomaszewski, J.; González, F.A.; Madabhushi, A. Accurate and reproducible invasive breast cancer detection in whole-slide images: A Deep Learning approach for quantifying tumor extent. *Sci. Rep.* **2017**, *7*, 46450. [CrossRef]
14. Ravì, D.; Wong, C.; Deligianni, F.; Berthelot, M.; Andreu-Perez, J.; Lo, B.; Yang, G.Z. Deep learning for health informatics. *IEEE J. Biomed. Health Inform.* **2016**, *21*, 4–21. [CrossRef] [PubMed]
15. Litjens, G.; Kooi, T.; Bejnordi, B.E.; Setio, A.A.A.; Ciompi, F.; Ghafoorian, M.; Van Der Laak, J.A.; Van Ginneken, B.; Sánchez, C.I. A survey on deep learning in medical image analysis. *Med Image Anal.* **2017**, *42*, 60–88. [CrossRef]
16. Shen, D.; Wu, G.; Suk, H.I. Deep learning in medical image analysis. *Annu. Rev. Biomed. Eng.* **2017**, *19*, 221–248. [CrossRef]
17. Zha, Z.J.; Hua, X.S.; Mei, T.; Wang, J.; Qi, G.J.; Wang, Z. Joint multi-label multi-instance learning for image classification. In Proceedings of the 2008 IEEE Conference on Computer Vision and Pattern Recognition, Anchorage, AK, USA, 23–28 June 2008; pp. 1–8.
18. Zhou, Z.H.; Xu, J.M. On the relation between multi-instance learning and semi-supervised learning. In Proceedings of the 24th International Conference on Machine Learning, Corvallis, OR, USA, 20–24 June 2007; pp. 1167–1174.
19. Zhou, Z.H.; Zhang, M.L. Neural networks for multi-instance learning. In Proceedings of the International Conference on Intelligent Information Technology, Beijing, China, 22–25 September 2002; pp. 455–459.
20. Zhou, Z.H. Multi-instance learning: A survey. *Dep. Comput. Sci. Technol. Nanjing Univ. Tech. Rep.* **2004**, 2.
21. Zhou, Z.H.; Zhang, M.L. Ensembles of multi-instance learners. In Proceedings of the 14th European Conference on Machine Learning, Cavtat-Dubrovnik, Croatia, 22–26 September 2003; Springer: Berlin/Heidelberg, Germany, 2003; pp. 492–502.
22. Sze, V.; Chen, Y.H.; Emer, J.; Suleiman, A.; Zhang, Z. Hardware for machine learning: Challenges and opportunities. In Proceedings of the 2017 IEEE Custom Integrated Circuits Conference (CICC), Austin, TX, USA, 30 April–3 May 2017; pp. 1–8.
23. Carbonneau, M.A.; Cheplygina, V.; Granger, E.; Gagnon, G. Multiple Instance Learning: A Survey of Problem Characteristics and Applications. *Pattern Recognit.* **2016**. [CrossRef]

24. Herrera, F.; Ventura, S.; Bello, R.; Cornelis, C.; Zafra, A.; Sanchez Tarrago, D.; Vluymans, S. *Multiple Instance Learning. Foundations and Algorithms*; Springer: Berlin/Heidelberg, Germany, 2016. [CrossRef]
25. Foulds, J.; Frank, E. A Review of Multi-Instance Learning Assumptions. *Knowl. Eng. Rev.* **2010**, *25*. [CrossRef]
26. Campanella, G.; Hanna, M.; Geneslaw, L.; Miraflor, A.; Silva, V.; Busam, K.; Brogi, E.; Reuter, V.; Klimstra, D.; Fuchs, T. Clinical-grade computational pathology using weakly supervised deep learning on whole slide images. *Nat. Med.* **2019**, *25*, 1. [CrossRef]
27. P J, S.; Petitjean, C.; Spanhol, F.; Oliveira, L.; Heutte, L.; Honeine, P. Multiple Instance Learning for Histopathological Breast Cancer Image Classification. *Expert Syst. Appl.* **2018**. [CrossRef]
28. Couture, H.D.; Williams, L.A.; Geradts, J.; Nyante, S.J.; Butler, E.N.; Marron, J.S.; Perou, C.M.; Troester, M.A.; Niethammer, M. Image analysis with deep learning to predict breast cancer grade, ER status, histologic subtype, and intrinsic subtype. *NPJ Breast Cancer* **2018**. [CrossRef]
29. Qaiser, T.; Mukherjee, A.; Reddy Pb, C.; Munugoti, S.D.; Tallam, V.; Pitkäaho, T.; Lehtimäki, T.; Naughton, T.; Berseth, M.; Pedraza, A.; et al. HER2 challenge contest: A detailed assessment of automated HER2 scoring algorithms in whole slide images of breast cancer tissues. *Histopathology* **2017**, *72*, 227–238. [CrossRef] [PubMed]
30. Jakobsen, M.R.; Teerapakpinyo, C.; Shuangshoti, S.; Keelawat, S. Comparison between digital image analysis and visual assessment of immunohistochemical HER2 expression in breast cancer. *Pathol.-Res. Pract.* **2018**, *214*, 2087–2092. [CrossRef] [PubMed]
31. Mukundan, R. Analysis of Image Feature Characteristics for Automated Scoring of HER2 in Histology Slides. *J. Imaging* **2019**, *5*, 35. [CrossRef]
32. Qaiser, T.; Rajpoot, N.M. Learning Where to See: A Novel Attention Model for Automated Immunohistochemical Scoring. *IEEE Trans. Med. Imaging* **2019**, *38*, 2620–2631. [CrossRef]
33. Yim, K.; Park, H.S.; Kim, D.M.; Lee, Y.S.; Lee, A. Image Analysis of HER2 Immunohistochemical Staining of Surgical Breast Cancer Specimens. *Yonsei Med. J.* **2019**, *60*, 158. [CrossRef]
34. Li, A.C.; Zhao, J.; Zhao, C.; Ma, Z.; Hartage, R.; Zhang, Y.; Li, X.; Parwani, A.V. Quantitative digital imaging analysis of HER2 immunohistochemistry predicts the response to anti-HER2 neoadjuvant chemotherapy in HER2-positive breast carcinoma. *Breast Cancer Res. Treat.* **2020**, *180*, 321–329. [CrossRef]
35. Güneş, A.; Kalkan, H.; Durmuş, E. Optimizing the color-to-grayscale conversion for image classification. *Signal Image Video Process.* **2016**, *10*, 853–860. [CrossRef]
36. Della Mea, V.; Pilutti, D. Classification of Histologic Images Using a Single Staining: Experiments With Deep Learning on Deconvolved Images. *Stud. Health Technol. Inform.* **2020**, *270*, 1223–1224.
37. Iandola, F.; Moskewicz, M.; Karayev, S.; Girshick, R.; Darrell, T.; Keutzer, K. Densenet: Implementing efficient convnet descriptor pyramids. *arXiv* **2014**, arXiv:1404.1869.
38. Yu, X.; Zeng, N.; Liu, S.; Zhang, Y.D. Utilization of DenseNet201 for diagnosis of breast abnormality. *Mach. Vis. Appl.* **2019**, *30*, 1135–1144. [CrossRef]
39. Yilmaz, F.; Kose, O.; Demir, A. Comparison of two different deep learning architectures on breast cancer. In Proceedings of the 2019 Medical Technologies Congress (TIPTEKNO), Izmir, Turkey, 3–5 October 2019; pp. 1–4.
40. Deng, J.; Dong, W.; Socher, R.; Li, L.J.; Li, K.; Fei-Fei, L. Imagenet: A large-scale hierarchical image database. In Proceedings of the 2009 IEEE Conference on Computer Vision and Pattern Recognition, Miami, FL, USA, 20–25 June 2009; pp. 248–255.
41. Aresta, G.; Araújo, T.; Kwok, S.; Chennamsetty, S.S.; Safwan, M.; Alex, V.; Marami, B.; Prastawa, M.; Chan, M.; Donovan, M. Bach: Grand challenge on breast cancer histology images. *Med. Image Anal.* **2019**, *56*, 122–139. [CrossRef] [PubMed]
42. Della Mea, V.; Baroni, G.L.; Pilutti, D.; Loreto, C.D. SlideJ: An ImageJ plugin for automated processing of whole slide images. *PLoS ONE* **2017**, *12*, e0180540. [CrossRef]
43. He, K.; Zhang, X.; Ren, S.; Sun, J. Deep residual learning for image recognition. In Proceedings of the 29th IEEE Conference on Computer Vision and Pattern Recognition, Las Vegas, NV, USA, 27–30 June 2016; pp. 770–778.
44. Szegedy, C.; Ioffe, S.; Vanhoucke, V.; Alemi, A.A. Inception-v4, inception-resnet and the impact of residual connections on learning. In Proceedings of the Thirty-First AAAI Conference on Artificial Intelligence, San Francisco, CA, USA, 4–9 February 2017.

45. Targ, S.; Almeida, D.; Lyman, K. Resnet in resnet: Generalizing residual architectures. *arXiv* **2016**, arXiv:1603.08029.
46. Wu, Z.; Shen, C.; Van Den Hengel, A. Wider or deeper: Revisiting the resnet model for visual recognition. *Pattern Recognit.* **2019**, *90*, 119–133. [CrossRef]
47. Smith, L.N. A disciplined approach to neural network hyper-parameters: Part 1—Learning rate, batch size, momentum, and weight decay. *arXiv* **2018**, arXiv:1803.09820.
48. Nguyen, L.D.; Lin, D.; Lin, Z.; Cao, J. Deep CNNs for microscopic image classification by exploiting transfer learning and feature concatenation. In Proceedings of the 2018 IEEE International Symposium on Circuits and Systems (ISCAS), Florence, Italy, 27–30 May 2018; pp. 1–5.

9

Applications of Computational Methods in Biomedical Breast Cancer Imaging Diagnostics

Kehinde Aruleba [1], George Obaido [1], Blessing Ogbuokiri [1], Adewale Oluwaseun Fadaka [2,*], Ashwil Klein [2], Tayo Alex Adekiya [3] and Raphael Taiwo Aruleba [4,*]

1 School of Computer Science and Applied Mathematics, University of the Witwatersrand, Johannesburg 2001, South Africa; arulebak@gmail.com (K.A.); rabeshi.george@gmail.com (G.O.); ogbuokiriblessing@gmail.com (B.O.)

2 Department of Biotechnology, Faculty of Natural Sciences, University of the Western Cape, Private Bag X17, Bellville, Cape Town 7535, South Africa; aklein@uwc.ac.za

3 Department of Pharmacy and Pharmacology, School of Therapeutic Science, Faculty of Health Sciences, University of the Witwatersrand, Johannesburg, 7 York Road, Parktown 2193, South Africa; adekiyatalex@gmail.com

4 Department of Molecular and Cell Biology, Faculty of Science, University of Cape Town, Cape Town 7701, South Africa

* Correspondence: afadaka@uwc.ac.za (A.O.F.); arulebataiwo@yahoo.com (R.T.A.);

Abstract: With the exponential increase in new cases coupled with an increased mortality rate, cancer has ranked as the second most prevalent cause of death in the world. Early detection is paramount for suitable diagnosis and effective treatment of different kinds of cancers, but this is limited to the accuracy and sensitivity of available diagnostic imaging methods. Breast cancer is the most widely diagnosed cancer among women across the globe with a high percentage of total cancer deaths requiring an intensive, accurate, and sensitive imaging approach. Indeed, it is treatable when detected at an early stage. Hence, the use of state of the art computational approaches has been proposed as a potential alternative approach for the design and development of novel diagnostic imaging methods for breast cancer. Thus, this review provides a concise overview of past and present conventional diagnostics approaches in breast cancer detection. Further, we gave an account of several computational models (machine learning, deep learning, and robotics), which have been developed and can serve as alternative techniques for breast cancer diagnostics imaging. This review will be helpful to academia, medical practitioners, and others for further study in this area to improve the biomedical breast cancer imaging diagnosis.

Keywords: cancer; breast cancer; diagnostics; imaging; computation; artificial intelligence

1. Introduction

Cancer is a non-communicable disease characterized by abnormal cell proliferation or cell division, with the ability to spread to other parts of the body [1]. Cancer continues to be a major public health problem and has been labeled as a global threat exacerbated by poor lifestyle choices and environmental factors [2,3]. Generally, cancer is classified according to the affected body part or tissue of origin. The most common cancer diseases include but are not limited to lung cancer, ovarian cancer, prostate cancer, head and neck cancer, breast cancer, etc. [4]. Indeed, breast cancer has been considered as one of the most common cancers diagnosed among women around the world. Breast cancer comprises 18% of the total cases of female cancer and approximately a million new cases are reported in the world every year [5]. Due to the ability of this type of cancer to metastasize to distant organs or lymph nodes, it has been considered to be the leading cause of mortality in females [5,6].

Due to the increase in the numbers of breast cancer over the years, there has been a rise in the number of computational models and algorithms for diagnosis and treatment to assist medical practitioners. A commonly, and frequently, used computational method is artificial intelligence (AI). Many AI related models have been developed for detecting and diagnosing diseases not only for breast cancer or mammography image analysis and classification [7] but for other diseases such as hycobacterium tuberculosis classification (MTC) [8], human immunodeficiency virus (HIV) therapy, screening, identification, and prediction [9], coronavirus disease 2019 (COVID-19) detection and diagnosis [10], etc. These AI models include machine learning, deep learning, and robotics. Rapid improvement in classification and learning algorithms is one of the main reasons these models have been widely used for these purposes with good and efficient results. Therefore, the contribution of this review is to provide a concise overview of past and present conventional diagnostics approaches in breast cancer detection and diagnosis. Further, we gave an account of several AI related computational models that have been developed and can serve as alternative models for breast cancer diagnosis. The remaining part of this paper is organized as follows: The types of biomedical imaging is presented in Section 2. The computational techniques used in breast cancer imaging diagnostics are outlined in Section 3. This section discusses the AI models used in breast cancer diagnosis. Finally, the paper is concluded in Section 4, where some points of future work are recommended.

2. Types of Biomedical Imaging

2.1. Mammography

Mammography is an excellent method used in primary breast imaging. It is used for early detection of abnormalities in the breast, especially those suspicious for breast cancer before it becomes apparent clinically, by using low-dose X-ray imaging to generate the images of the breast [11,12]. According to the United States of America preventive services task force (USPSTF), this type of breast imaging has been helpful in the earlier and better treatment for women over 40 years of age and has decreased breast cancer mortality by at least 30% [13]. Although this imaging approach remains the key for early breast cancer detection and screening, the overall accuracy of the test remains low and second-line accurate imaging techniques are required in some instances to lessen the number of unnecessary excisional biopsies [14,15].

Screening mammography is credited with the examination of an asymptomatic woman and decreases the risk of breast cancer-related death [16,17]. Conventional mammography has limitations in specificity and sensitivity, especially in dense breasts. The sensitivity of this type of imaging in breast cancer diagnostics is about 50 to 85%, depending on the density of the breast. Meanwhile, the sensitivity is below 50% in the dense breast due to tissue superposition; this is a major reason for the false-positive result, which leads to additional imagining and cost and false-negative results due to masking of true lesions [18–20].

In the breast, the normal internal mammary lymph node chain is usually below 5 mm in diameter. Metastases to this chain cannot be easily detected by mammography or ultrasonography clinical examination because they are normally covered by cartilaginous and bony structures of the chest wall [21,22]. The use of mammography in the detection of recurrent breast cancer is a challenging task due to changes in the architecture of the breast, mainly in fibrosis and scarring secondary to radiotherapy and surgery, resulting in difficulties to interpret mammograms. Breast compression is another major challenge faced by this modality due to accompanied pain which could lead to delayed diagnosis. Hence, considering all of the aforementioned mammography limitations, there is a call for alternative and more accurate methods that can resolve the imaging of dense breasts [19,20].

2.2. *Tomosynthesis*

Due to the limitations of mammography, breast tomosynthesis was introduced to the clinic because of its ability to produce three-dimensional information at a lower dose and its relative cost-effectiveness. Consequently, there has been an upsurge in interest in tomosynthesis. The Food and Drug Administration (FDA) has approved some products that are now in use and on the market [23]. This technique involves using X-ray projection images acquired over an arc to generate image slices for a partially 3D image [24]. Tomosynthesis allows for the generation of an arbitrary number of in-focus planes retrospectively from a series of radiograph projections obtained in a single motion of the X-ray tube [25]. Notably, a combination of tomosynthesis and digital mammography increases the brightness of invasive cancers while at the same time decreasing the likelihood of false-positive data [24]. Tomosynthesis has been applied to several clinical tasks, including dental imaging, angiography, breast imaging, bone imaging, and chest imaging [23]. In breast cancer, tomosynthesis increases the sensitivity of mammography, which could enhance the early detection of breast cancer due to the improved lesion margin conspicuity [25]. This is very beneficial to breast cancer patients, especially those with radiographically dense breasts. However, Poplack et al. [26] showed that breast tomosynthesis has a comparable or superior image when compared with diagnostic film-screen mammography in 89% of recruited subjects. More recently, this was supported by another study where one-view stand-alone digital breast tomosynthesis (DBT) detected more breast cancer than digital mammogram (DM) [27]. This suggests that the use of one-view DBT alone could be feasible in breast cancer screening. Although the acquisition procedures of tomosynthesis mimic standard mammography, the X-ray tube of tomosynthesis takes several low-dose exposures as it travels within a limited arc of motion unlike conventional mammography [26]. Sechopoulos [28] has written an excellent review of all aspects of tomosynthesis, including doses and reconstruction processes. When the overall dose used for visualization is constant, the quality of the image improves with a wider angular range [29]. However, the quality of image degenerates once the maximum is attained at a particular number of projections.

2.3. *Ultrasound Imaging*

Ultrasound (US) imaging diagnostics, otherwise known as sonography or ultrasound scanning, is a painless and safe approach. US makes use of 1 to 10 MHz sound waves to produce pictures that reveal the movement and structure of the breast, and other soft tissue [30,31]. It can also reveal the movements of blood and other materials within the blood vessels and body [31]. It is a cross-sectional technique that uses a small probe, known as a transducer, and gel that is directly placed on the breast/skin; it displays the tissues without overlap [31–33]. The high-frequency soundwaves travel from the probe via the gel into the body, and the probe receives the sounds that bounce back, which in turn produces an image on a computer. This type of imaging technique does not make use of radiation because it captures images in real-time [31–33].

In recent times, the development of high-resolution US technique has greatly improved the diagnosis of breast cancer because, in the past, US was thought to only be suitable for the diagnosis of cysts [34,35]. It has been shown to enhance the differential diagnosis of both benign and malignant lesions during guided interventional and local preoperative staging diagnosis. Due to the higher sensitivity of this type of imaging technique, it has been adopted as a complementary technique to mammography with limited sensitivity to identify early, node-negative cancer in dense breasts [36,37].

However, the use of US imaging techniques is diminishing due to the time and skill required to detect small tumors with hand-held imaging, and non-palpable cancers. The implementation of this imaging technique in breast cancer diagnostics has been hampered by limited numbers of qualified personnel and lack of uniformity in the results; this has caused low specificity that can lead to the generation of high numbers of false-positive results [38]. This assertion is corroborated by findings of some previous studies which revealed that US can identify and detect the presence of carcinoma in dense breasts. Some other studies have shown low detection of cancerous cells in dense breasts, but have proposed the addition of this imaging method to negate mammography which seems to have limited cost-efficiency and is controversial for women with dense breasts without any other major risk factors. In addition, due to the high scattering ability of the soundwaves at bone and air interfaces, various parts of the body are invisible, which limits the effectiveness of depth imaging in most organs to about 10 cm [39,40].

2.4. Dedicated Breast Computed Tomography

Dedicated breast computed tomography (DBCT) is a recently used and fastest-growing imaging technique that allows for true isotropic and provides three-dimensional (3D) information which can be reconstructed or rebuilt into several imaging planes. Although DBCT is comparable to breast magnetic resonance imaging (MRI), the process involved can be carried out without breast compression, and is not limited by breast implants or the density of the breast [41–43]. The radiation dose in this type of imaging technique is similar to that of a conventional two-view mammogram [42]. Boone et al. [44] investigated the feasibility of low dose radiation on the image quality of DBCT. The findings from their average glandular dose for 80-kVp breast CT study, when compared to two-view mammography, revealed that the breast CT dose for thicker breasts is approximately one-third lower than that of two-view mammography. For a typical breast of 5 cm 50% glandular, it was discovered that the maximum dose of mammography in 1 mm^3 voxel is far greater (20.0 mGy) than that of breast CT with 5.4 mGy. It was further stated that the CT images for 8 cm cadaveric breasts have an average glandular dose of 6.32 mGy, which is superior to the estimated dose of 5.06 mGy for the craniocaudal view, with an average glandular dose of 10.1 mGy for standard two-view mammography of the same specimen [44]. The invention, improvement, and development of DBCT with dedicated scanners with novel technology has been documented in the literature by Sarno et al. [45]. Studies further reported the development of low radiation dose scanners with improved spatial resolution and rapid image acquisition times, which is aimed at addressing the issue of imaging dense breasts and painful breast compression [41–43].

Kuzmiak et al. [42] investigated the confidence of radiology experts in the characterization of suspicious breast lesions with a DBCT system compared with the conventional diagnostics of two-dimensional (2D) digital mammography in terms of overall lesion visibility and dose. It was discovered that DBCT is superior in the characterization of the masses and radiologists' visualizations, although it is inferior to calcifications when diagnostic mammography is used. It was further averred that the DBCT application could help eliminate the 2D mammography drawback of overlapping tissue. Their study concluded that the technical challenges in breast imaging remain, but 3D DBCT could have a promising clinical application in breast cancer diagnosis or screening, however, this needs further investigation.

In 2008, Lindfors et al. [41] carried out a comparative study between the DBCT and screen-films mammograms where it was discovered, in the study of the selected group of women, that the visualization of breast lesions with both the DBCT and screen-film mammography is approximately the same. Although, DBCT was reported to be superior in the visualization of the masses, while in the imaging of microcalcification lesions screen-film mammography shows to be better. It was further deduced in their study that women are more comfortable with DBCT screening when compared to screen-film mammography. Hence, it was assumed that DBCT is a potential technology and may be a promising clinical application in diagnostic and screening for breast cancer investigation. Additionally, it was further presumed that DBCT is more accessible and could be a replacement for breast MRI or act as a control technique for tumor ablation procedures or robotic breast biopsy, all of this calls for further studies.

Recently, Shah et al. [43] investigated the characterization of computed tomography (CT). Hounsfield units were used in clinical settings for the purpose of tissue differentiation in a reconstructed CT image in 3D acquisition trajectories on a DBCT system. It was depicted in their statistical study that the approach has a better performance in the saddle orbit, mostly when close to the chest and the nipple areas of dense breast. It was further discovered that the saddle orbit functions significantly well and provides a tighter distribution of Hounsfield unit values in the reconstructed volumes. In addition, the study demonstrated the significance of the application of 3D acquisition for breast CT trajectories and other uses through the establishment of the robustness in Hounsfield unit values in the large reconstructed volumes.

2.5. Magnetic Resonance Imaging

Since the beginning of the third millennium, magnetic resonance imaging (MRI) has developed into a paramount tool in breast cancer screening, diagnosing, staging, and follow-up [46]. This imaging tool has played a vital role in the screening of high-risk breast cancer patients. Breast MRI uses an intravenous contrast agent such as gadolinium, which allows for the visualization of lesions. The sensitivity of this tool in breast cancer has been documented to be over 90% while the specificity is still about 72%; hence, the distinction between benign and malignant lesions is still challenging [46]. Although mammography is the basic imaging tool for breast tumor identification, it has been indicated that MRI has a higher sensitivity for detection of breast cancer, and the breast density does not affect it [47]. In most cases, the sensitivity of mammography in the detection of multiple malignant foci is below 50%. It is important to note that breast MRI is not meant to replace mammography particularly in ductal carcinoma in situ, which is not detectable by MRI but rather by mammography [48]. The MRI screening in women with genetic susceptibility to breast cancer has proved to be beneficial [49,50]. In a prospective cohort study, the sensitivity of MRI in women with a high risk of breast cancer but who were asymptomatic was between 93–100%, the 10-year survival was 95.3% [50]. Similarly, the sensitivity of MRI in contralateral breast tumor detection was documented to be 91%, and specificity was 88% [51]. In women with a known BRCA1/2 mutation, MRI surveillance detected breast cancer at early stages; encouragingly, there was no distant recurrence after 8.4 years follow-up since diagnosis [52]. This tool can be used in identifying the size and degree of the tumor towards achieving better surgery procedures. Nevertheless, the use of MRI before surgery continues to be controversial with extensive variations in the outcome; however, it helps in planning conservation in patients that respond to chemotherapy where feasible [46]. Despite the high sensitivity of this imaging tool in breast cancer, the cost involved in MRI makes it difficult to be employed in the general population. Conclusively, the invention and development of new imaging techniques such as diffusion-weighted imaging offer an added advantage in breast cancer management.

2.6. Diffusion-Weighted Imaging

Since the early years of the 21st century, diffusion-weighted imaging (DWI) has been at the forefront of cancer imaging attaining widespread recognition due to its ability in the diagnosis of stroke [53,54]. DWI is a noninvasive MRI technique that relies on the principle of random molecular motion of free water in tissues (Brownian movement). With the development of stronger diffusion gradients and application in whole-body imaging, DWI has attracted attention in oncology [55]. In breast cancer, Sinha et al. [56] demonstrated that DWI is reliable in a clinical setting with an echo-planar sequence and possesses potential in breast lesion characterization as either benign or malignant using apparent diffusion coefficient (ADC) values. Generally, breast lesions classified as malignant have a high-cellular level with limited water diffusion and lower ADC values when compared to benign lesions [57]. An earlier clinical study that recruited women with breast lesions stated that ADC values and the tumor biological aggressiveness correlate; hence, ADC is a promising factor in the evaluation and analysis of the degree of the malignancy [58]. In most clinical settings, DWI is interpreted in combination with dynamic contrast-enhanced (DCE)-MRI to increase the specificity. However, more recently, lesions in the breast (31 = malignant; 13 = benign) were analyzed using quantitative diffusion-weighted sequence on 3T MRI with b-values of 500 and 1000 s/mm^2 [59]. The ADC cut-off value for benign and malignant lesions was set to 1.21×10^{-3} mm^2/s for b = 500 s/mm^2 and 1.22×10^{-3} mm^2/s for b = 1000 s/mm^2, respectively. The sensitivity of DCE-MRI was 100% with a specificity of 66.7%, when DCE-MRI was combined with b = 1000 s/mm^2, 100% specificity was attained and sensitivity of 90.6%; there was no significant difference between the ADC and prognostic factors [59]. Non-contrast (NC)-MRI can be an alternative for DCE-MRI for breast cancer diagnosis, though its inferior lesion conspicuity and lower inter-reader agreement should be considered [60]. This study and many more have documented explanatory results for DWI as a tool for diagnosing breast lesion and aids the orthodox breast MRI procedures. Several pitfalls, which include but are not limited to motion artifacts, ADC value accuracy, image quality, and signal-to-noise ratio, are associated with DWI [61,62]. These challenges are bothersome and lay emphasis on the need to incorporate computer science into breast cancer diagnosis, for example, robotics could significantly decrease time in DWI MRI and create improved breast cancer detection.

2.7. Computed Tomography

CT scan is a method that exposes the pictures of cross-sections or 2D slices of the body's organs via a connected computer [63,64]. The use of a contrast solution (iodine), injected into the body via the arm, dramatically improves and aids in the visualization of the cancerous cells in organs. In 2003, the use of CT for breast cancer imaging was proposed by Suga et al. [65], after a surgical issue in patients, to obtain interstitial lymphography that can map and present sentinel lymph nodes of the breast. The use of CT in breast cancer has some advantages, which includes patient comfort and fast scanning time. However, CT has not been widely used in breast cancers due to the risks involved in radiation exposure and poor quality of the image produced.

Due to the dynamic technique of CT, it can be used in the detection and characterization of breast tumors, investigation of neoadjuvant chemotherapy effects, and local staging of cancerous cells in the breast. In 2015, Foo et al. [66] employed this imaging scan method to evaluate the staging of cancer cells in newly diagnosed breast cancer patients that are in a locally advanced stage. It was revealed that a limited number of patients involved in this study had some pelvic significance with relation to a patient who had peritoneal cancer with widespread metastasis, and a patient with a presumed gene carrier of a concurrent primary ovarian malignancy. It was further stated that 50% of all pelvic results required additional radiological examinations.

Although the CT scan technique in breast cancer examinations may not replace the conventional mammography routine, based on improvements carried out in some studies [67,68], it can be used to overcome several limitations associated with mammography such as detection of cancers in premenopausal, dysplastic, and dense breasts. The mean glandular dose of 8.2 ± 1.2 mGy has also been documented for different types of breast shapes and sizes [69]. As documented by Park et al. [68], in prone positions, low-dose perfusion CT is possible for imaging with regards to the quantification of tumor vascularity and radiation doses. CT can be used in the detection of unsuspected very small cancers in the breast that cannot be identified or seen by physical examinations or conventional mammography. It is useful in definitive diagnostic evaluation in a situation where physical examinations and mammography are inconclusive, and it can also be helpful in recognition of precancerous and high-risk lesions. More so, CT can be used in the discrimination of tumor tissue from normal tissue in breast cancer patients without the use of a contrast medium.

2.8. Near-Infrared (NIR) Fluorescence

During human surgery, X-ray fluoroscopy and ultrasound have been used widely. However, during X-ray fluoroscopy, patients and caregivers are exposed to ionizing radiation; in an ultrasound, only a thin surgical field-of-view is seen and requires direct contact with tissue, in this case, breast. Interestingly, none of the methods can be amended by target contrast agents to guide imaging during oncologic surgery due to the number of procedures required [70,71]. Thus, near-infrared (NIR) light, with a wavelength range of about 700 to 900 nm, has offered diverse significant advantages over some widely used tools including relatively high penetration of photon in and out of living tissue (breast) due to the reduction in the rate of absorbance and scatter. Owing to lower tissue autofluorescence, NIR has a higher signal-to-background ratio [71,72]. This technique has a great potential to interrogate deep tissues (breast) for molecular-based imaging. The NIR light is visible to the human eyes when conjugated with NIR excitable fluorophore or dyes. These are chemical compounds which convert light generated from one NIR wavelength into the NIR light of diverse wavelength. It has been recommended that the mapping of sentinel lymph nodes (SLN) is a standard approach for the management of breast cancer and care staging of the axilla [71].

NIR fluorescence imaging, which uses indocyanine green (ICG), has been shown to improve the procedure of the SLN mapping by facilitating percutaneous incisions and identifying the intraoperative ability of lymphatic channels and SLNs [71,72]. The safety and accuracy of NIR fluorescence imaging applications for identifying SLNs in patients suffering from breast cancer were demonstrated by Verbeek et al. [73]. The use of the Mini-FLARE camera system and 1.6 mL of 0.5 mM ICG showed the excellent identification of the SLN in patients with breast cancer. Although, the technique which should be used as the gold standard in future analyses, was raised as a question [73]. In a similar study by Mieog et al. [74], the clinical translation of a novel NIR fluorescence imaging system and the optimal ratio of ICG to the human serum albumin (HSA) dose for mapping of SLN in breast cancer was described. It was stated that 400 and 800 μM is the optimal dose of the injection ratio of ICG:HSA and this can be chosen based on the preferences of local preparation. For instance, a dose of 500 μM was depicted to be the most convenient in the United States due to the minimal requirement in the manipulation of albumin volumes. Other studies that have employed this approach in mapping SLNs in breast cancer patients include Sevick-Muraca et al. [75] which demonstrated the prospective feasibility in the use of the minimal dose of ICG in noninvasive optical imaging of lymph nodes in the breast cancer patients undergoing SLNs mapping. In 2008, Altınoğlu et al. [76]. demonstrated the synthesis and bioresorbable use of calcium phosphate nanoparticles (CPNPs) which incorporated the molecule of the NIR emitted fluorophore and ICG. In their study, the in vivo and ex vivo studies demonstrated the potentiality of the NIR CPNPs in diagnostic imaging of early breast solid tumors. Although, the result from their ex situ imaging of deep tissue showed that the depths of NIR CPNPs in porcine muscle tissue is 3 cm. Poellinger et al. [77] employed the use of NIR fluorescence imaging with the late and early enhancement of ICG, which corresponds to extravascular and vascular phases of contrast agent enhancement to distinguish between malignant and benign breast lesions as well as to detect breast cancer. Ke et al. [78] assessed the specificity of continuous-wave NIR fluorescence imaging by an intensified charge-coupled device (CDD) camera on a novel epidermal growth factor (EGF)-Cy5.5 to detect EGF receptors in breast cancer xenografts.

2.9. *Single-Photon Emission Computed Tomography*

Single-photon emission computed tomography (SPECT) is a medical imaging tool based on tomographic reconstruction protocols and routinely used in a clinical decision in cancer [79], coronary artery disease, left ventricular dysfunction [80], and Parkinson disease [81]. In fact, it is the most used tool in myocardial ischemia assessment. SPECT aims at getting a perfect 3D radioactivity distribution resulting from the uptake of a radiotracer in humans. One or more photons are released in random directions when a SPECT radioisotope decays [82]. However, collimators are used to focus the angle of the emitted photons that reach the detector because conventional lenses cannot restrict high-energy photons, and only 0.02% of the decay events is measured [82]. SPECT, coupled with CT, can be used when conventional images are complex to interpret, for example, suspicion of contamination [83]. Clinically, SPECT/CT provides more value in anatomical localization of sentinel nodes. This highlights a relevant role for this tool in the surgical approach and may improve staging [84]. The sentinel lymph node biopsy is a well-known procedure used in evaluating the status of the axillary lymph node in patients with early stages of breast cancer [85]. Markedly, SPECT/CT improved visualization from 84% to 92% in patients, but it only showed sentinel nodes in 11 out of 22 breast cancer patients (50%) with non-visualization on planar imaging [84]. Similarly, Lerman et al. [86] documented that the addition of SPECT/CT to lymphoscintigraphy enhances sentinel node identification in breast cancer patients who are overweight. Notably, SPECT/CT identified hot nodes in 91% of patients and sentinel nodes in 29 of 49 patients (59%) who were negative on planar imaging (planar lymphoscintigraphy) [86]. Hence, this technique is of high relevance in overweight breast cancer patients because intraoperative techniques have failed in the identification of draining nodes. Another SPECT/CT evaluation study demonstrated a sentinel node in 91.1% of breast cancer patients, and localization was more precise on SPECT/CT fusion images than on the planar views [87]. Mann et al. [88] documented that the use of dedicated SPECT identifies regions of interest at a global lower-level threshold within dense breast tissue without any negative effects, which in turn betters patient care. Additionally, dedicated breast positron emission tomography (PET)/CT can accurately visualize uncompressed breast suspected lesions in 3D [89]. However, this scanner was unable to generate a full quantitative image. Recently, Tornai et al. [90] developed a fully 3D CT in a hybrid SPECT/CT breast imaging system that facilitated complex trajectories, which improved the quality of the image when compared with simple circular breast CT acquisitions. The SPECT-subsystem allows viewing of the chest wall for pendant breast imaging [90]. Recently, it was shown that the hybrid SPECT/CT provides precise anatomical data that enables clear assessment of patients contaminated with radionuclide during the procedure [83]. Such precise data can assist surgeons towards a better surgical plan. Non-visualization of sentinel nodes, unexpected lymphatic drainage, and complicated planar imaging interpretation are challenges faced by these imaging techniques. However, this can be amended by incorporating AI, such as deep learning and machine learning algorithms, with currently available breast cancer imaging tools. Overall, such combinations will improve breast cancer diagnosis, predict treatment outcome and ultimately, improve the patient quality of life. The dose in the dedicated SPECT-CT system using both the geometric and anthropomorphic phantoms showed that the average doses absorbed in 100% fibroglandular-equivalent was 4.5 ± 0.4 mGy, while 100% adipose-equivalent tissues was 3.8 ± 0.2 mGy. More so, the dose measured in a cadaver breast using a radiochromic film in the same study yielded an average dose of 4.3 ± 0.3 mGY and 4.2 ± 0.3 mGy along two orthogonal planes [91].

3. Computational Techniques Used in Breast Cancer Imaging Diagnostics

A correct diagnosis of mammograms containing malignant tumors is a complex task for even the most experienced medical practitioner. To circumvent this complexity, several computational models have been developed to assist medical practitioners to distinguish between benign and malignant breast tumors. The models described in this paper are based on machine learning, deep learning, and robotics which have been shown to be useful in breast cancer diagnosis. In this section, we present some studies that have applied these models.

3.1. Machine Learning Algorithms

Several machine learning algorithms have been proposed for the detection and diagnosis of breast cancer. Despite this, the development of new algorithms and models for this purpose is still an active research area, especially in the detection of abnormalities in mammograms. In the following, we review machine learning models that have been used in diagnosing this type of cancer, such as artificial neural network (ANN) and support vector machine (SVM).

3.1.1. Support Vector Machines

SVMs are supervised learning models that aim at formulating a computationally effective approach of learning to separate hyperplanes in high-dimensional feature space [92]. It has been used and proven to be an efficient learning technique for several real-world problems such as image recognition [93], bioinformatics [94], and classification problems [95], among others. SVMs are one of the earliest machine learning techniques used for cancer diagnosis. Acharya et al. [96] focused on detecting breast abnormalities or cancer automatically by using infrared imaging. The approach used texture features and SVMs to detect breast cancer based on thermography. Texture features were obtained from a run-length matrix and co-occurrence matrix from 25 cancerous and 25 normal infra-red breast images. These features were then fed to an SVM for automatic classification and detection of malignant and normal breast conditions. A comparison of SVMs based classifiers with ANNs and Bayesian classifiers for the prognosis and diagnosis of breast cancer was done in Maglogiannis et al. [97]. The implementation of the comparison was performed on the Wisconsin prognostic breast cancer and the Wisconsin diagnostic breast cancer datasets. The expected result of the implementation was to predict a class that corresponds to a likely tumor recurrence in four-time intervals. The result also shows that SVM outperforms the other classifiers. Huang et al. [98] used SVM to evaluate several pathologically proven breast tumors. The study presented a computer-aided diagnosis (CAD) system with textural features for classifying malignant and benign breast tumors on medical ultrasound systems. The aim of the CAD is to assist medical practitioners and radiologists in identifying lesions and also to differentiate malignant lesions from benign lesions on the basis of medical images. The proposed SVM technique was able to identify solid breast nodules at very high accuracy. Recently, Wang et al. [7] proposed an approach to solving the limitations of machine learning models' performance in diagnosing breast cancer. The approach was based on an SVM-based ensemble learning algorithm; this approach reduces the diagnosis variance and increases diagnosis accuracy. In doing this, 12 different SVMs were hybrid using the proposed weight area under the receiver operating characteristics curve ensemble (WAUCE) approach.

3.1.2. Artificial Neural Network

ANN is a computational-intelligent model that uses different optimization tools to learn from the data available in the past and use that prior training to identify or predict new patterns or to classify new data. Several research works have applied ANN for medical purposes [99], such as cancer treatments [100]. The Memetic Pareto ANN (MPANN) approach was proposed by Abbass [101]. The approach was based on a pareto-differential evolution algorithm. This algorithm was augmented with a local search for the prediction and diagnosis of breast cancer. Tourassi et al. [102] proposed a new approach for breast cancer diagnosis based on the constraint satisfaction neural network (CSNN) technique using mammographic and breast cancer patient history findings. The main advantage of this technique is that it has a non-hierarchical architecture and flexibility that allows it to work as a predictive tool and as an analysis or data mining tool to discover the knowledge of association rules among clinical diagnosis and historical findings. In this work, the authors used two different datasets of breast cancer, each containing 250 patient cases. The CSNN was first used to train the first 250 datasets and the other 250 datasets were used to test the predictive strength of the CSNN. The result of the analysis was done based on the kind of mammographic lesions seen in each patient. The result of this study shows that CSNN is a very efficient CAD tool for predicting and diagnosing breast cancer from mammographic and historical findings. A study by Janghel et al. [103] implemented a model using ANN to assist medical practitioners in diagnosing breast cancer. The model has four phases, namely radial basis function networks (RBFN), back propagation algorithm (BPA), competitive learning network (CLN), and learning vector quantization (LVQ). The dataset used in this study consisted of 55 malignant cases and 184 benign cases. The result of the experiment showed that the LVQ output was the best result during testing then CLN, BPA, and RBFN in order. Figure 1 presents a simple ANN diagnosis for breast cancer.

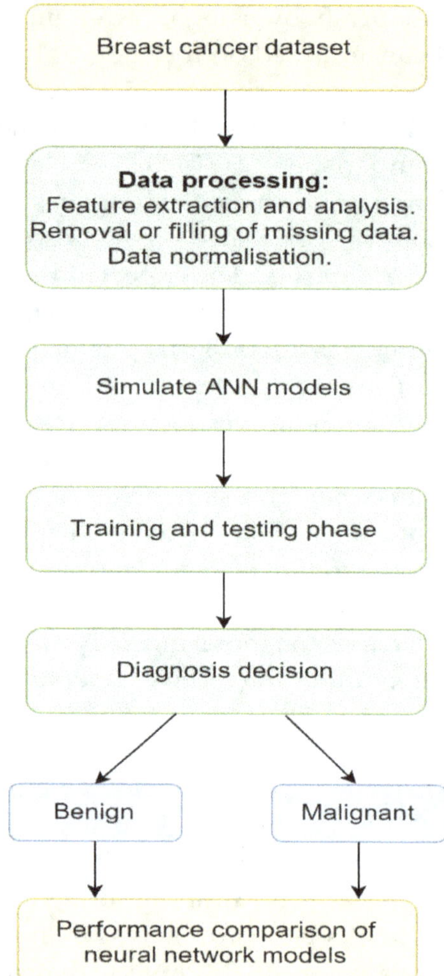

Figure 1. A simple artificial neural network (ANN) method on breast cancer [103].

Other works in the literature used data mining methods in diagnosing breast cancer [104,105]. Data mining is the process of extracting useful data from a larger set of raw data using one or more software. Çakır et al. [106] used Weka, a data mining tool to analyze 462 breast cancer patients data obtained from the Ankara Oncology Hospital. Classification algorithms are applied to each of the datasets and the outputs of the classification were compared to find the most effective treatment method. This work assists oncology doctors to suggest the best treatment method for a patient. Şahan et al. [107] proposed a hybrid system of a fuzzy-artificial immune system with the k-nearest neighbor (KNN) algorithm. This method was used to solve diagnosis problems through classifying the Wisconsin breast cancer dataset (WBCD). The system has a high classification accuracy on large datasets and can be used for any type of breast cancer diagnosis. Additionally, it can be used for other medical condition diagnoses. The Table 1 below presents an overview of machine learning (ML) techniques in breast cancer diagnosis that are explained in this section. The evaluation results presented in the table are the 50–50% training–test partition for the reference with three different training-test partitions.

Table 1. An overview of machine learning (ML) techniques in breast cancer diagnosis.

Reference	Computation Technique	Scope	Evaluation Results	Datasets
Acharya et al. [96]	Texture features + SVM	Breast cancer detection using thermal imaging	Accuracy = 88.10%, specificity = 90.48%, sensitivity = 85.71%	25 normal and 25 cancerous collected from Singapore General Hospital, Singapore
Maglogiannis et al. [97]	SVM	Diagnosis and prognosis	Accuracy = 96.91%, specificity = 97.67%, Sensitivity = 97.84%	Wisconsin prognostic breast cancer (WPBC)
Huang et al. [98]	SVM	Classifying benign and malignant	Accuracy = 94.4%, specificity = 94.4%, Sensitivity = 94.3%	250 images of benign breast tumors from 215 patients and carcinomas from 35 patients.
Wang et al. [7]	SVM	Reduce the diagnosis variance and increase the diagnostic accuracy of breast cancer	Variance = 97.89%, increase in accuracy by 33.34%	Wisconsin Breast Cancer, Wisconsin Diagnostic Breast Cancer, and the U.S. National Cancer Institute's Surveillance, Epidemiology, and End Results (SEER) program
Abbass [101]	EANN	Diagnosis	Average accuracy = 0.981 ± 0.005	Wisconsin
Bhardwaj et al. [108]	Genetically optimized neural network	Classification	Accuracy of 98.24%, 99.63% and 100% for 50–50, 60–40, 70–30 training–testing partition, respectively	WBCD
Tourassi et al. [102]	CSNN	Diagnosis	CSNN ROC area index = 0.84 ± 0.02	500 private images
Çakır et al. [106]	Weka	Treatment methods	Accuracy = 92%	462 patients data
Karabatak [109]	Weighted Naïve Bayesian	Detection	Sensitivity = 99.11%, specificity = 98.25%, accuracy = 98.54%	WBCD
Şahan et al. [107]	Fuzzy + KNN	Diagnosis	Accuracy = 99.14%	WBCD
Bagui et al. [110]	Rank nearest neighbor	Diagnosis	Accuracy = 98.1%	WBCD
Chen et al. [111]	Rough set_SVM	Distinguishing benign breast tumour from malignant one	Accuracy = 99.41%, Sensitivity = 100%, specificity = 100%	WBCD
Polat et al. [112]	Least square SVM	Classification	Accuracy = 94.87%, Sensitivity = 96.42%, specificity = 95.86%	WBCD

3.2. Deep Learning

In recent years, deep learning has set an exciting trend in the fields of machine learning and AI [113]. Deep learning techniques utilize computational models, composed of multiple processing layers that are used to learn data representations and applied to many real-world applications. These applications range from image recognition, object detection, power systems, breast cancer detection, speech recognition to drug discovery and genomics, etc. [114–117]. In the following sections, deep learning models for breast cancer diagnosis are presented.

3.2.1. Convolutional Neural Network

The convolutional neural network (CNN), often called ConvNet, is a type of deep learning model that has become dominant for many computer vision tasks, ranging from image classification, object tracking and detection to semantic segmentation [118,119]. CNN was designed to adaptively learn hierarchies of features, usually from low-level to high-level patterns [120]. Indolia et al. [121] explained that the CNN overcomes limitations as seen in traditional machine learning approaches; it has shown to be widely used for solving complex problems, especially in the medical imaging domain. Recent studies have adopted the CNN model for effective breast cancer diagnosis [122–124]. An example of CNN segmentation tasks for breast cancer diagnosis is presented in Figure 2.

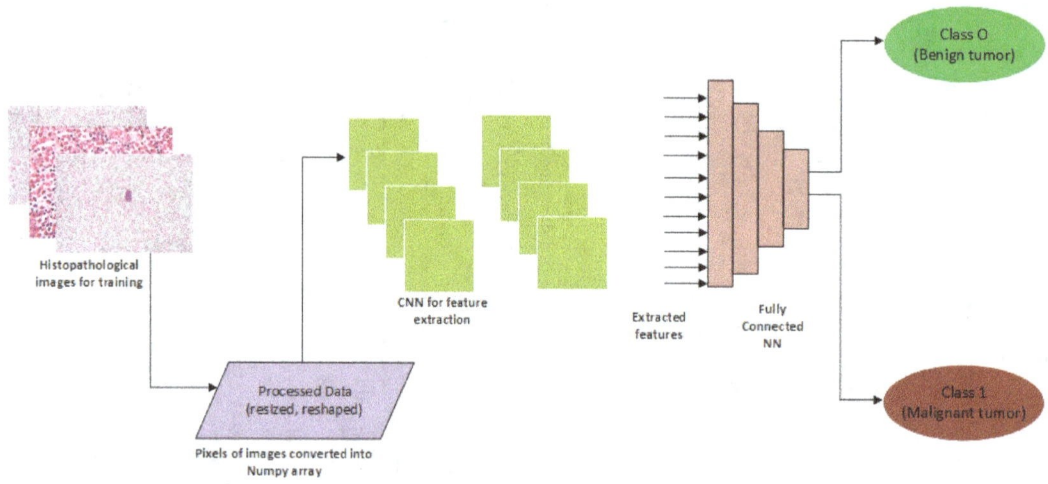

Figure 2. A convolutional neural network (CNN)-based approach for screening mammography [125].

For an improved diagnosis, Tan et al. [126] developed an imaging system called breast cancer detection using convolutional neural networks (BCDCNN) aimed at assisting medical practitioners to classify mammographic images into malignant or benign. The results showed that the BCDCNN system improved the accuracy of the classification tasks on the mini-Mammographic Image Analysis Society (mini-MIAS) database. Amit et al. [122] proposed an approach for dynamic contrast-enhanced (DCE) imaging that uses the CNN to correctly classify medical images and a pre-trained classifier to extract features in the images. The study showed that CNN outperformed the pre-trained classifier and accuracy improved significantly. In another study, Byra et al. [127] described a CAD approach that uses the Nakagami imaging method to train a CNN model, aimed at breast cancer diagnosis. The study was tested on 458 RF data matrices of breast lesions. The study showed that better area under the curve (AUC) results that amounts to 0.912 were obtained. Gao et al. [128] extended the use of CNN using the INbreast dataset to overcome the challenges faced with the contrast-enhanced digital mammography (CEDM), which is prone to a high false-positive rate. CNN was effective at differentiating benign cases from malignant lesions, which is the main challenge faced with a breast cancer diagnosis.

In a similar study, Wang et al. [129] explored a CAD method that utilizes feature fusion with CNN using a private dataset. The method uses CNN for feature extraction based on several image sub-regions. After the feature extraction tasks, the images were then classified into benign or malignant.

The study concluded that this task outperformed other existing methods. Murtaza et al. [124] applied the use of CNN on the BreakHis dataset to improve the detection of breast cancer. The study reported a high accuracy with the use of the CNN model. Other interesting areas of application of CNN to breast cancer diagnosis are found in the following references [126,130–136].

3.2.2. Generative Adversarial Networks

The advent of generative adversarial networks (GANs) by Goodfellow [137] has opened a new area of research within the image segmentation domain. According to Kazeminia et al. [138], GANs have been shown to generate realistic-looking images in the large, unlabelled corpus. One of the many challenges faced within the CV and medical image analysis (MIA) community is the heavy reliance on labelled training data, which can be a major limitation [7]. The communities have recognized the potential of GANs and have eagerly investigated in its efficacy to tackle many problems. Recently, a good deal of research has leveraged the use of GANs for image-to-image translation [139,140]. GANs have found many applications in generative modelling and distribution learning [139]. Furthermore, GANs unique generation and identification network is increasingly used for image segmentation and has achieved good results. GANs create outputs using its discriminator and generator [141]. Figure 3 shows the structure of GANs.

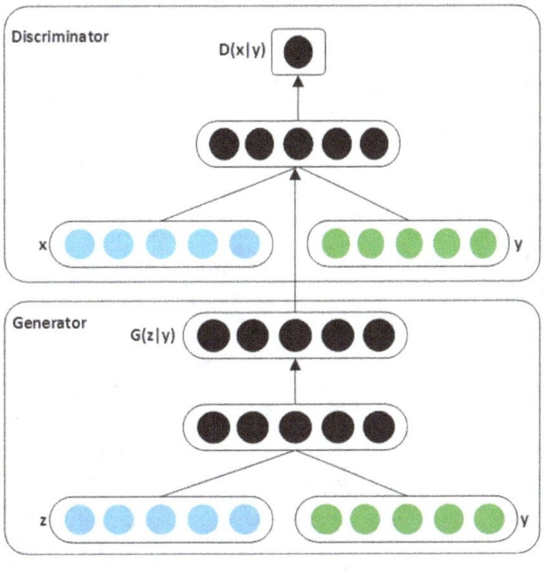

Figure 3. Structure of a generative adversarial networks (GANs) [142].

Shams et al. [143] developed DiaGRAM (deep GenerRAtive multi-task), which is based on GANs and CNN in a mammography study to detect early signs of breast cancer. The study concluded that feature learning with GANs led to high classification performance and an effective end-to-end scheme. A study by Singh et al. [144] applied GANs to segment mammographic images from regions of interests (ROIs) with varying length and sizes. GANs helped eliminate issues of overfitting on the datasets (INbreast and digital database for screening mammography (DDSM)) and showed effectiveness in the screening of cases. Wu et al. [145] addressed the issue of limited data and class imbalance for breast cancer classification using GANs. The classification performance of GANs was compared with other augmentation methods. The results showed that GANs improved the classification task. Guan et al. [146] applied GANs to generate synthetic images from a digital database for screening mammography. The authors opined that GANs performed better in augmenting the training dataset, which was useful for the study. Together, we have discussed the CNN and GANs approaches to breast cancer detection. Most of the works presented in this section are summarised in Table 2. In the table, we present the deep learning techniques, and scope of work that are used for breast cancer diagnosis. In addition, the performance metrics for each technique and the type of dataset used were presented.

Table 2. Summary of deep learning models in breast cancer diagnosis.

Reference	Deep Learning Technique	Scope	Evaluation Results	Datasets
Tan et al. [126]	CNN	Classification	Accuracy = 82%	mini-Mammographic Image Analysis Society (mini-MIAS)
Amit et al. [122]	CNN	Classification	Accuracy = 83%, Area under the curve = 0.91	ED (MRI)
Byra et al. [127]	CNN	Classification	Accuracy = 83%, Area under the curve = 0.912	ED (US, Nakagami)
Gao et al. [128]	CNN	Classification	Accuracy = 90% Area under the curve = 0.92	INbreast
Wang et al. [129]	CNN	Classification	Accuracy = 76.5%	Private
Tan et al. [126]	CNN	Classification	Accuracy = 95%, Area under the curve = 0.97	BreakHis
Litjens et al. [130]	CNN	Classification	Area under the curve = 0.99	Private
Araújo et al. [132]	CNN	Classification	Accuracy = 77.8% (four classes), Accuracy = 83.3% (two classes)	BICBH
Ragab et al. [135]	CNN with SVM	Feature extraction	Accuracy = 73%, Area under the curve = 0.94	Digital Database for Screening Mammography (DDSM), CBIS-DDSM
Acharya et al. [136]	CNN with K-means	Feature extraction	Accuracy = 97%	Private
Karthik et al. [147]	DNN	Classification	Accuracy = 98%	WBC
Yu et al. [134]	DNN + CNN	Classification	Accuracy = 81%, Area under the curve = 0.88	BCDR
Sun et al. [131]	CNN	Classification	Accuracy = 82.43%, Area under the curve = 0.8818	ED(Mg)
Hadad et al. [148]	CNN	Classification	Accuracy = 94%, Area under the curve = 0.98	ED(Mg, MRI)
Nahid et al. [123]	CNN	Classification	Accuracy = 91%	BreakHis
Shams et al. [143]	GANs	Classification	Area under the curve = 0.88, Area under the curve = 0.925	DDSM, INbreast
Singh et al. [144]	GANs + CNN	Classification	Accuracy = 72%	DDSM and Private
Wu et al. [149]	GANs	Classification	Accuracy = 89%	DDSM
Guan et al. [146]	GANs	Classification	Accuracy = 79.8%	DDSM

3.3. Robotics

With the improvements in medical robots' accuracy, robots in healthcare now assist by relieving medical practitioners from their routine tasks and also make medical procedures less costly and safer for patients [129]. These could be the reasons research into creating robots to detect and diagnose breast cancer in patients have been gaining popularity in the last decade. Robotics as a branch of AI, is developed based on some machine learning algorithms [129,150]. Such algorithms include but are not limited to reinforcement learning and deep reinforcement learning [150].

3.3.1. Reinforcement Learning

Reinforcement learning is an approach to machine learning that involves computational learning by interaction. It involves learning about what to do and how to map situations to actions to maximize a numerical solution. Unlike other machine learning approaches, reinforcement learning does not directly demonstrate how to perform a task but works through the problem on its own [129,150].

Examples of systems that are built based on the unsupervised learning approach of reinforcement learning are self-driving cars, a program playing chess (e.g., Alphago), etc. These systems interact with their environment, such that, when they complete a task successfully, they receive a reward state. Such tasks could be driving to a destination safely or winning a game. On the other hand, when the system does not complete a task successfully, they receive a penalty for performing incorrectly. Such a task could also be going off the road or being checkmated [150].

These systems, over time, make decisions to maximize their reward and minimize their penalty using dynamic programming. The advantage of this approach to AI is that it allows an AI program to learn without a programmer spelling out how a system should perform the task; this type of approach is popularly called unsupervised learning [150].

3.3.2. Robotic Tools for Breast Cancer Diagnosis

In the research reported by Kato et al. [151], a robotic system called WAPRO-4 was developed for the automatic palpation of breast cancer. The study aimed at palpating and diagnosing breast cancer without the assistance of medical personnel. The major objective was to aid the early detection of breast cancer. Additionally, WAPRO-4 consists of three parts which include the measuring instrument, the locomotion unit, and the microcomputer system [151]. The WAPRO-4 was constructed to detect tumors while ignoring breathing and the configuration of the chest wall. Kobayashi et al. [152] developed a palpation-based needle insertion method for diagnostic biopsy and treatment of breast cancer. The system locates cancerous tissues from force information and reduces tissue during needle insertion. Kobayashi et al. [152] compared the palpation-based needle insertion approach to the normal needle insertion approach using a numerical simulation of a breast tissue model. The outcome showed that palpation-based needle insertion had a smaller error which suggests that the procedure could be a safe and effective alternative [152].

Larson et al. [153] developed a robotic device to perform minimally invasive breast interventions with real-time MRI guidance for the early diagnosis and treatment of breast cancer. In this work, five computer-controlled degrees of freedom were used to perform minimally invasive interventions inside a closed MRI scanner. According to Larson et al. [153], the intervention consists of a biopsy of the suspicious lesion for diagnosis, which involves the therapies to destroy or remove malignant tissue in the breast. As a result, the procedure includes conditioning of the breast along with a prescribed orientation, the definition of an insertion vector by its height and pitch angle, and insertion into the breast. The entire device is made of materials compatible with an MRI machine, avoiding artefacts and distortion of the local magnetic field. This device was built to be remotely controlled via a graphical user interface.

Meanwhile, automated detection of breast lesions from DCE-MRI volumes was implemented based on deep reinforcement learning [154]. The method significantly reduces the inference time for lesion detection compared to an exhaustive search, while retaining state-of-the-art accuracy. The authors demonstrated their results on a dataset containing 117 DCE-MRI volumes, validating runtime and accuracy of lesion detection [154,155].

Moreover, Tsekos et al. [155] implemented a robotic device with haptic, tactile, and ultrasound capabilities, that can acquire and render the information of breast pathology remotely. In this work, the device is designed to screen for breast cancer by examination for the patient in a remote area without convenient access to medical personnel. The device was said to be more accurate than human medical personnel [155]. Further, a robotic based device designed to assist medical personnel in placing the instrument on the tumor location and automatically acquiring tumor images in real-time was implemented in [153,156]. This device has the potential to increase targeting accuracy while reducing the level of skill required to perform minimally invasive breast interventional procedures.

4. Conclusions

Breast cancer has shown to be one of the leading causes of female mortality in the world. Recent studies have shown that early diagnosis is the first step towards a successful treatment, which can help save many lives. This review presented a brief overview of past and present conventional diagnostics approaches as well as recent computational techniques that have contributed immensely to the diagnosis of breast cancer. Articles on breast cancer classification published from 2006 to 2020 were extensively reviewed. In total, 55 were carefully reviewed from different academic repositories. Several criteria were used for the review, such as conventional diagnostics approaches, the computational technique used, scope, evaluation results, and different types of datasets were used for these studies. We noticed that researchers preferred publicly available datasets over exclusive ones. For example, WBC and DDSM were seen to be popular among researchers. For computational approaches, we reviewed three areas: Machine learning, deep learning, and robotics. Out of these approaches, the deep learning techniques appear to be increasingly popular for most researchers. Among these techniques, we noticed that CNN was a popular choice, used for classification. Currently, GANs have shown to be a promising deep learning algorithm for breast cancer diagnosis due to its ability to give convincingly good results. Performance metrics such as AUC, accuracy, sensitivity, specificity, and measure were used for evaluating deep learning approaches.

Finally, this review provides a roadmap for future conversations about building better techniques for early detection, which could help save millions of lives. We believe that this comprehensive review will offer a better understanding of the breast cancer classification domain and provide valuable insights to researchers in this field.

Author Contributions: K.A., G.O., B.O., T.A.A., and R.T.A. conceived the idea; K.A., G.O., B.O., T.A.A., A.O.F., A.K., and R.T.A. designed and wrote the manuscript. All authors have read and agreed to the published version of the manuscript.

References

1. Adekiya, T.A.; Aruleba, R.T.; Khanyile, S.; Masamba, P.; Oyinloye, B.E.; Kappo, A.P. Structural analysis and epitope prediction of MHC class-1-chain related protein-a for cancer vaccine development. *Vaccines* **2018**, *6*, 1. [CrossRef]
2. Aruleba, R.T.; Adekiya, T.A.; Oyinloye, B.E.; Kappo, A.P. Structural studies of predicted ligand binding sites and molecular docking analysis of Slc2a4 as a therapeutic target for the treatment of cancer. *Int. J. Mol. Sci.* **2018**, *19*, 386. [CrossRef]
3. Oyinloye, B.E.; Adekiya, T.A.; Aruleba, R.T.; Ojo, O.A.; Ajiboye, B.O. Structure-Based Docking Studies of GLUT4 Towards Exploring Selected Phytochemicals from Solanum xanthocarpum as a Therapeutic Target for the Treatment of Cancer. *Curr. Drug Discov. Technol.* **2019**, *16*, 406–416. [CrossRef]
4. Shapiro, C.L. Cancer survivorship. *N. Engl. J. Med.* **2018**, *379*, 2438–2450. [CrossRef]
5. Akram, M.; Iqbal, M.; Daniyal, M.; Khan, A.U. Awareness and current knowledge of breast cancer. *Biol. Res.* **2017**, *50*, 33. [CrossRef]
6. Singh, S.K.; Singh, S.; Lillard, J.W., Jr.; Singh, R. Drug delivery approaches for breast cancer. *Int. J. Nanomed.* **2017**, *12*, 6205. [CrossRef]
7. Wang, H.; Zheng, B.; Yoon, S.W.; Ko, H.S. A support vector machine-based ensemble algorithm for breast cancer diagnosis. *Eur. J. Oper. Res.* **2018**, *267*, 687–699. [CrossRef]
8. Dande, P.; Samant, P. Acquaintance to artificial neural networks and use of artificial intelligence as a diagnostic tool for tuberculosis: A review. *Tuberculosis* **2018**, *108*, 1–9. [CrossRef]
9. Lengauer, T.; Sing, T. Bioinformatics-assisted anti-HIV therapy. *Nat. Rev. Genet.* **2006**, *4*, 790–797. [CrossRef]

10. Vaishya, R.; Javaid, M.; Khan, I.H.; Haleem, A. Artificial Intelligence (AI) applications for COVID-19 pandemic. *Diabet. Metab. Syndr. Clin. Res. Rev.* **2020**, *14*, 337–339. [CrossRef]
11. Nover, A.B.; Jagtap, S.; Anjum, W.; Yegingil, H.; Shih, W.Y.; Shih, W.-H.; Brooks, A.D. Modern breast cancer detection: A technological review. *Int. J. Biomed. Imaging* **2009**, *2009*, 1–14. [CrossRef] [PubMed]
12. Kolb, T.M.; Lichy, J.; Newhouse, J.H. Comparison of the performance of screening mammography, physical examination, and breast US and evaluation of factors that influence them: An analysis of 27825 patient evaluations. *Radiology* **2002**, *225*, 165–175. [CrossRef] [PubMed]
13. Nelson, H.D.; Tyne, K.; Naik, A.; Bougatsos, C.; Chan, B.K.; Humphrey, L. Screening for breast cancer: An update for the US Preventive Services Task Force. *Ann. Intern. Med.* **2009**, *151*, 727–737. [CrossRef] [PubMed]
14. Bagni, B.; Franceschetto, A.; Casolo, A.; De Santis, M.; Bagni, I.; Pansini, F.; Di Leo, C. Scintimammography with 99mTc-MIBI and magnetic resonance imaging in the evaluation of breast cancer. *Eur. J. Nucl. Med. Mol. Imaging* **2003**, *30*, 1383–1388. [CrossRef]
15. Lladó, X.; Oliver, A.; Freixenet, J.; Martí, R.; Martí, J. A textural approach for mass false positive reduction in mammography. *Comput. Med. Imaging Graph.* **2009**, *33*, 415–422. [CrossRef] [PubMed]
16. Aiken, L.S.; West, S.G.; Woodward, C.K.; Reno, R.R. Health beliefs and compliance with mammography-screening recommendations in asymptomatic women. *Health Psychol.* **1994**, *13*, 122. [CrossRef]
17. Kennedy, D.A.; Lee, T.; Seely, D. A comparative review of thermography as a breast cancer screening technique. *Integr. Cancer Ther.* **2009**, *8*, 9–16. [CrossRef]
18. Schillaci, O.; Buscombe, J.R. Breast scintigraphy today: Indications and limitations. *Eur. J. Nucl. Med. Mol. Imaging* **2004**, *31*, S35–S45. [CrossRef]
19. Cherel, P.; Hagay, C.; Benaim, B.; De Maulmont, C.; Engerand, S.; Langer, A.; Talma, V. Mammographic evaluation of dense breasts: Techniques and limits. *J. Radiol.* **2008**, *89*, 1156. [CrossRef]
20. Mori, M.; Akashi-Tanaka, S.; Suzuki, S.; Daniels, M.I.; Watanabe, C.; Hirose, M.; Nakamura, S. Diagnostic accuracy of contrast-enhanced spectral mammography in comparison to conventional full-field digital mammography in a population of women with dense breasts. *Breast Cancer* **2017**, *24*, 104–110. [CrossRef]
21. Jung, J.I.; Kim, H.H.; Park, S.H.; Song, S.W.; Chung, M.H.; Kim, H.S.; Kim, K.J.; Ahn, M.I.; Seo, S.B.; Hahn, S.T. Thoracic manifestations of breast cancer and its therapy. *Radiographics* **2004**, *24*, 1269–1285. [CrossRef] [PubMed]
22. Savaridas, S.L.; Spratt, J.D.; Cox, J. Incidence and potential significance of internal mammary lymphadenopathy on computed tomography in patients with a diagnosis of primary breast cancer. *Breast Cancer Basic Clin. Res.* **2015**, *9*. [CrossRef] [PubMed]
23. Dobbins, J.T. Tomosynthesis imaging: At a translational crossroads. *Med. Phys.* **2009**, *36*, 1956–1967. [CrossRef] [PubMed]
24. Friedewald, S.M.; Rafferty, E.A.; Rose, S.L.; Durand, M.A.; Plecha, D.M.; Greenberg, J.S.; Hayes, M.K.; Copit, D.S.; Carlson, K.L.; Cink, T.M. Breast cancer screening using tomosynthesis in combination with digital mammography. *JAMA* **2014**, *311*, 2499–2507. [CrossRef] [PubMed]
25. Niklason, L.T.; Christian, B.T.; Niklason, L.E.; Kopans, D.B.; Castleberry, D.E.; Opsahl-Ong, B.; Landberg, C.E.; Slanetz, P.J.; Giardino, A.A.; Moore, R. Digital tomosynthesis in breast imaging. *Radiology* **1997**, *205*, 399–406. [CrossRef] [PubMed]
26. Poplack, S.P.; Tosteson, T.D.; Kogel, C.A.; Nagy, H.M. Digital breast tomosynthesis: Initial experience in 98 women with abnormal digital screening mammography. *Am. J. Roentgenol.* **2007**, *189*, 616–623. [CrossRef] [PubMed]
27. Lång, K.; Andersson, I.; Rosso, A.; Tingberg, A.; Timberg, P.; Zackrisson, S. Performance of one-view breast tomosynthesis as a stand-alone breast cancer screening modality: Results from the Malmö Breast Tomosynthesis Screening Trial, a population-based study. *Eur. Radiol.* **2016**, *26*, 184–190. [CrossRef]
28. Sechopoulos, I. A review of breast tomosynthesis. Part I. The image acquisition process. *Med. Phys.* **2013**, *40*, 014301. [CrossRef]
29. Van de Sompel, D.; Brady, M.; Boone, J. Task-based performance analysis of FBP, SART and ML for digital breast tomosynthesis using signal CNR and Channelised Hotelling Observers. *Med. Image Anal.* **2011**, *15*, 53–70. [CrossRef]
30. O'Brien, W.D., Jr. Ultrasound–biophysics mechanisms. *Prog. Biophys. Mol. Biol.* **2007**, *93*, 212–255.
31. Mason, T.J. Therapeutic ultrasound an overview. *Ultrason. Sonochem.* **2011**, *18*, 847–852. [CrossRef]

32. Dewall, R.J. Ultrasound elastography: Principles, techniques, and clinical applications. *Crit. Rev. Biomed. Eng.* **2013**, *41*, 1–19. [CrossRef] [PubMed]
33. Guo, R.; Lu, G.; Qin, B.; Fei, B. Ultrasound Imaging Technologies for Breast Cancer Detection and Management: A Review. *Ultrasound Med. Biol.* **2018**, *44*, 37–70. [CrossRef]
34. Thornton, G.D.; McPhail, M.J.W.; Nayagam, S.; Hewitt, M.J.; Vlavianos, P.; Monahan, K.J. Endoscopic ultrasound guided fine needle aspiration for the diagnosis of pancreatic cystic neoplasms: A meta-analysis. *Pancreatology* **2013**, *13*, 48–57. [CrossRef]
35. Liu, R.; Adler, D.G. Duplication cysts: Diagnosis, management, and the role of endoscopic ultrasound. *Endosc. Ultrasound* **2014**, *3*, 152–160. [CrossRef]
36. Park, M.K.; Jo, J.; Kwon, H.; Cho, J.H.; Oh, J.Y.; Noh, M.H.; Nam, K.J. Usefulness of acoustic radiation force impulse elastography in the differential diagnosis of benign and malignant solid pancreatic lesions. *Ultrasonography* **2014**, *33*, 26. [CrossRef] [PubMed]
37. Xie, X.-H.; Xu, H.-X.; Xie, X.-Y.; Lu, M.-D.; Kuang, M.; Xu, Z.-F.; Liu, G.-J.; Wang, Z.; Liang, J.-Y.; Chen, L.-D. Differential diagnosis between benign and malignant gallbladder diseases with real-time contrast-enhanced ultrasound. *Eur. Radiol.* **2010**, *20*, 239–248. [CrossRef] [PubMed]
38. Masroor, I.; Afzal, S.; Suffian, S.N. Imaging guided breast interventions. *J. Coll. Physicians Surg. Pak.* **2016**, *26*, 521–526.
39. Giuliano, V.; Giuliano, C. Improved breast cancer detection in asymptomatic women using 3D-automated breast ultrasound in mammographically dense breasts. *Clin. Imaging* **2013**, *37*, 480–486. [CrossRef]
40. Bachawal, S.V.; Jensen, K.C.; Lutz, A.M.; Gambhir, S.S.; Tranquart, F.; Tian, L.; Willmann, J.K. Earlier detection of breast cancer with ultrasound molecular imaging in a transgenic mouse model. *Cancer Res.* **2013**, *73*, 1689–1698. [CrossRef]
41. Lindfors, K.K.; Boone, J.M.; Nelson, T.R.; Yang, K.; Kwan, A.L.; Miller, D.F. Dedicated breast CT: Initial clinical experience. *Radiology* **2008**, *246*, 725–733. [CrossRef]
42. Kuzmiak, C.M.; Cole, E.B.; Zeng, D.; Tuttle, L.A.; Steed, D.; Pisano, E.D. Dedicated three-dimensional breast computed tomography: Lesion characteristic perception by radiologists. *J. Clin. Imaging Sci.* **2016**, *6*, 14. [CrossRef]
43. Shah, J.P.; Mann, S.D.; McKinley, R.L.; Tornai, M.P. Characterization of CT Hounsfield units for 3D acquisition trajectories on a dedicated breast CT system. *J. X-ray Sci. Technol.* **2018**, *26*, 535–551. [CrossRef]
44. Boone, J.M.; Nelson, T.R.; Lindfors, K.K.; Seibert, J.A. Dedicated breast CT: Radiation dose and image quality evaluation. *Radiology* **2001**, *221*, 657–667. [CrossRef]
45. Sarno, A.; Mettivier, G.; Russo, P. Dedicated breast computed tomography: Basic aspects. *Med. Phys.* **2015**, *42*, 2786–2804. [CrossRef]
46. Radhakrishna, S.; Agarwal, S.; Parikh, P.M.; Kaur, K.; Panwar, S.; Sharma, S.; Dey, A.; Saxena, K.; Chandra, M.; Sud, S. Role of magnetic resonance imaging in breast cancer management. *South Asian J. Cancer* **2018**, *7*, 69–71. [CrossRef]
47. Sardanelli, F.; Giuseppetti, G.M.; Panizza, P.; Bazzocchi, M.; Fausto, A.; Simonetti, G.; Lattanzio, V.; Del Maschio, A. Sensitivity of MRI versus mammography for detecting foci of multifocal, multicentric breast cancer in fatty and dense breasts using the whole-breast pathologic examination as a gold standard. *Am. J. Roentgenol.* **2004**, *183*, 1149–1157. [CrossRef]
48. Lee, C.H.; Dershaw, D.D.; Kopans, D.; Evans, P.; Monsees, B.; Monticciolo, D.; Brenner, R.J.; Bassett, L.; Berg, W.; Feig, S. Breast cancer screening with imaging: Recommendations from the Society of Breast Imaging and the ACR on the use of mammography, breast MRI, breast ultrasound, and other technologies for the detection of clinically occult breast cancer. *J. Am. Coll. Radiol.* **2010**, *7*, 18–27. [CrossRef]
49. Morrow, M.; Waters, J.; Morris, E. MRI for breast cancer screening, diagnosis, and treatment. *Lancet* **2011**, *378*, 1804–1811. [CrossRef]
50. Gareth, E.D.; Nisha, K.; Yit, L.; Soujanye, G.; Emma, H.; Massat, N.J.; Maxwell, A.J.; Sarah, I.; Rosalind, E.; Leach, M.O. MRI breast screening in high-risk women: Cancer detection and survival analysis. *Breast Cancer Res. Treat.* **2014**, *145*, 663–672. [CrossRef]
51. Lehman, C.D.; Gatsonis, C.; Kuhl, C.K.; Hendrick, R.E.; Pisano, E.D.; Hanna, L.; Peacock, S.; Smazal, S.F.; Maki, D.D.; Julian, T.B. MRI evaluation of the contralateral breast in women with recently diagnosed breast cancer. *N. Engl. J. Med.* **2007**, *356*, 1295–1303. [CrossRef] [PubMed]

52. Passaperuma, K.; Warner, E.; Causer, P.; Hill, K.; Messner, S.; Wong, J.; Jong, R.; Wright, F.; Yaffe, M.; Ramsay, E. Long-term results of screening with magnetic resonance imaging in women with BRCA mutations. *Br. J. Cancer* **2012**, *107*, 24–30. [CrossRef] [PubMed]
53. Bang, O.Y.; Li, W. Applications of diffusion-weighted imaging in diagnosis, evaluation, and treatment of acute ischemic stroke. *Precis. Future Med.* **2019**, *3*, 69–76. [CrossRef]
54. Chung, J.W.; Park, S.H.; Kim, N.; Kim, W.J.; Park, J.H.; Ko, Y.; Yang, M.H.; Jang, M.S.; Han, M.K.; Jung, C. Trial of ORG 10172 in Acute Stroke Treatment (TOAST) classification and vascular territory of ischemic stroke lesions diagnosed by diffusion-weighted imaging. *J. Am. Heart Assoc.* **2014**, *3*, e001119. [CrossRef] [PubMed]
55. Malayeri, A.A.; El Khouli, R.H.; Zaheer, A.; Jacobs, M.A.; Corona-Villalobos, C.P.; Kamel, I.R.; Macura, K.J. Principles and applications of diffusion-weighted imaging in cancer detection, staging, and treatment follow-up. *Radiographics* **2011**, *31*, 1773–1791. [CrossRef] [PubMed]
56. Sinha, S.; Lucas-Quesada, F.A.; Sinha, U.; De Bruhl, N.; Bassett, L.W. In vivo diffusion-weighted MRI of the breast: Potential for lesion characterization. *J. Magn. Reson. Imaging* **2002**, *15*, 693–704. [CrossRef]
57. Menezes, G.L.; Knuttel, F.M.; Stehouwer, B.L.; Pijnappel, R.M.; van den Bosch, M.A. Magnetic resonance imaging in breast cancer: A literature review and future perspectives. *World J. Clin. Oncol.* **2014**, *5*, 61. [CrossRef]
58. Costantini, M.; Belli, P.; Rinaldi, P.; Bufi, E.; Giardina, G.; Franceschini, G.; Petrone, G.; Bonomo, L. Diffusion-weighted imaging in breast cancer: Relationship between apparent diffusion coefficient and tumour aggressiveness. *Clin. Radiol.* **2010**, *65*, 1005–1012. [CrossRef]
59. Tan, S.; Rahmat, K.; Rozalli, F.; Mohd-Shah, M.; Aziz, Y.; Yip, C.; Vijayananthan, A.; Ng, K. Differentiation between benign and malignant breast lesions using quantitative diffusion-weighted sequence on 3 T MRI. *Clin. Radiol.* **2014**, *69*, 63–71. [CrossRef]
60. Baltzer, P.A.; Bickel, H.; Spick, C.; Wengert, G.; Woitek, R.; Kapetas, P.; Clauser, P.; Helbich, T.H.; Pinker, K. Potential of noncontrast magnetic resonance imaging with diffusion-weighted imaging in characterization of breast lesions: Intraindividual comparison with dynamic contrast-enhanced magnetic resonance imaging. *Investig. Radiol.* **2018**, *53*, 229–235. [CrossRef]
61. Chilla, G.S.; Tan, C.H.; Xu, C.; Poh, C.L. Diffusion weighted magnetic resonance imaging and its recent trend—A survey. *Quant. Imaging Med. Surg.* **2015**, *5*, 407. [PubMed]
62. Baliyan, V.; Das, C.J.; Sharma, R.; Gupta, A.K. Diffusion weighted imaging: Technique and applications. *World J. Radiol.* **2016**, *8*, 785. [CrossRef] [PubMed]
63. Scarfe, W.C.; Li, Z.; Aboelmaaty, W.; Scott, S.; Farman, A. Maxillofacial cone beam computed tomography: Essence, elements and steps to interpretation. *Aust. Dent. J.* **2012**, *57*, 46–60. [CrossRef] [PubMed]
64. Sun, W.; Lal, P. Recent development on computer aided tissue engineering—A review. *Comput. Methods Programs Biomed.* **2002**, *67*, 85–103. [CrossRef]
65. Suga, K.; Yuan, Y.; Ogasawara, N.; Okada, M.; Matsunaga, N. Localization of breast sentinel lymph nodes by MR lymphography with a conventional gadolinium contrast agent: Preliminary observations in dongs and humans. *Acta Radiol.* **2003**, *44*, 35–42. [CrossRef] [PubMed]
66. Foo, S.Y.; Gray, K. Computed tomography (CT) staging in breast cancer. *Clin. Radiol.* **2015**, *70*, S13. [CrossRef]
67. Okamura, Y.; Yoshizawa, N.; Yamaguchi, M.; Kashiwakura, I. Application of dual-energy computed tomography for breast cancer diagnosis. *Int. J. Med. Phys. Clin. Eng. Radiat. Oncol.* **2016**, *5*, 288–297. [CrossRef]
68. Park, E.K.; Seo, B.K.; Kwon, M.; Cho, K.R.; Woo, O.H.; Song, S.E.; Cha, J.; Lee, H.Y. Low-dose perfusion computed tomography for breast cancer to quantify tumor vascularity: Correlation with prognostic biomarkers. *Investig. Radiol.* **2019**, *54*, 273–281. [CrossRef] [PubMed]
69. Shah, J.P.; Mann, S.D.; McKinley, R.L.; Tornai, M.P. Three dimensional dose distribution comparison of simple and complex acquisition trajectories in dedicated breast CT. *Med. Phys.* **2015**, *42*, 4497–4510. [CrossRef]
70. Hawrysz, D.J.; Sevick-Muraca, E.M. Developments toward diagnostic breast cancer imaging using near-infrared optical measurements and fluorescent contrast agents1. *Neoplasia* **2000**, *2*, 388–417. [CrossRef]
71. Troyan, S.L.; Kianzad, V.; Gibbs-Strauss, S.L.; Gioux, S.; Matsui, A.; Oketokoun, R.; Ngo, L.; Khamene, A.; Azar, F.; Frangioni, J.V. The FLARE™ intraoperative near-infrared fluorescence imaging system: A first-in-human clinical trial in breast cancer sentinel lymph node mapping. *Ann. Surg. Oncol.* **2009**, *16*, 2943–2952. [CrossRef] [PubMed]

72. Tagaya, N.; Yamazaki, R.; Nakagawa, A.; Abe, A.; Hamada, K.; Kubota, K.; Oyama, T. Intraoperative identification of sentinel lymph nodes by near-infrared fluorescence imaging in patients with breast cancer. *Am. J. Surg.* **2008**, *195*, 850–853. [CrossRef] [PubMed]
73. Verbeek, F.P.; Troyan, S.L.; Mieog, J.S.D.; Liefers, G.-J.; Moffitt, L.A.; Rosenberg, M.; Hirshfield-Bartek, J.; Gioux, S.; van de Velde, C.J.; Vahrmeijer, A.L. Near-infrared fluorescence sentinel lymph node mapping in breast cancer: A multicenter experience. *Breast Cancer Res. Treat.* **2014**, *143*, 333–342. [CrossRef] [PubMed]
74. Mieog, J.S.D.; Troyan, S.L.; Hutteman, M.; Donohoe, K.J.; Van Der Vorst, J.R.; Stockdale, A.; Liefers, G.-J.; Choi, H.S.; Gibbs-Strauss, S.L.; Putter, H. Toward optimization of imaging system and lymphatic tracer for near-infrared fluorescent sentinel lymph node mapping in breast cancer. *Ann. Surg. Oncol.* **2011**, *18*, 2483–2491. [CrossRef] [PubMed]
75. Sevick-Muraca, E.M.; Sharma, R.; Rasmussen, J.C.; Marshall, M.V.; Wendt, J.A.; Pham, H.Q.; Bonefas, E.; Houston, J.P.; Sampath, L.; Adams, K.E. Imaging of lymph flow in breast cancer patients after microdose administration of a near-infrared fluorophore: Feasibility study. *Radiology* **2008**, *246*, 734–741. [CrossRef]
76. Altınoğlu, E.I.; Russin, T.J.; Kaiser, J.M.; Barth, B.M.; Eklund, P.C.; Kester, M.; Adair, J.H. Near-infrared emitting fluorophore-doped calcium phosphate nanoparticles for in vivo imaging of human breast cancer. *ACS Nano* **2008**, *2*, 2075–2084. [CrossRef] [PubMed]
77. Poellinger, A.; Burock, S.; Grosenick, D.; Hagen, A.; Lüdemann, L.; Diekmann, F.; Engelken, F.; Macdonald, R.; Rinneberg, H.; Schlag, P.-M. Breast cancer: Early-and late-fluorescence near-infrared imaging with indocyanine green—A preliminary study. *Radiology* **2011**, *258*, 409–416. [CrossRef]
78. Ke, S.; Wen, X.; Gurfinkel, M.; Charnsangavej, C.; Wallace, S.; Sevick-Muraca, E.M.; Li, C. Near-infrared optical imaging of epidermal growth factor receptor in breast cancer xenografts. *Cancer Res.* **2003**, *63*, 7870–7875.
79. Vallabhajosula, S.; Polack, B.D.; Babich, J.W. Molecular Imaging of Prostate Cancer: Radiopharmaceuticals for Positron Emission Tomography (PET) and Single-Photon Emission Computed Tomography (SPECT). In *Precision Molecular Pathology of Prostate Cancer*; Springer: Berlin/Heidelberg, Germany, 2018; pp. 475–501.
80. Pellikka, P.A.; She, L.; Holly, T.A.; Lin, G.; Varadarajan, P.; Pai, R.G.; Bonow, R.O.; Pohost, G.M.; Panza, J.A.; Berman, D.S. Variability in ejection fraction measured by echocardiography, gated single-photon emission computed tomography, and cardiac magnetic resonance in patients with coronary artery disease and left ventricular dysfunction. *JAMA Netw. Open* **2018**, *1*, e181456. [CrossRef]
81. Noyce, A.J.; Dickson, J.; Rees, R.N.; Bestwick, J.P.; Isaias, I.U.; Politis, M.; Giovannoni, G.; Warner, T.T.; Lees, A.J.; Schrag, A. Dopamine reuptake transporter-single-photon emission computed tomography and transcranial sonography as imaging markers of prediagnostic Parkinson's disease. *Mov. Disord.* **2018**, *33*, 478–482. [CrossRef]
82. Frangioni, J.V. New technologies for human cancer imaging. *J. Clin. Oncol.* **2008**, *26*, 4012. [CrossRef] [PubMed]
83. Koizumi, M.; Koyama, M. Comparison between single photon emission computed tomography with computed tomography and planar scintigraphy in sentinel node biopsy in breast cancer patients. *Ann. Nucl. Med.* **2019**, *33*, 160–168. [CrossRef] [PubMed]
84. Van der Ploeg, I.M.; Nieweg, O.E.; Kroon, B.B.; Rutgers, E.J.; Baas-Vrancken Peeters, M.J.; Vogel, W.V.; Hoefnagel, C.A.; Olmos, R.A. The yield of SPECT/CT for anatomical lymphatic mapping in patients with breast cancer. *Eur. J. Nucl. Med. Mol. Imaging* **2009**, *36*, 903–909. [CrossRef] [PubMed]
85. Maza, S.; Valencia, R.; Geworski, L.; Zander, A.; Guski, H.; Winzer, K.J.; Munz, D.L. Peritumoural versus subareolar administration of technetium-99m nanocolloid for sentinel lymph node detection in breast cancer: Preliminary results of a prospective intra-individual comparative study. *Eur. J. Nucl. Med. Mol. Imaging* **2003**, *30*, 651–656. [CrossRef] [PubMed]
86. Lerman, H.; Lievshitz, G.; Zak, O.; Metser, U.; Schneebaum, S.; Even-Sapir, E. Improved sentinel node identification by SPECT/CT in overweight patients with breast cancer. *J. Nucl. Med.* **2007**, *48*, 201–206.
87. Pecking, A.P.; Wartski, W.; Cluzan, R.; Bellet, D.; Albérini, J. SPECT–CT fusion imaging radionuclide lymphoscintigraphy: Potential for limb lymphedema assessment and sentinel node detection in breast cancer. In *Cancer Metastasis and the Lymphovascular System: Basis for Rational Therapy*; Springer: Berlin/Heidelberg, Germany, 2007; pp. 79–84.
88. Mann, S.D.; Perez, K.L.; McCracken, E.K.; Shah, J.P.; Wong, T.Z.; Tornai, M.P. Initial in vivo quantification of Tc-99m sestamibi uptake as a function of tissue type in healthy breasts using dedicated breast SPECT-CT. *J. Oncol.* **2012**, *2012*, 1–7. [CrossRef]

89. Bowen, S.L.; Wu, Y.; Chaudhari, A.J.; Fu, L.; Packard, N.J.; Burkett, G.W.; Yang, K.; Lindfors, K.K.; Shelton, D.K.; Hagge, R. Initial characterization of a dedicated breast PET/CT scanner during human imaging. *J. Nucl. Med.* **2009**, *50*, 1401–1408. [CrossRef]
90. Tornai, M.P.; Shah, J.P.; Mann, S.D.; McKinley, R.L. Development of Fully-3D CT in a Hybrid SPECT-CT Breast Imaging System. In Proceedings of the 13th International Workshop on Breast Imaging, Malmo, Sweden, 19–22 June 2016; pp. 567–575.
91. Crotty, D.J.; Brady, S.L.; Jackson, D.V.C.; Toncheva, G.I.; Anderson, C.E.; Yoshizumi, T.T.; Tornai, M.P. Evaluation of the absorbed dose to the breast using radiochromic film in a dedicated CT mammotomography system employing a quasi-monochromatic X-ray beam. *Med. Phys.* **2011**, *38*, 3232–3245. [CrossRef]
92. Suthaharan, S. Machine learning models and algorithms for big data classification. *Integr. Ser. Inf. Syst.* **2016**, *36*, 1–12.
93. Tsai, H.-H.; Chang, Y.-C. Facial expression recognition using a combination of multiple facial features and support vector machine. *Soft Comput.* **2018**, *22*, 4389–4405. [CrossRef]
94. Manavalan, B.; Shin, T.H.; Lee, G. PVP-SVM: Sequence-based prediction of phage virion proteins using a support vector machine. *Front. Microbiol.* **2018**, *9*, 476. [CrossRef]
95. Chen, S.; Wu, X.; Zhang, R. A novel twin support vector machine for binary classification problems. *Neural Process. Lett.* **2016**, *44*, 795–811. [CrossRef]
96. Acharya, U.R.; Ng, E.Y.-K.; Tan, J.-H.; Sree, S.V. Thermography based breast cancer detection using texture features and support vector machine. *J. Med. Syst.* **2012**, *36*, 1503–1510. [CrossRef]
97. Maglogiannis, I.; Zafiropoulos, E.; Anagnostopoulos, I. An intelligent system for automated breast cancer diagnosis and prognosis using SVM based classifiers. *Appl. Intell.* **2009**, *30*, 24–36. [CrossRef]
98. Huang, Y.-L.; Wang, K.-L.; Chen, D.-R. Diagnosis of breast tumors with ultrasonic texture analysis using support vector machines. *Neural Comput. Appl.* **2006**, *15*, 164–169. [CrossRef]
99. Abu-Elanien, A.E.; Salama, M.; Ibrahim, M. Determination of transformer health condition using artificial neural networks. In Proceedings of the 19th International Symposium on Innovations in Intelligent Systems and Applications, Warsaw, Poland, 28–30 June 2011; pp. 1–5.
100. Lisboa, P.J.; Taktak, A.F. The use of artificial neural networks in decision support in cancer: A systematic review. *Neural Netw.* **2006**, *19*, 408–415. [CrossRef] [PubMed]
101. Abbass, H.A. An evolutionary artificial neural networks approach for breast cancer diagnosis. *Artif. Intell. Med.* **2002**, *25*, 265–281. [CrossRef]
102. Tourassi, G.D.; Markey, M.K.; Lo, J.Y.; Floyd, C.E., Jr. A neural network approach to breast cancer diagnosis as a constraint satisfaction problem. *Med. Phys.* **2001**, *28*, 804–811. [CrossRef] [PubMed]
103. Janghel, R.; Shukla, A.; Tiwari, R.; Kala, R. Breast cancer diagnosis using artificial neural network models. In Proceedings of the 3rd International Conference on Information Sciences and Interaction Sciences, Chengdu, China, 23–25 June 2010; pp. 89–94.
104. Delen, D.; Walker, G.; Kadam, A. Predicting breast cancer survivability: A comparison of three data mining methods. *Artif. Intell. Med.* **2005**, *34*, 113–127. [CrossRef]
105. Sarvestani, A.S.; Safavi, A.; Parandeh, N.; Salehi, M. Predicting breast cancer survivability using data mining techniques. In Proceedings of the 2nd International Conference on Software Technology and Engineering, San Juan, PR, USA, 3–5 October 2010; p. V2-227.
106. Çakır, A.; Demirel, B. A software tool for determination of breast cancer treatment methods using data mining approach. *J. Med. Syst.* **2011**, *35*, 1503–1511. [CrossRef]
107. Şahan, S.; Polat, K.; Kodaz, H.; Güneş, S. A new hybrid method based on fuzzy-artificial immune system and k-nn algorithm for breast cancer diagnosis. *Comput. Biol. Med.* **2007**, *37*, 415–423. [CrossRef] [PubMed]
108. Bhardwaj, A.; Tiwari, A. Breast cancer diagnosis using genetically optimized neural network model. *Expert Syst. Appl.* **2015**, *42*, 4611–4620. [CrossRef]
109. Karabatak, M. A new classifier for breast cancer detection based on Naïve Bayesian. *Measurement* **2015**, *72*, 32–36. [CrossRef]
110. Bagui, S.C.; Bagui, S.; Pal, K.; Pal, N.R. Breast cancer detection using rank nearest neighbor classification rules. *Pattern Recognit.* **2003**, *36*, 25–34. [CrossRef]
111. Chen, H.-L.; Yang, B.; Liu, J.; Liu, D.-Y. A support vector machine classifier with rough set-based feature selection for breast cancer diagnosis. *Expert Syst. Appl.* **2011**, *38*, 9014–9022. [CrossRef]

112. Polat, K.; Güneş, S. Breast cancer diagnosis using least square support vector machine. *Digit. Signal Process.* **2007**, *17*, 694–701. [CrossRef]
113. Le Cun, Y.; Bengio, Y.; Hinton, G. Deep learning. *Nature* **2015**, *521*, 436–444. [CrossRef]
114. Zhao, R.; Yan, R.; Chen, Z.; Mao, K.; Wang, P.; Gao, R.X. Deep learning and its applications to machine health monitoring. *Mech. Syst. Signal Process.* **2019**, *115*, 213–237. [CrossRef]
115. Zou, J.; Huss, M.; Abid, A.; Mohammadi, P.; Torkamani, A.; Telenti, A. A primer on deep learning in genomics. *Nat. Genet.* **2019**, *51*, 12–18. [CrossRef]
116. Lee, S.M.; Seo, J.B.; Yun, J.; Cho, Y.-H.; Vogel-Claussen, J.; Schiebler, M.L.; Gefter, W.B.; Van Beek, E.J.; Goo, J.M.; Lee, K.S. Deep Learning Applications in Chest Radiography and Computed Tomography. *J. Thorac. Imaging* **2019**, *34*, 75–85. [CrossRef]
117. Mishra, S.; Glaws, A.; Palanisamy, P. Predictive Analytics in Future Power Systems: A Panorama and State-Of-The-Art of Deep Learning Applications. In *Optimization, Learning, and Control for Interdependent Complex Networks*; Springer: Berlin/Heidelberg, Germany, 2020; pp. 147–182.
118. Kalchbrenner, N.; Grefenstette, E.; Blunsom, P. A convolutional neural network for modelling sentences. *arXiv* **2014**, arXiv:1404.2188.
119. Cong, I.; Choi, S.; Lukin, M.D. Quantum convolutional neural networks. *Nat. Phys.* **2019**, *15*, 1273–1278. [CrossRef]
120. Coley, C.W.; Jin, W.; Rogers, L.; Jamison, T.F.; Jaakkola, T.S.; Green, W.H.; Barzilay, R.; Jensen, K.F. A graph-convolutional neural network model for the prediction of chemical reactivity. *Chem. Sci.* **2019**, *10*, 370–377. [CrossRef] [PubMed]
121. Indolia, S.; Goswami, A.K.; Mishra, S.; Asopa, P. Conceptual understanding of convolutional neural network-a deep learning approach. *Procedia Comput. Sci.* **2018**, *132*, 679–688. [CrossRef]
122. Amit, G.; Ben-Ari, R.; Hadad, O.; Monovich, E.; Granot, N.; Hashoul, S. Classification of breast MRI lesions using small-size training sets: Comparison of deep learning approaches. In Proceedings of the Medical Imaging: Computer-Aided Diagnosis Conference, Orlando, FL, USA, 11–16 February 2017; p. 101341H.
123. Nahid, A.-A.; Mehrabi, M.A.; Kong, Y. Histopathological breast cancer image classification by deep neural network techniques guided by local clustering. *BioMed Res. Int.* **2018**. [CrossRef] [PubMed]
124. Murtaza, G.; Shuib, L.; Mujtaba, G.; Raza, G. Breast cancer multi-classification through deep neural network and hierarchical classification approach. *Multimed. Tools Appl.* **2019**. [CrossRef]
125. Dabeer, S.; Khan, M.M.; Islam, S. Cancer diagnosis in histopathological image: CNN based approach. *Inform. Med. Unlocked* **2019**, *16*, 100231. [CrossRef]
126. Tan, Y.; Sim, K.; Ting, F. Breast cancer detection using convolutional neural networks for mammogram imaging system. In Proceedings of the 27th International Conference on Robotics, Automation and Sciences (ICORAS), Melaka, Malaysia, 27–29 November 2017; pp. 1–5.
127. Byra, M.; Piotrzkowska-Wróblewska, H.; Dobruch-Sobczak, K.; Nowicki, A. Combining Nakagami imaging and convolutional neural network for breast lesion classification. In Proceedings of the 2017 IEEE International Ultrasonics Symposium (IUS), Washington, DC, USA, 6–9 September 2017; pp. 1–4.
128. Gao, F.; Wu, T.; Li, J.; Zheng, B.; Ruan, L.; Shang, D.; Patel, B. SD-CNN: A shallow-deep CNN for improved breast cancer diagnosis. *Comput. Med. Imaging Graph.* **2018**, *70*, 53–62. [CrossRef]
129. Wang, Z.; Li, M.; Wang, H.; Jiang, H.; Yao, Y.; Zhang, H.; Xin, J. Breast cancer detection using extreme learning machine based on feature fusion with CNN deep features. *IEEE Access* **2019**, *7*, 105146–105158. [CrossRef]
130. Litjens, G.; Sánchez, C.I.; Timofeeva, N.; Hermsen, M.; Nagtegaal, I.; Kovacs, I.; Hulsbergen-Van De Kaa, C.; Bult, P.; Van Ginneken, B.; Van Der Laak, J. Deep learning as a tool for increased accuracy and efficiency of histopathological diagnosis. *Sci. Rep.* **2016**, *6*, 26286. [CrossRef]
131. Sun, W.; Tseng, T.-L.B.; Zhang, J.; Qian, W. Enhancing deep convolutional neural network scheme for breast cancer diagnosis with unlabeled data. *Comput. Med. Imaging Graph.* **2017**, *57*, 4–9. [CrossRef] [PubMed]
132. Araújo, T.; Aresta, G.; Castro, E.; Rouco, J.; Aguiar, P.; Eloy, C.; Polónia, A.; Campilho, A. Classification of breast cancer histology images using convolutional neural networks. *PLoS ONE* **2017**, *12*, e0177544. [CrossRef] [PubMed]
133. Hernández-Julio, Y.F.; Prieto-Guevara, M.J.; Nieto-Bernal, W.; Meriño-Fuentes, I.; Guerrero-Avendaño, A. Framework for the development of data-driven Mamdani-type fuzzy clinical decision support systems. *Diagnostics* **2019**, *9*, 52. [CrossRef] [PubMed]

134. Yu, S.; Liu, L.; Wang, Z.; Dai, G.; Xie, Y. Transferring deep neural networks for the differentiation of mammographic breast lesions. *Sci. China Technol. Sci.* **2019**, *62*, 441–447. [CrossRef]
135. Ragab, D.A.; Sharkas, M.; Marshall, S.; Ren, J. Breast cancer detection using deep convolutional neural networks and support vector machines. *PeerJ* **2019**, *7*, e6201. [CrossRef]
136. Acharya, S.; Alsadoon, A.; Prasad, P.; Abdullah, S.; Deva, A. Deep convolutional network for breast cancer classification: Enhanced loss function (ELF). *J. Supercomput.* **2020**. [CrossRef]
137. Goodfellow, I.J. On distinguishability criteria for estimating generative models. *arXiv* **2014**, arXiv:1412.6515.
138. Kazeminia, S.; Baur, C.; Kuijper, A.; van Ginneken, B.; Navab, N.; Albarqouni, S.; Mukhopadhyay, A. GANs for medical image analysis. *Artif. Intell. Med.* **2020**. [CrossRef]
139. Odena, A.; Olah, C.; Shlens, J. Conditional image synthesis with auxiliary classifier gans. In Proceedings of the 34th International Conference on Machine Learning (ICML), Sydney, Australia, 6–11 August 2017; pp. 2642–2651.
140. Son, J.; Park, S.J.; Jung, K.-H. Retinal vessel segmentation in fundoscopic images with generative adversarial networks. *arXiv* **2017**, arXiv:1706.09318.
141. Pan, Z.; Yu, W.; Yi, X.; Khan, A.; Yuan, F.; Zheng, Y. Recent progress on generative adversarial networks (GANs): A survey. *IEEE Access* **2019**, *7*, 36322–36333. [CrossRef]
142. Mirza, M.; Osindero, S. Conditional generative adversarial nets. *arXiv* **2014**, arXiv:1411.1784.
143. Shams, S.; Platania, R.; Zhang, J.; Kim, J.; Lee, K.; Park, S.-J. Deep generative breast cancer screening and diagnosis. In Proceedings of the 21st International Conference on Medical Image Computing and Computer-Assisted Intervention, Granada, Spain, 16–20 September 2018; pp. 859–867.
144. Singh, V.K.; Romani, S.; Rashwan, H.A.; Akram, F.; Pandey, N.; Sarker, M.M.K.; Abdulwahab, S.; Torrents-Barrena, J.; Saleh, A.; Arquez, M. Conditional generative adversarial and convolutional networks for X-ray breast mass segmentation and shape classification. In Proceedings of the 21st International Conference on Medical Image Computing and Computer-Assisted Intervention, Granada, Spain, 16–20 September 2018; pp. 833–840.
145. Wu, E.; Wu, K.; Cox, D.; Lotter, W. Conditional infilling GANs for data augmentation in mammogram classification. In *Image Analysis for Moving Organ, Breast, and Thoracic Images*; Springer: Berlin/Heidelberg, Germany, 2018; pp. 98–106.
146. Guan, S.; Loew, M. Breast cancer detection using synthetic mammograms from generative adversarial networks in convolutional neural networks. *J. Med. Imaging* **2019**, *6*, 031411. [CrossRef] [PubMed]
147. Karthik, S.; Perumal, R.S.; Mouli, P.C. Breast cancer classification using deep neural networks. In *Knowledge Computing and Its Applications*; Springer: Berlin/Heidelberg, Germany, 2018; pp. 227–241.
148. Hadad, O.; Bakalo, R.; Ben-Ari, R.; Hashoul, S.; Amit, G. Classification of breast lesions using cross-modal deep learning. In Proceedings of the IEEE 14th International Symposium on Biomedical Imaging (ISBI 2017), Melbourne, Australia, 18–21 April 2017; pp. 109–112.
149. Wu, E.; Wu, K.; Lotter, W. Synthesizing lesions using contextual GANs improves breast cancer classification on mammograms. *arXiv* **2020**, arXiv:2006.00086.
150. Sutton, S.R.; Barto, G.A. Reinforcement Learning: An Introduction. In *A Bradford Book*; The MIT Press: Cambridge, MA, USA, 2015.
151. Kato, I.; Koganezawa, K.; Takanishi, A. Automatic breast cancer palpation robot: WAPRO-4. *Adv. Robot.* **1988**, *3*, 251–261. [CrossRef]
152. Kobayashi, Y.; Suzuki, M.; Kato, A.; Konishi, K.; Hashizume, M.; Fujie, M.G. A robotic palpation-based needle insertion method for diagnostic biopsy and treatment of breast cancer. In Proceedings of the IEEE/RSJ International Conference on Intelligent Robots and Systems, St Louis, MO, USA, 11–15 October 2009; pp. 5534–5539.
153. Larson, B.T.; Tsekos, N.V.; Erdman, A.G. A robotic device for minimally invasive breast interventions with real-time MRI guidance. In Proceedings of the Third IEEE Symposium on Bioinformatics and Bioengineering, Bethesda, MD, USA, 10–12 March 2003; pp. 190–197.
154. Maicas, G.; Carneiro, G.; Bradley, A.P.; Nascimento, J.C.; Reid, I. Deep reinforcement learning for active breast lesion detection from DCE-MRI. In Proceedings of the 20th International Conference on Medical Image Computing and Computer-Assisted Intervention, Quebec City, QC, Canada, 10–14 September 2017; pp. 665–673.

155. Tsekos, N.V.; Shudy, J.; Yacoub, E.; Tsekos, P.V.; Koutlas, I.G. Development of a robotic device for MRI-guided interventions in the breast. In Proceedings of the 2nd Annual IEEE International Symposium on Bioinformatics and Bioengineering (BIBE 2001), Bethesda, MD, USA, 4–6 November 2001; pp. 201–208.
156. Mallapragada, V.; Sarkar, N.; Podder, T.K. Toward a robot-assisted breast intervention system. *IEEE/ASME Trans. Mechatron.* **2010**, *16*, 1011–1020. [CrossRef]

10

Fully 3D Active Surface with Machine Learning for PET Image Segmentation

Albert Comelli

Ri.MED Foundation, 90133 Palermo, Italy; acomelli@fondazionerimed.com;

Abstract: In order to tackle three-dimensional tumor volume reconstruction from Positron Emission Tomography (PET) images, most of the existing algorithms rely on the segmentation of independent PET slices. To exploit cross-slice information, typically overlooked in these 2D implementations, I present an algorithm capable of achieving the volume reconstruction directly in 3D, by leveraging an active surface algorithm. The evolution of such surface performs the segmentation of the whole stack of slices simultaneously and can handle changes in topology. Furthermore, no artificial stop condition is required, as the active surface will naturally converge to a stable topology. In addition, I include a machine learning component to enhance the accuracy of the segmentation process. The latter consists of a forcing term based on classification results from a discriminant analysis algorithm, which is included directly in the mathematical formulation of the energy function driving surface evolution. It is worth noting that the training of such a component requires minimal data compared to more involved deep learning methods. Only eight patients (i.e., two lung, four head and neck, and two brain cancers) were used for training and testing the machine learning component, while fifty patients (i.e., 10 lung, 25 head and neck, and 15 brain cancers) were used to test the full 3D reconstruction algorithm. Performance evaluation is based on the same dataset of patients discussed in my previous work, where the segmentation was performed using the 2D active contour. The results confirm that the active surface algorithm is superior to the active contour algorithm, outperforming the earlier approach on all the investigated anatomical districts with a dice similarity coefficient of 90.47 ± 2.36% for lung cancer, 88.30 ± 2.89% for head and neck cancer, and 90.29 ± 2.52% for brain cancer. Based on the reported results, it can be claimed that the migration into a 3D system yielded a practical benefit justifying the effort to rewrite an existing 2D system for PET imaging segmentation.

Keywords: 3D segmentation; machine learning; active surface; discriminant analysis; PET imaging

---

1. Introduction

In oncological studies, the main motivation to image segmentation is to recognize the portions of ill tissues so that treatment can be better directed (e.g., radio-therapy, [1–3]) and chances of survival improved [4–7]. Furthermore, segmentation is a pre-requisite to advanced studies such as radiomics feature extraction [8–10]. The present study discusses the segmentation of Positron Emission Tomography images leveraging a fully 3D hybrid algorithm which combines traditional segmentation (e.g., active surface) with machine learning (ML). Unlike several algorithms based on the segmentation of independent Positron Emission Tomography (PET) slices, the present algorithm is capable of segmenting all the slices in a PET data set simultaneously with the immediate advantage of exploiting valuable cross-slice information which would be ignored otherwise (e.g., [11–13]). In addition, in order to improve the accuracy of the final result, I included a machine learning component. A term based on information from a classifier (i.e., discriminant analysis) is included in the formulation of the energy function driving the surface evolution. The main advantage brought by artificial intelligence is that these approaches are designed to "learn" a non-obvious input–output relation directly from data. In the clinical context, artificial intelligence is used to obtain the morphology of organs or for the delineation of pathological tissue. Examples include the identification of cancer within the head and the neck using deep learning [14,15], classification using a kernel support vector machine [16], thyroid volume computation in 3D ultrasound imaging using random forest and convolutional neural network (CNN) [17], etc. It could be observed that deep learning techniques are more efficient than classical statistical approaches and, consequently, they are applied in many biomedical image segmentation tasks [18]. Nevertheless, while such methods are commonly used in magnetic resonance or computerized tomography imaging, their application on PET is still rather scarce and not much is found in the literature [19]. The reason is that in order to be successful, deep learning approaches require datasets containing hundreds of labelled examples, which is rarely the case in nuclear medicine. Vice versa, deep learning is largely used to classify patients in terms of outcome based on quantitative features extracted from previously delineated tumors for radiomics analyses of PET images [20]. Furthermore, to date, artificial intelligence algorithms are often employed as a stand-alone tool. Conversely, such a class of algorithms can be leveraged to improve the performance of more traditional approaches as well. For example, in [11], the k-means clustering technique was used to support a random walk segmentation algorithm, while, in [21], a convolutional neural network was used to obtain an initial delineation, successively refined by threshold segmentation and morphological methods. Moreover, an enhanced active contour (AC) algorithm has been proposed to delineate tumor in PET datasets in a semi-automatic way [22]. In detail, Comelli et al. [22] developed a 2D algorithm based on an AC enhanced by the inclusion of tissue classification information [23–25]. In these studies, authors reconstructed the 3D tumor shape by separately segmenting 2D PET slices because the main goal was to obtain a delineation method capable of being efficient, repeatable and real time. The core of such volume reconstruction was an active contour segmentation of PET images (i.e., 2D), performed marching through the PET slices and where the converged segmentation of one slice was used to initialize segmentation on the next. Nevertheless, the distance between consecutive PET slices is typically much greater than their voxel size. This feature introduces a sort of preferential direction in the data which may influence the reconstructed volume. In addition, the 2D contour evolution on one PET slice does not retain memory of what actually happened in the previous slice, nor does it takes into account what is the information in the slice that will come next.

Based on these considerations, the present study proposes a fully 3D active surface (AS) driven by a 3D machine learning component (i.e., 3D tissue classification). Starting from a region placed around the target, the AS deforms and moves to fit the target minimizing an "energy", defined as a multi-parameter function. In addition, the ML component, trained trough examples generated by expert human operators, learns to classify the PET data (i.e., the voxels in the slices) and introduces insight into the AS on which tissue portions are to be considered tumor or healthy. Therefore, to some extent, the algorithm learns to "mimic" how a human would perform this complex task and to avoid false positives. Although several classifiers were considered in previous publications (k-nearest neighbors, Naive Bayes, and Discriminant Analysis [23–25]), it is worth noting that the discriminant analysis provided consistently better performances [24]. As such, since a quite large comparative work was performed in [23–25], and since a full investigation on which classification approach would perform best within the new 3D framework is beyond the scope of the present study, the discriminant analysis is the algorithm of choice for this publication as well.

Summarizing, the key aspect of the proposed study is the evolution of a 3D surface embedded in the data volume, henceforth referred to as active surface, the evolution of which is driven by the minimization of a cost function specifically built to take into account information contained in the data and from 3D tissue classification. To evaluate the performance of the algorithm, fifty-eight patient studies are considered. In detail, eight studies are used for training and testing of the artificial intelligence component and fifty to test the full 3D reconstruction algorithm.

2. Materials and Methods

2.1. Overview of the 3D as Proposed Method and Differences with the Previous 2D AC Method

This study proposes a re-engineering of the algorithm from my previous work and focuses on the development of a 3D AS for the volume delineation augmented with the inclusion of a discriminant analysis (DA) component for 3D tissue classification. Figure 1 compares the 2D DA system proposed in [24] and the new 3D DA implementation discussed here to highlight differences and improvements.

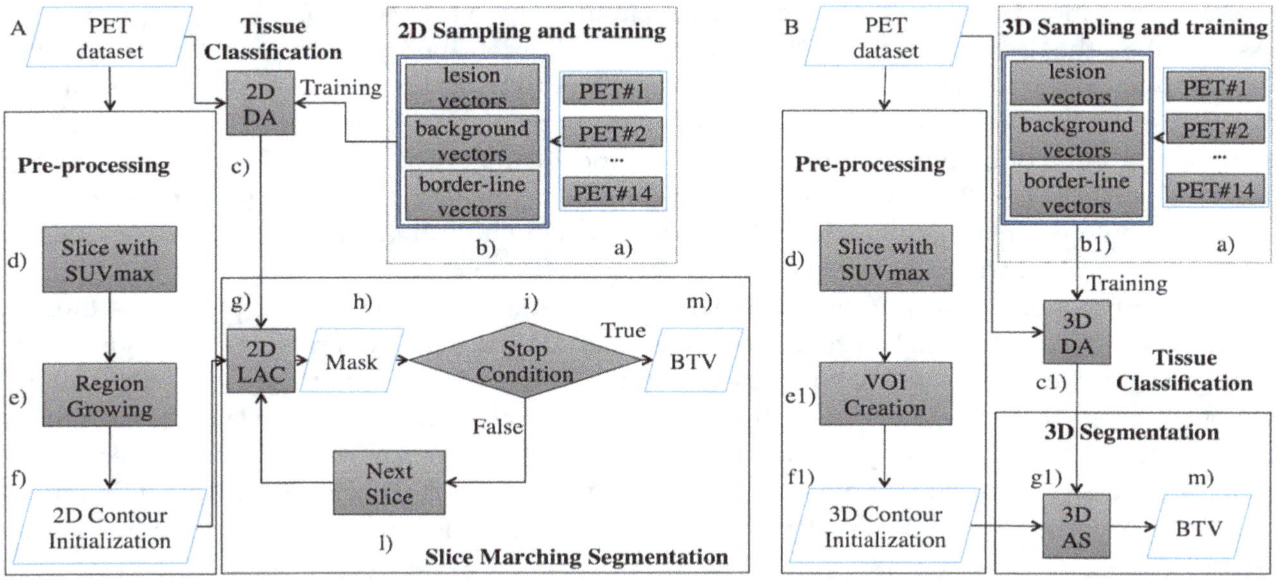

Figure 1. Comparison of the Positron Emission Tomography (PET) system proposed in the previous work (**A**) [24], and the implementation set out here (**B**). The proposed implementation substitutes the 'Slice Marching Segmentation' block (**A**) with the fully "3D Segmentation" block (**B**). Therefore, cross-slice information previously ignored is now being completely exploited. Moreover, the artificial stopping condition (step i) is no longer necessary. Additionally, (steps b, c, f, and g) were modified in order to provide a 3D sampling and training (step b1), a 3D tissue classification (step c1), 3D contour initialization (step f1), and 3D AS (step g1).

Figure 1A describes the system from my previous work [24]. Here, the "Pre-processing" block consisted of a pre-segmentation where the user draws, on a single PET slice, a contour roughly encircling the cancer area. This input is required to minimize the risk of incurring in false positives. Such an input was used to generate a user-independent mask which could be located on a different slice from the one chosen by the operator. By construction, this mask belonged to the same anatomical anomaly and included the radio-tracer maximum absorption area. After this step, the initial mask was fed to the next block of the workflow ("Slice Marching Segmentation" step), where the segmentation was obtained using a local region-based AC in which the contour evolved while minimizing its energy function. Information from the "2D Sampling and training" block consisted of labels associated to the PET image's pixels which identified each pixel as "lesion", "background", or "border-line" tissue. The different tissues in the PET slices were automatically identified using a 2D floating window (3 × 3 voxels). Finally, this algorithm used a slice-by-slice marching strategy to obtain an accurate segmentation, which began at the slice containing the user-independent mask and propagated upward and downward. Every time a slice segmentation was completed, the contour was propagated to the nearest adjacent slice until the stop condition was finally met. The final 3D shape consisted of the union of all contours obtained on each slice.

The algorithm presented here (Figure 1B) inherits the same pre-segmentation workflow of [24], although a 3D shape is required as the output of the pre-segmentation step. Specifically, to initialize the AS (step "g1" in Figure 1B), the pre-segmentation step (step "f1" in Figure 1B) must output a 3D shape transforming the user independent mask (step "f" in Figure 1A) in an ellipsoid (the 3D shape needed to start the 3D AS method). It is worth noting that the only requirement for the ellipsoid is that it envelops a portion of the tumor, including the voxel with the maximum intensity value (requirement already satisfied in [24] and naturally inherited from the ellipsoid). The energy function being minimized depends on the shape of the curves generated by the intersection of the AS with the planes containing the PET slices. Consequently, the ellipsoid around the tumor changes shape and moves towards the tumor borders with the aim of minimizing the energy function. Information from the 3D classifier is now included in the energy function in terms of labelled voxels combining, during the classification process, information involving multiple slices. As in the previous 2D classifier [24], the proposed 3D classifier labels the tissue as "lesion", "background" or "border-line" and drives the 3D AS algorithm ("3D Sampling and training" block), although the classification occurs now in terms of voxels and not pixels. This task comprises the training and validation steps of the DA classifier. Different tissues (i.e., lesion, background, or border-line tissue) are automatically identified in the PET data volume using a 3D floating window (i.e., $3 \times 3 \times 3$ voxels). The highlighted values are then arranged for every window into 27-element vectors describing the volume sample being investigated. The "training and testing" step needs to be performed only once. When completed, the classifier is capable of labelling new tissue and, subsequently, this information will be used to guide the segmentation process. A thorough explanation of this aspect will be provided in Section 2.1.1. The main advantage of leveraging a AS is that it is free to intersect the whole volume of PET images (i.e., all slices) and therefore segments them all at once, using cross-slice information, both in terms of data volume and tissue labels, that could not be leveraged before (i.e., in the system of Figure 1A). Details of this part will be given in Section 2.1.2. Finally, an operator-independent biological tumor volume (BTV) is obtained (step "m" in Figure 1B).

The following subsections will provide detailed discussion of the various components of system 1-A.

2.1.1. The 3D Discriminant Analysis

The DA was used to classify PET tissues into three clusters: background, lesion, and border-line tissues. The training needs to be done only once, after which DA is able to classify newly encountered tissues and can be re-used at any time.

Three clinicians with different expertise segmented 58 patients [24] (see Section 2.2 for more details). The STAPLE tool [26] was used to combine the three manual segmentations and to define a consolidated reference to be used as gold standard. Only eight patients (considering multiple PET slices for each study) were used for the training and testing of the 3D tissue classification algorithm. These comprised 2 with brain metastases, 4 with head and neck cancers, and 2 with lung cancers, respectively. The sampling process produced 13,762,560 vectors divided into 28,152 lesion vectors, 16,107 border-line vectors, and 13,718,301 background vectors. Specifically, in order to extract such samples, each PET slice was processed using a 3D floating window (i.e., $3 \times 3\times 3$ voxels). The values in every window were arranged into 27-element vectors. Such a sample size was empirically determined to provide the best results on the current data set.

Of the generated samples, 80% were used for the training step, while the remaining 20% were used for the testing step (as stated by the Pareto principle, also known as the 80/20 rule). The K-Fold cross-validation was used to obtain a robust classification and to eliminate over-fitting. Accordingly, the dataset was split into K equal folds, and the holdout method repeated K times. Every time one of the K folds was used as a validation set, and the remaining K-1 subsets were assembled to form a training set. The variance of the resulting estimate decreased as K increased. Samples with no more than 17 lesion voxels or totally outside the gold standard were labelled as "border-line" and "background" tissue, respectively. In all other instances, the label "lesion" was assigned. Once the training process was completed, a validation stage to test the efficiency of the classification followed.

2.1.2. The Active Surface Algorithm

Starting from the model proposed by Lankton et al. [27], which benefits purely local edge-based active contours and more global region-based active contours, I propose a more efficient segmentation technique that segments all slices simultaneously by developing a single surface inside the corresponding 3D PET volume [28], and a new mathematical formulation of the active surface energy including the 3D classifier information.

Summarizing, the obtained algorithm possesses the following novelty and improvements:

- A new active surface volumetric energy formulation.
- A full 3D development so leveraging cross-slice information.
- Inclusion of 3D tissue information.

These aspects are further detailed below.

First, a new formulation of the energy driving the AS by the inclusion of information from the 3D classifier is introduced.

In view of the fact that the tumor and the background regions are not easily split into two distinct regions, the energy was modified to include a new energy term based on tissue classes generated by the 3D classifier:

$$\chi_{lesion}(x) = \begin{cases} 1 & when \quad 3D\ DA(x) = lesion; \\ 0 & otherwise; \end{cases} \tag{1}$$

$$\chi_{border-line}(x) = \begin{cases} 1 & when \quad 3D\ DA(x) = borderline; \\ 0 & otherwise; \end{cases} \tag{2}$$

$$\chi_{\mathrm{background}}(x) = \begin{cases} 1 & when \quad 3D\ DA(x) = background; \\ 0 & otherwise; \end{cases} \tag{3}$$

where the characteristic functions $\chi_{lesion}(x)$, $\chi_{border-line}(x)$ and $\chi_{\mathrm{background}}(x)$ represent the 3D tissue's classification for lesion, border-line, and background, respectively.

In Functional Energy Equation (4), the first term is basically a prior term penalizing the overlap between regions which are classified in a conflicting way by the 3D AS and the 3D classifier (in regions classified as "border-line" no penalty is applied).

To integrate the standardized uptake value (SUV) and to insert this new prior term in the mathematical model and formulate it in a fully 3D setup, the active surface energy to be minimized for PET image segmentation is defined as:

$$E = \int_S \lambda \left(\int_{R_{in}} \chi_l(x,s) \overline{\mathrm{Pout}}_l(x)\, dx + \int_{R_{out}} \chi_l(x,s) \overline{\mathrm{Pin}}_l(x)\, dx \right) + (1-\lambda) \left(\int_{R_{in}} \chi_l(x,s)(\mathrm{SUV}(x) - u_l(s))^2 dx + \int_{R_{out}} \chi_l(x,s)(\mathrm{SUV}(x) - v_l(s))^2 dx \right) dS \tag{4}$$

- $\lambda \in R^+$ was chosen equal to 0.01, because such value proved to yield the best result;
- $\overline{\mathrm{Pin}}_l(x)$ and $\overline{\mathrm{Pout}}_l(x)$ indicate the 3D local mean DA classification within the portions of the local neighborhood $\chi_l(x)$ inside and outside the surface, respectively (within Ω);
- S is the 3D AS and dS is the surface area measure;
- s is the 3D surface parameter;
- x is a point within the 3D volume and dx the volume measure;
- R_{in} and R_{out} are the corresponding 3D regions inside and outside the surface;
- $\chi_l(x, s)$ is the indicator function around the surface point $S(s)$ of a local neighborhood.

Such neighborhoods are spheres of radius l centered around each point of the surface S. It was equal to 3 as proposed in [19].

$$\overline{\text{Pin}}_l(x) = \frac{\int_\Omega \chi_l(x)\chi_{lesion}(x)\,dx}{\int_\Omega \chi_l(x)\,dx}, \quad \overline{\text{Pout}}_l(x) = \frac{\int_\Omega \chi_l(x)\chi_{\text{background}}(x)\,dx}{\int_\Omega \chi_l(x)\,dx} \tag{5}$$

In practice, the 3D surface obtained after pre-segmentation is used as initialization to the AS and evolved to minimize the energy E until it finally fits the tumor silhouette.

2.2. The Clinical Dataset

In order to compare the performance of this new algorithm to its 2D predecessor, I considered the same dataset discussed in [24], which comprises 12 lung, 29 head and neck, and 17 brain cancers for a total of 58 PET studies. Eight PET datasets (2 with brain metastases, 4 with head and neck cancers, 2 with lung cancers) were used to train and test the 3D DA classifier while the remaining fifty PET datasets (i.e., 10 lung, 25 head and neck, and 15 brain cancers) were used to evaluate the performance of the proposed segmentation method.

Segmentations were done off-line and the findings did not affect either the treatment plan or the care of the patient. No personal information on patients has been released. Concerning the use of dataset, written consent was released by patients.

The PET investigation protocol was approved by the institutional Hospital Medical Ethics Review Board. Acquisitions were performed on a Discovery 690 PET/CT scanner with time of flight (General Electric Medical Systems, Milwaukee, WI, USA) and produced PET images with resolution of 256 $\times$ 256 voxels with grid spacing of 2.73 mm^3, thickness of 3.27 mm^3 and voxel size 2.73 $\times$ 2.73 $\times$ 3.27 mm^3.

2.3. Framework for Performance Evaluation

The following parameters are used here for performance evaluation:

$$Sensitivity = \frac{True\ Positive}{True\ Positive + False\ Negative} \tag{6}$$

$$Specificity = \frac{True\ Negative}{True\ Negative + False\ Positive} \tag{7}$$

$$positive\ predictive\ value\ (PPV) = \frac{True\ Positive}{True\ Positive + False\ Positive} \tag{8}$$

$$Accuracy(ACC) = \frac{True\ Positive + True\ Negative}{True\ Positive + False\ Positive + False\ Negative + True\ Negative} \tag{9}$$

$$Dice\ similarity\ coefficient\ (DSC) = \frac{2 \times True\ Positive}{2 \times True\ Positive + False\ Positive + False\ Negative} \tag{10}$$

$$Hausdorff\ distance\ (HD) = max\{d(A,B), d(B,A)\} \tag{11}$$

$$Pearson\ correlation\ coefficient\ (PCC) = \frac{COV(X,Y)}{\sigma X \sigma Y} \tag{12}$$

The PCC can take a value between +1 and −1, where +1 and −1 show total correlation (no difference between two segmentations), while 0 means no correlation (totally difference between two segmentations).

The proposed fully 3D DA segmentation method was implemented in Matlab R2019a and run on MacBook Pro computer with a 2.5 GHz Intel Core i7 processor, 16 GB 1600 MHz DDR3 memory, and OS X Sierra.

3. Results

Segmentation Results

To train and test the classifier, tumor, background and border-line tissues were automatically identified on PET images using the strategy described in Section 2.1.1. Starting from eight patient cases, the sampling process produced 13,762,560 vectors divided into 28,152 lesion vectors, 16,107 border-line vectors, and 13,718,301 background vectors. In total, 80% of the samples were used for training, while the remaining 20% were used for testing. Concerning the K-Fold cross-validation, the optimal k value was determined through the trial-and-error method (k ranged: 5–15, step size of 5), k = 5 corresponded to the highest classification accuracy. The capability of the 3D DA classifier in discerning different tissues achieved excellent result with a sensitivity of 99.09%, a specificity of 90.58%, a precision of 98.53%, and an accuracy of 96.46%. Figure 2 shows the receiver operating characteristic (ROC) analysis performed to assess the efficiency of 3D DA classification after the training phase. The area under the curve (AUC) is 0.99538. The maximum AUC is 1, which corresponds to the perfect classifier. After this training, the classifier is able to label new tissues and is ready to be integrated in the segmentation process (as described in Section 2.1.2).

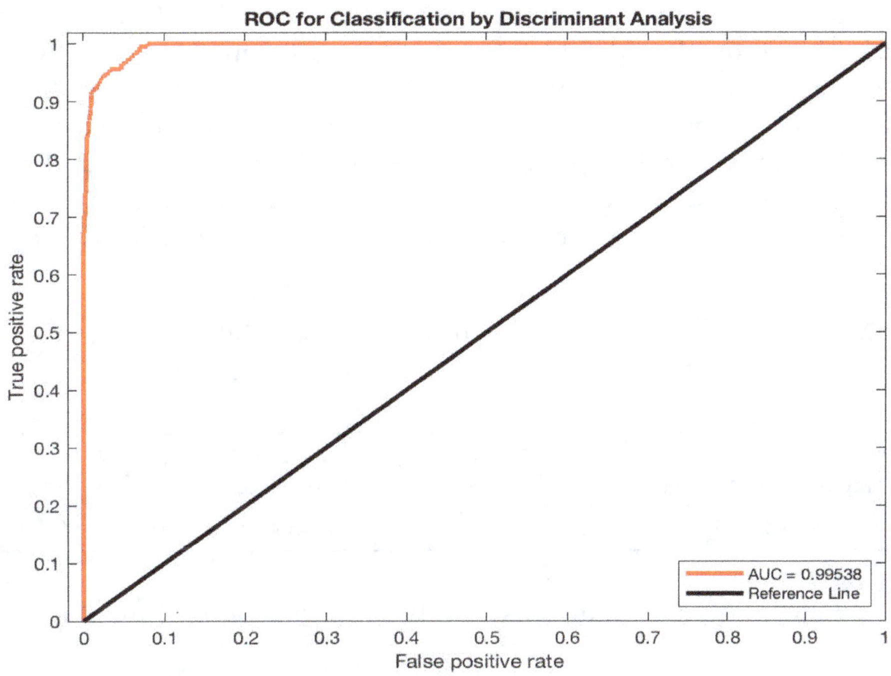

Figure 2. Classification performance of the 3D DA classifier was evaluated by calculating the area under the receiver operating characteristic (ROC) curve (AUC) using the ROC analysis.

To assess the performance of the segmentation method, ten patient studies with lung cancer (^{18}F-fluorodeoxyglucose PET), 25 with head and neck cancer (^{18}F-fluorodeoxyglucose PET), and 15 with brain cancer (^{11}C-methionine PET) were considered. Table 1 summarizes the results of the three previous anatomical districts including the results from the previous study [24]. Since the 2D slice-by-slice approach worked better than several other state-of-the-art approaches [24], I felt judged comparison with additional approaches to be unnecessary.

Table 1. Sensitivities, PPVs, DSCs and HDs for cancer studies using the 3D and 2D algorithms.

	3D Active Surface with 3D Discriminant Analysis		
	Lung	**Head and Neck**	**Brain**
	Mean ± std	Mean ± std	Mean ± std
Sensitivity	90.09 ± 6.50%	86.05 ± 5.70%	89.61 ± 4.29%
PPV	91.36 ± 3.89%	91.19 ± 5.30%	91.27 ± 4.52%
DSC	90.47 ± 2.36%	88.30 ± 2.89%	90.29 ± 2.52%
HD	1.40 ± 0.72	1.33 ± 0.57	1.04 ± 0.49
	2D Active Contour with 2D Discriminant Analysis		
	Lung	**Head and Neck**	**Brain**
	Mean ± std	Mean ± std	Mean ± std
Sensitivity	88.00 ± 5.41%	89.28 ± 5.70%	89.58 ± 3.40%
PPV	88.19 ± 4.73%	85.53 ± 5.13%	89.76 ± 3.31%
DSC	88.01 ± 4.23%	87.15 ± 3.23%	89.58 ± 2.37%
HD	1.53 ± 0.54	1.18 ± 0.39	1.07 ± 0.61

As confirmed by the analysis of variance (ANOVA) (see Table 2), the proposed 3D AS DA algorithm generated better results than the previous 2D algorithm. This was further demonstrated by the statistical difference (ANOVA p-value < 0.047) in the DSC comparison. In addition, Pearson correlation coefficient (PCC) analysis has been performed to evaluate the similarity of the proposed segmentation with the previous method [24], across all the fifty cases. The fully 3D AS DA approach, with a mean DSC of 89.69 ± 1.21%, not only performed overall better than the old method (DSC = 87.24 ± 4.59%), but with PCC~0.53 provided significantly different results as well (p-value = 0.000044).

Table 2. ANOVA and PCC on the DSC showed statistical differences between 2D and 3D segmentation methods.

Active Surface with Discriminant Analysis	**ANOVA p-Value**	**Mean DSC Difference**	**PCC**	**PCC p-Value**
2D vs. 3D	0.046	2.45%	0.53	0.000044

Figure 3 shows the qualitative comparison between the proposed method and the algorithm proposed in [24].

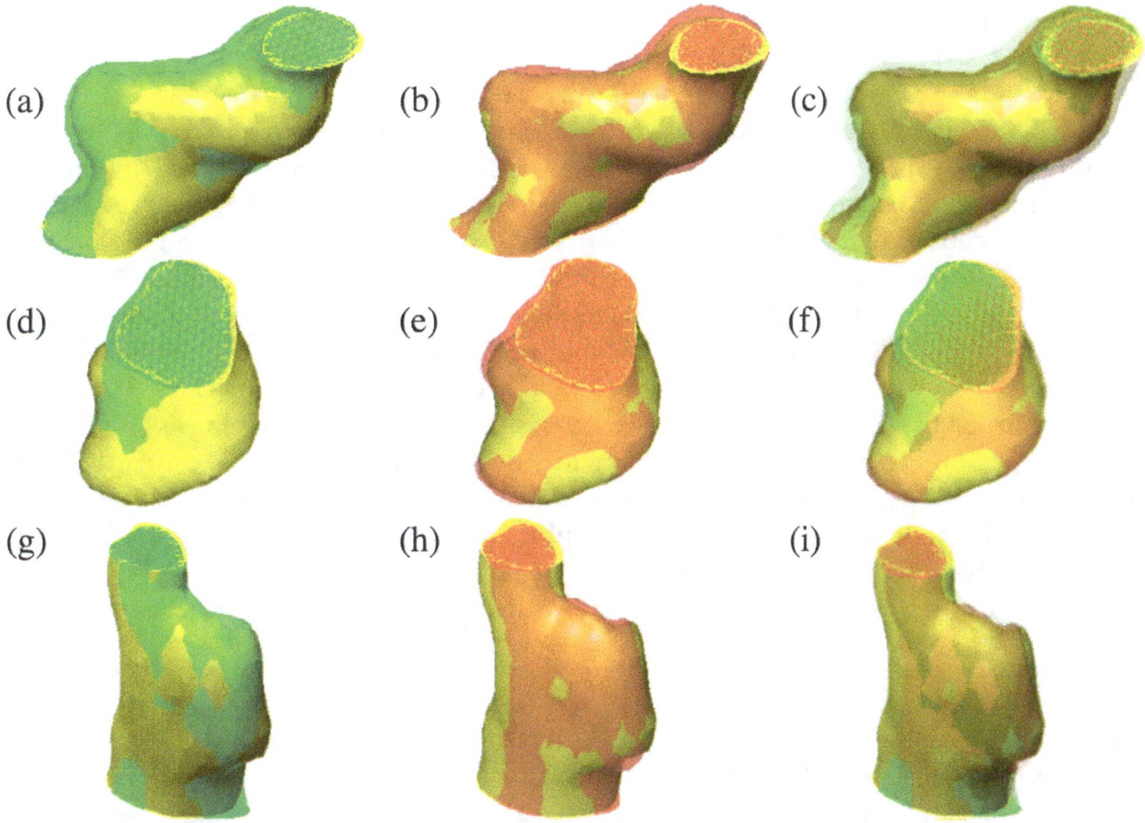

Figure 3. Three different tumors reported in the figure show the difference between 2D active contours (**a**,**d**,**g**) [24] and 3D active surface (**b**,**e**,**h**) segmentations guided by the 3D classifier. The reconstructed surfaces (green and red) and the gold standards (in yellow) are rendered partially transparent for better comparison. In the last column, the overlap of both methods and the gold standard is shown (**c**,**f**,**i**). Specifically, an over-segmentation of the 2D approach compared to 3D can be observed. (Color images can be found on the electronic version of this article).

4. Discussion

In this study, I discuss the inclusion of 3D tissue labelling with in the energy to be minimized during the 3D segmentation based on AS. The key improvement over the previous work [24] is a new segmentation algorithm obtained by evolving a 3D active surface, not only according to the PET data itself, but also leveraging information conveyed by a purposely-trained 3D DA classifier. Such information is included directly in the energy formulation. Previously [24], the 3D shape reconstruction challenge was addressed by using a reconstruction strategy based on a 2D approach, where the tumor segmentation was performed on each slice independently, and marching from one slice to the next until a stop condition is satisfied. While this represented an important step toward 3D delineation, it introduced a preferential direction (the direction of the marching) in the algorithm. In addition, the presence of a preferential direction is an embedded feature of PET data itself, being the distance between pet slices much greater than their planar resolution. While this particular aspect did not seem to influence the outcome of [24], it is nevertheless possible to conceive tumor topologies for which the marching 2D algorithm could actually ignore part of the tumor. To remove such a risk, I wanted to perform the shape reconstruction using an algorithm capable of handling any topology and where no preferential direction is present, either implicitly or explicitly. For this reason, the BTV delineation in this work is obtained through the evolution of a fully 3D surface. While some key features of the present system remained unchanged with respect to the previous version [24], such as (i) input is minimal and consist of just one manual delineation on one pet slice (see Section 2.1.), (ii) conversion of PET images into SUV images (see Section 2.1.2), and (iii) an optimal mask is retrieved during the pre-segmentation step, the core approach to segmentation, the initialization strategy and the DA labelling underwent consistent changes. In particular, initialization is now provided in form of a 3D shape and the DA has been re implemented to handle voxels, as opposed to pixels.

Finally, for better comparison, I used the same PET dataset as in Comelli et al. [24] where I demonstrated that the 2D approach already performed better than many commonly employed delineation methods. My results clearly show that both the migration from assembled 2D to full 3D, and the inclusion of tissue classification contributed to improve performance regardless of the anatomical district considered. In particular, in terms of DSC the improvement can be summarized as follows: 90.47 ± 2.36% versus 88.01 ± 4.23% for lung cancer, 88.30 ± 2.89% versus 87.15 ± 3.23% for head and neck cancer, and 90.29 ± 2.52% versus 89.58 ± 2.37% for brain cancer. Moreover, it is worth noting that, with the active surface, no stopping condition is needed and any preferential direction is removed. The converged active surface delivers a final, fully operator-independent 3D segmentation. In addition, I included the tissue classification, which was implemented in 3D as well. In this way, both the evolving shape and the tissue classification included in the energy, and consequently in the shape evolution, exploit cross-slice information that has never been exploited before. Despite (from a surficial search of the literature) the impression that the combination of ML with the active surface approach has been investigated by many authors, most studies have instead kept active surface and ML as independent entities. In contrast, I integrated ML directly in the energy of the active surface approach.

5. Conclusions

In this study, I discussed the inclusion of 3D tissue classification into fully 3D segmentation based on the evolution of an active surface. The obtained algorithm outperforms my previous formulation in which the tumor delineation was achieved using a 2D active contour approach. As an immediate advantage, the active surface is capable of segmenting all volume at once. Additionally, I enriched such an algorithm with the inclusion of a machine learning component, which consists of a 3D tissue classification based on discriminant analysis and compared the results with previous work. Noteworthy, both shape evolution and tissue classification can now leverage cross-slice information that was not available before. Based on the reported results, I can claim that migrating the system into 3D yielded a practical benefit justifying the effort to rewrite an existing 2D system for PET imaging segmentation.

Acknowledgments: I would like to thank Alessandro Stefano, Samuel Bignardi, Anthony Yezzi, Giorgio Russo, Maria Gabriella Sabini, and Massimo Ippolito, who provided crucial suggestions and high-quality observations during the preparation of this study. Additionally, I would like to acknowledge my family, for their continuous support and encouragement.

References

1. Niyazi, M.; Landrock, S.; Elsner, A.; Manapov, F.; Hacker, M.; Belka, C.; Ganswindt, U. Automated biological target volume delineation for radiotherapy treatment planning using FDG-PET/CT. *Radiat. Oncol.* **2013**, *8*, 180. [CrossRef]
2. Borasi, G.; Russo, G.; Alongi, F.; Nahum, A.; Candiano, G.C.; Stefano, A.; Gilardi, M.C.; Messa, C. High-intensity focused ultrasound plus concomitant radiotherapy: A new weapon in oncology? *J. Ther. Ultrasound* **2013**, *1*, 6. [CrossRef] [PubMed]
3. Guo, Z.; Guo, N.; Gong, K.; Zhong, S.; Li, Q. Gross tumor volume segmentation for head and neck cancer radiotherapy using deep dense multi-modality network. *Phys. Med. Biol.* **2019**, *64*, 205015. [CrossRef] [PubMed]
4. Wahl, R.L.; Jacene, H.; Kasamon, Y.; Lodge, M.A. From RECIST to PERCIST: Evolving Considerations for PET response criteria in solid tumors. *J. Nucl. Med.* **2009**, *50*, 122S. [CrossRef] [PubMed]
5. Cegla, P.; Kazmierska, J.; Gwozdz, S.; Czepczynski, R.; Malicki, J.; Cholewinski, W. Assessment of biological parameters in head and neck cancer based on in vivo distribution of 18F-FDG-FLT-FMISO-PET/CT images. *Tumori* **2019**, *106*, 33–38. [CrossRef] [PubMed]

6. Banna, G.L.; Anile, G.; Russo, G.; Vigneri, P.; Castaing, M.; Nicolosi, M.; Strano, S.; Gieri, S.; Spina, R.; Patanè, D.; et al. Predictive and Prognostic Value of Early Disease Progression by PET Evaluation in Advanced Non-Small Cell Lung Cancer. *Oncology* **2017**, *92*, 39–47. [CrossRef]
7. Stefano, A.; Porcino, N.; Banna, G.; Russoa, G.; Mocciaro, V.; Anile, G.; Gieri, S.; Cosentino, S.; Murè, G.; Baldari, S.; et al. Metabolic response assessment in non-small cell lung cancer patients after platinum-based therapy: A preliminary analysis. *Curr. Med. Imaging Rev.* **2015**, *11*, 218–227. [CrossRef]
8. Gillies, R.J.; Kinahan, P.E.; Hricak, H. Radiomics: Images Are More than Pictures, They Are Data. *Radiology* **2016**, *278*, 563–577. [CrossRef]
9. Stefano, A.; Gioè, M.; Russo, G.; Palmucci, S.; Torrisi, S.E.; Bignardi, S.; Basile, A.; Comelli, A.; Benfante, V.; Sambataro, G.; et al. Performance of Radiomics Features in the Quantification of Idiopathic Pulmonary Fibrosis from HRCT. *Diagnostics* **2020**, *10*, 306. [CrossRef]
10. Comelli, A.; Stefano, A.; Coronnello, C.; Russo, G.; Vernuccio, F.; Cannella, R.; Salvaggio, G.; Lagalla, R.; Barone, S. Radiomics: A New Biomedical Workflow to Create a Predictive Model. In *Annual Conference on Medical Image Understanding and Analysis*; Springer: Cham, Switzerland, 2020; pp. 280–293.
11. Stefano, A.; Vitabile, S.; Russo, G.; Ippolito, M.; Sabini, M.G.; Sardina, D.; Gambino, O.; Pirrone, R.; Ardizzone, E.; Gilardi, M.C. An enhanced random walk algorithm for delineation of head and neck cancers in PET studies. *Med. Biol. Eng. Comput.* **2017**, *55*, 897–908. [CrossRef]
12. Abdoli, M.; Dierckx, R.A.J.O.; Zaidi, H. Contourlet-based active contour model for PET image segmentation. *Med. Phys.* **2013**, *40*, 082507. [CrossRef]
13. Foster, B.; Bagci, U.; Mansoor, A.; Xu, Z.; Mollura, D.J. A review on segmentation of positron emission tomography images. *Comput. Biol. Med.* **2014**, *50*, 76–96. [CrossRef] [PubMed]
14. Guo, Z.; Guo, N.; Li, Q.; Gong, K. Automatic multi-modality segmentation of gross tumor volume for head and neck cancer radiotherapy using 3D U-Net. In *Medical Imaging 2019: Computer-Aided Diagnosis*; San Diego, CA, USA, 16–21 February 2019; International Society for Optics and Photonics: Bellingham, WA, USA, 2009.
15. Huang, B.; Chen, Z.; Wu, P.M.; Ye, Y.; Feng, S.T.; Wong, C.Y.O.; Zheng, L.; Liu, Y.; Wang, T.; Li, Q.; et al. Fully Automated Delineation of Gross Tumor Volume for Head and Neck Cancer on PET-CT Using Deep Learning: A Dual-Center Study. *Contrast Media Mol. Imaging* **2018**, *2018*. [CrossRef] [PubMed]
16. Comelli, A.; Terranova, M.C.; Scopelliti, L.; Salerno, S.; Midiri, F.; Lo Re, G.; Petrucci, G.; Vitabile, S. A Kernel Support Vector Machine Based Technique for Crohn's Disease Classification in Human Patients. In *Conference on Complex, Intelligent, and Software Intensive Systems*; Springer: Cham, Switzerland, 2018; pp. 262–273.
17. Poudel, P.; Illanes, A.; Sheet, D.; Friebe, M. Evaluation of Commonly Used Algorithms for Thyroid Ultrasound Images Segmentation and Improvement Using Machine Learning Approaches. *J. Healthc. Eng.* **2018**, *2018*. [CrossRef]
18. Çiçek, Ö.; Abdulkadir, A.; Lienkamp, S.S.; Brox, T.; Ronneberger, O. 3D U-net: Learning dense volumetric segmentation from sparse annotation. In Proceedings of the Lecture Notes in Computer Science (including subseries Lecture Notes in Artificial Intelligence and Lecture Notes in Bioinformatics), 25 January 2016; Springer: Cham, Switzerland, 2016; Volume 9901, pp. 424–432.
19. Hatt, M.; Lee, J.A.; Schmidtlein, C.R.; El Naqa, I.; Caldwell, C.; De Bernardi, E.; Lu, W.; Das, S.; Geets, X.; Gregoire, V.; et al. Classification and evaluation strategies of auto-segmentation approaches for PET: Report of AAPM task group No. 211. *Med. Phys.* **2017**, *44*, e1–e42. [CrossRef]
20. Avanzo, M.; Wei, L.; Stancanello, J.; Vallières, M.; Rao, A.; Morin, O.; Mattonen, S.A.; El Naqa, I. Machine and deep learning methods for radiomics. *Med. Phys.* **2020**, *47*, e185–e202. [CrossRef] [PubMed]
21. Feng-Ping, A.; Zhi-Wen, L. Medical image segmentation algorithm based on feedback mechanism convolutional neural network. *Biomed. Signal Process. Control* **2019**, *53*, 101589. [CrossRef]
22. Comelli, A.; Stefano, A.; Russo, G.; Sabini, M.G.; Ippolito, M.; Bignardi, S.; Petrucci, G.; Yezzi, A. A smart and operator independent system to delineate tumours in Positron Emission Tomography scans. *Comput. Biol. Med.* **2018**, *102*, 1–15. [CrossRef] [PubMed]
23. Comelli, A.; Stefano, A.; Russo, G.; Bignardi, S.; Sabini, M.G.; Petrucci, G.; Ippolito, M.; Yezzi, A. K-nearest neighbor driving active contours to delineate biological tumor volumes. *Eng. Appl. Artif. Intell.* **2019**, *81*, 133–144. [CrossRef]
24. Comelli, A.; Stefano, A.; Bignardi, S.; Russo, G.; Sabini, M.G.; Ippolito, M.; Barone, S.; Yezzi, A. Active contour algorithm with discriminant analysis for delineating tumors in positron emission tomography. *Artif. Intell. Med.* **2019**, *94*, 67–78. [CrossRef]

25. Comelli, A.; Stefano, A.; Bignardi, S.; Coronnello, C.; Russo, G.; Sabini, M.G.; Ippolito, M.; Yezzi, A. Tissue Classification to Support Local Active Delineation of Brain Tumors. In *Proceedings of the Communications in Computer and Information Science*; Springer: Cham, Switzerland, 2020; Volume 1065, pp. 3–14.
26. Warfield, S.K.; Zou, K.H.; Wells, W.M. Simultaneous truth and performance level estimation (STAPLE): An algorithm for the validation of image segmentation. *IEEE Trans. Med. Imaging* **2004**, *23*, 903–921. [CrossRef] [PubMed]
27. Lankton, S.; Nain, D.; Yezzi, A.; Tannenbaum, A. Hybrid geodesic region-based curve evolutions for image segmentation. In *Proceedings of the Medical Imaging 2007: Physics of Medical Imaging*; Hsieh, J., Flynn, M.J., Eds.; International Society for Optics and Photonics: Bellingham, WA, USA, 2007; Volume 6510, p. 65104U.
28. Comelli, A.; Bignardi, S.; Stefano, A.; Russo, G.; Sabini, M.G.; Ippolito, M.; Yezzi, A. Development of a new fully three-dimensional methodology for tumours delineation in functional images. *Comput. Biol. Med.* **2020**, *120*, 103701. [CrossRef] [PubMed]

11

Deep Learning-Based Pixel-Wise Lesion Segmentation on Oral Squamous Cell Carcinoma Images

Francesco Martino [1], Domenico D. Bloisi [2,*], Andrea Pennisi [3], Mulham Fawakherji [4], Gennaro Ilardi [1], Daniela Russo [1], Daniele Nardi [4], Stefania Staibano [1,†] and Francesco Merolla [5,†]

1 Department of Advanced Biomedical Sciences, University of Naples Federico II, 80131 Napoli, Italy; francesco.martino@unina.it (F.M.); gennaro.ilardi@unina.it (G.I.); daniela.russo@unina.it (D.R.); stefania.staibano@unina.it (S.S.)

2 Department of Mathematics, Computer Science, and Economics, University of Basilicata, 85100 Potenza, Italy

3 Allianz Benelux, 1000 Brussels, Belgium; andrea.pennisi@allianz.be

4 Department of Computer Science, Control, and Management Engineering, Sapienza University of Rome, 00185 Rome, Italy; fawakherji@diag.uniroma1.it (M.F.); nardi@diag.uniroma1.it (D.N.)

5 Department of Medicine and Health Sciences "V. Tiberio", University of Molise, 86100 Campobasso, Italy; francesco.merolla@unimol.it

* Correspondence: domenico.bloisi@unibas.it

† Co-senior authors.

Abstract: Oral squamous cell carcinoma is the most common oral cancer. In this paper, we present a performance analysis of four different deep learning-based pixel-wise methods for lesion segmentation on oral carcinoma images. Two diverse image datasets, one for training and another one for testing, are used to generate and evaluate the models used for segmenting the images, thus allowing to assess the generalization capability of the considered deep network architectures. An important contribution of this work is the creation of the Oral Cancer Annotated (ORCA) dataset, containing ground-truth data derived from the well-known Cancer Genome Atlas (TCGA) dataset.

Keywords: oral carcinoma; medical image segmentation; deep learning

1. Introduction

Malignant tumors of the head and neck region include a large variety of lesions, the great majority of which are squamous cell carcinomas of the oral cavity [1]. According to GLOBOCAN 2018 data on cancer [2], oral cavity malignant neoplasms, together with lip and pharynx malignancies, account for more than half-million new occurrences per year worldwide, with an estimated incidence of 5.06 cases per 100,000 inhabitants. Moreover, Oral Squamous Cell Carcinoma (OSCC) is characterized by high morbidity and mortality, and, in most countries, the survival rate after five years from the diagnosis is less than 50% of the patients [3].

The histology examination is the gold standard for the definition of these tumors. Surgical pathologists use both clinical and radiological evidence to complement their diagnoses, differentiating between benign and malignant lesions. In the last years, surgical pathology is witnessing a digital transformation thanks to (1) the increase of the processing speed of Whole Slide Images (WSI) scanners [4] and (2) the lower storage costs and better compression algorithm [5]. Consequently, WSI digital analysis is one of the most prominent and innovative topics in anatomical pathology, catching academic and industries attentions. An example of an image obtained using a WSI scanner is shown in Figure 1.

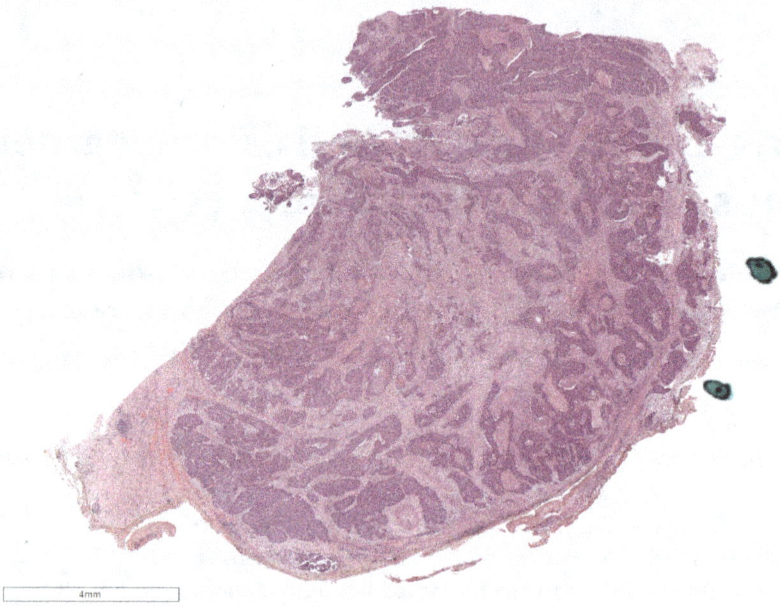

Figure 1. An example of image generated by a Whole Slide Images (WSI) scanner. The image has a dimension of 35,862 × 32,195 pixels and the file size is 213.3 MB.

However, WSI (and associated datasets) are characterized by three important limitations:

1. WSI are extremely large images, having a memory size of two gigabytes on average [6].
2. There are a few surgical pathology units that are fully digitalized and that can store a large amount of digitalized slides, although their number is increasing exponentially [7].
3. There is a small number of available image datasets and most of them are not annotated [8].

Due to the above-discussed limitations, the research activity based on Artificial Intelligence (AI) algorithms applied to WSI is still limited compared to other diagnostic imaging branches, such as radiology, but the scientific literature on the topic is growing fast and we are observing the appearance of public datasets of unannotated and annotated histopathology WSI.

In this paper, we present a performance evaluation of four different image segmentation architectures based on deep learning to obtain a pixel-wise separation between benign and malignant areas on WSI samples. In particular, we test four widely used Semantic Segmentation deep neural Networks (SSNs) on publicly available data for the detection of carcinomas. As a difference with respect to classification neural network, SSNs take as input images of arbitrary sizes and produce a correspondingly sized segmented output, without relying on local patches.

The contributions of this work are three-fold:

1. We compare four different supervised pixel-wise segmentation methods for detecting carcinoma areas in WSI using quantitative metrics. Different input formats, including separating the color channels in the RGB and Hue, Saturation, and Value (HSV) models, are taken into account in the experiments.
2. We use two different image datasets, one for training and another one for testing. This allows us to understand the real generalization capabilities of the considered SSNs.
3. We created a publicly available dataset, called Oral Cancer Annotated (ORCA) dataset, containing annotated data from the Cancer Genome Atlas (TCGA) dataset, which can be used by other researchers for testing their approaches.

The paper is organized as follows. Section 2 contains a discussion of similar approaches present in the literature. Section 3 describes the details of the proposed method, while Section 4 shows both qualitative and quantitative results obtained on publicly available data. Finally, conclusions are drawn in Section 5.

2. Related Work

Artificial intelligence (AI) algorithms have been proposed to address a wide variety of questions in medicine; e.g., for prostate Gleason score classification [9], renal cancer grading [10], breast cancer molecular subtyping [11] and their outcome prediction. Moreover, AI-based methods have been applied to the segmentation of various pathological lesions in the fields of neuropathology [12], breast cancer [13], hematopathology [14], and nephrology [15].

The above-cited studies have been conducted mainly on the most common tumors (i.e., breast or prostate), while AI-based methods have been scarcely adopted to deal with other types of cancer, despite their high incidence and mortality rates, as the Oral Squamous Cell Carcinoma (OSCC). The analysis of a recent systematic review by Mahmood et al. [16] shows that still few applications of automatic WSI analysis algorithms are available for OSCC. In particular, the survey reports 11 records about the employment of AI-based methods for the analysis of specific histological features of oral lesions: out of 11, only four papers refer to OSCCs, namely [17–20], one paper is about oral epithelial dysplasia [21], five about oral submucous fibrosis, i.e., [22–26], and one paper is about oropharyngeal squamous cell carcinoma [19]. Another recent application of machine learning algorithms on oral lesions histopathological is based on immunohistochemistry (IHC) positivity prediction [27].

Segmentation methods on WSI images have been developed mainly for nuclei segmentation [28–30], epithelium segmentation [19,24], microvessels and nerves [31], and colour-based tumour segmentation [17]. Recently, Shaban et al. [32] proposed an indirect segmentation method, through small tiles classification, with an accuracy of 95.12% (sensitivity 88.69%, specificity 97.37%).

To the best of our knowledge, there are no published results on direct OSCC segmentation using deep learning and none employing the TCGA as a source of histopathological images. This work represents a first attempt of applying well-known deep learning-based segmentation methods on the publicly available TCGA images, providing also annotations to quantitatively validate the proposed approach.

Datasets

Concerning WSI datasets, most of them have been made available for challenges, such as Camelyon [33] and HEROHE, on Kaggle or as part of larger databases. The Cancer Genome Atlas (TCGA) [34] contains publicly available data provided by the National Cancer Institute (NCI), which is the U.S. federal government's principal agency for cancer research and training, since 2006. In particular, it contains clinicopathological information and unannotated WSI of over 20,000 primary cancer covering 33 different cancer types [35].

3. Methods

Our aim is to use a supervised method to automatically segment an input WSI sample into three classes:

1. Carcinoma pixels;
2. Tissue pixels not belonging to a carcinoma;
3. Non-tissue pixels.

Figure 2 shows the functional architecture of our approach. We worked on input images having a large dimension of 4500 × 4500 pixels, which is an input dimension about ten times greater than the input dimension supported by existing segmentation SSNs. Thus, a preprocessing step is needed in order to fit the input format of the deep neural network. We tested two different pre-processing functions:

- Simple resizing, where the original input WSI sample is resized from 4500 × 4500 to 512 × 512 pixels without any other change in the color model.
- Color model change, where the WSI sample is resized to 512 × 512 pixels and the original color model is modified. For example, we tested as input for the deep neural network the use of the Red channel of the RGB model in combination with the Hue channel of the HSV model.

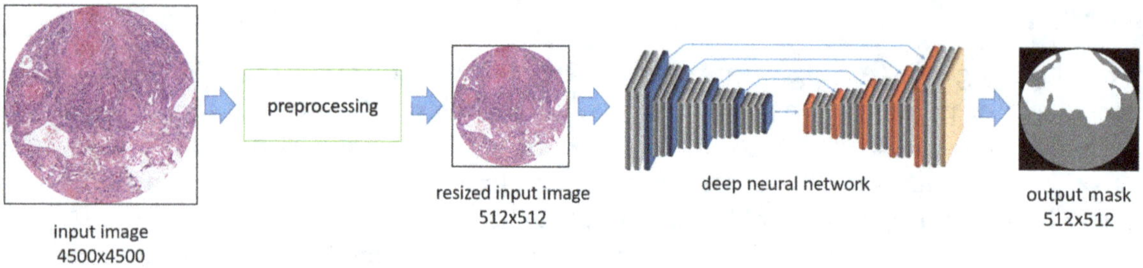

Figure 2. Functional architecture of the proposed approach.

Segmentation results obtained using the different pre-processing functions are discussed in Section 4.

3.1. Network Architectures

The core of the proposed approach consists in the use of a semantic segmentation network. We have selected four different network architectures among the most used ones:

1. SegNet [36].
2. U-Net [37].
3. U-Net with VGG16 encoder.
4. U-Net with ResNet50 encoder.

3.1.1. Segnet

SegNet is made of an encoder network and a corresponding decoder network, followed by a final pixel-wise classification layer (Figure 3). The encoder network consists of the first 13 convolutional layers of the VGG16 [38] network designed for object classification, without considering the fully connected layer in order to retain higher resolution feature maps at the deepest encoder output. In such a way, the number of parameters to train is significantly reduced. Each encoder layer has a corresponding decoder made of 13 layers. The final decoder output is fed to a multi-class soft-max classifier to produce class probabilities for each pixel independently.

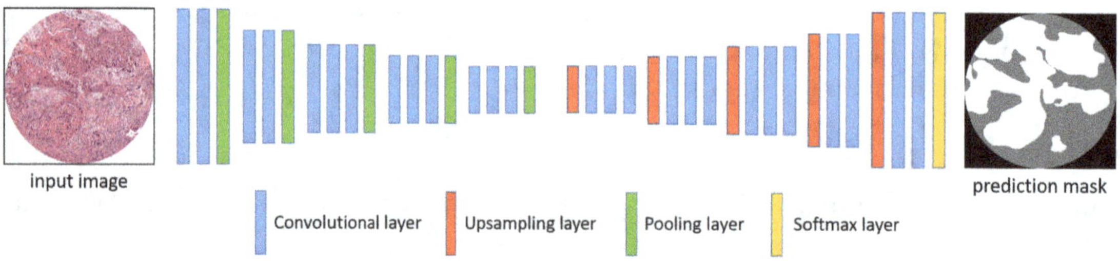

Figure 3. SegNet architecture.

3.1.2. U-Net

The architecture of the net is shown in Figure 4. The input image is downsampled to obtain a 512 × 512 resized image.

The encoding stage is needed to create a 512 feature vector and it is made of ten 3 × 3 convolutional layers, and by four 2 × 2 max pooling operations with stride 2. In particular, there is a repeated application of two unpadded convolutions, each followed by a rectified linear unit (ReLU) and a max pooling operation. The decoding stage (see the right side of Figure 4) is needed to obtain the predicted mask at 512 × 512 pixels. It is made of eight 3 × 3 convolutional layers and by four 2 × 2 transpose layers. There is a repeated application of two unpadded convolutions, each followed by a ReLU and a transpose operation. Figure 4 shows also the concatenation arcs from the encoding side to the decoding side of the network. Cropping is necessary due to the loss of border pixels in every convolution layer.

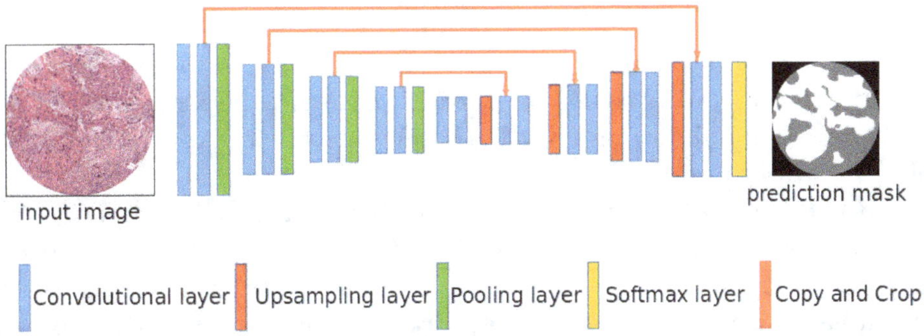

Figure 4. U-Net architecture.

3.1.3. U-Net with Different Encoders

The original U-Net consists of two paths, the first one (left side) composed of four blocks. Each block consists of a typical architecture of a convolution network, composed of repeated two 3×3 Convolutional layers followed by a rectified linear unit (ReLU) and a 2×2 max pooling layer with stride 2 as down-sampling steps. The second path (right side) represents the up-sampling path also composed of four blocks. Each block consists of an up-sampling feature map followed by concatenation with the corresponding cropped feature map from the first path followed by a double 3×3 Convolutional layer. Each convolution layer is composed of batch normalization. Between the first and the second path, there is a bottleneck block. This bottleneck is built from two convolution layers with batch normalization and dropout. In the models we applied, we replaced the first path, which is the encoder path of the network, with two different models, namely VGG16 [38] and ResNet50 [39], in order to obtain higher accuracy.

3.2. Training and Test

Two diverse datasets are used to train, validate, and test the networks. The training dataset consists of 188 annotated images of advanced OSCC derived from the digital data acquired in the Surgical Pathology Unit of the Federico II Hospital in Naples (Italy). The study was performed in agreement with Italian law. Moreover, according to the Declaration of Helsinki for studies based only on retrospective analyses on routine archival FFPE-tissue, written informed consent was acquired from the living patient at the time of surgery. The validation dataset consists of 100 annotated images from the newly created ORCA dataset (described below), while the test dataset consists of a further 100 images from the ORCA dataset also. All the images in the two datasets have been manually annotated by two of the authors of this paper that are expert pathologists (D. Russo and F. Merolla, both MD PhD and Board in Pathology) using three color labels:

1. Carcinoma pixels, colored in white.
2. Tissue pixels not belonging to a carcinoma, colored in grey.
3. Non-tissue pixels, colored in black.

The above-listed labels represent the classes learned by the deep network during the training stage. Figure 5 shows an example of annotation mask.

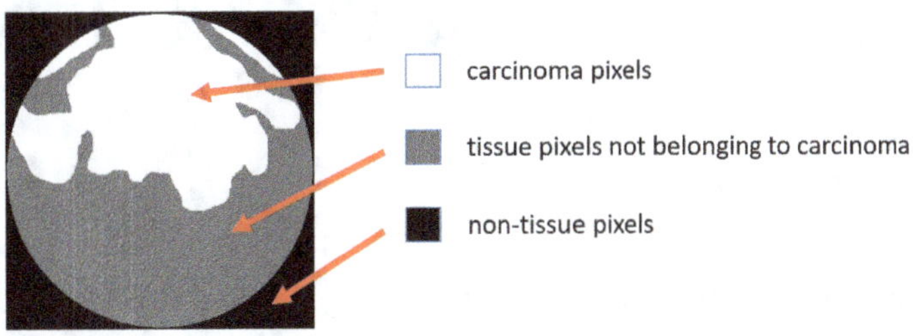

Figure 5. Example of annotation mask. Carcinoma pixels are colored in white, tissue pixels not belonging to a carcinoma are colored in grey, and non-tissue pixels are colored in black.

3.2.1. Training Data

The dataset used for training consists of a set of images collected by the Surgical Pathology Unit of the Federico II Hospital, in Naples (Italy). In particular, cases were assembled as four Tissue Micro Array and, after H&E staining, the slides were scanned with a Leica Aperio AT2 at 40× (20× optical magnification plus a 2× optical multiplier).

Slides were annotated using the Leica Aperio ImageScope software. In the first instance, to define each core, we used the ImageScope rectangle tool with a fixed size of 4500 × 4500 pixels, corresponding to nearly 1.125 mm, i.e., the size of each TMA core. Then, an expert pathologist used the pen tool to contour the tumor areas within each core. ImageScope provides an XML file as output for each WSI. RGB core images were extracted using OpenCV and OpenSlide libraries.

Concerning the annotation masks, we started by automatically detecting the tissue portion of each core using the OpenCV functions contouring and convex hull, to isolate the tissue pixels (colored in grey, as mentioned beforehand) from the background (non-tissue pixels colored in black). Then, the tumor masks (colored in white) were superimposed over the tissue pixels to draw carcinoma pixels. Finally, the masks were manually refined at pixel-size resolution.

An example of a couple <original image, annotated mask> used for the training stage is shown on the top of Figure 6.

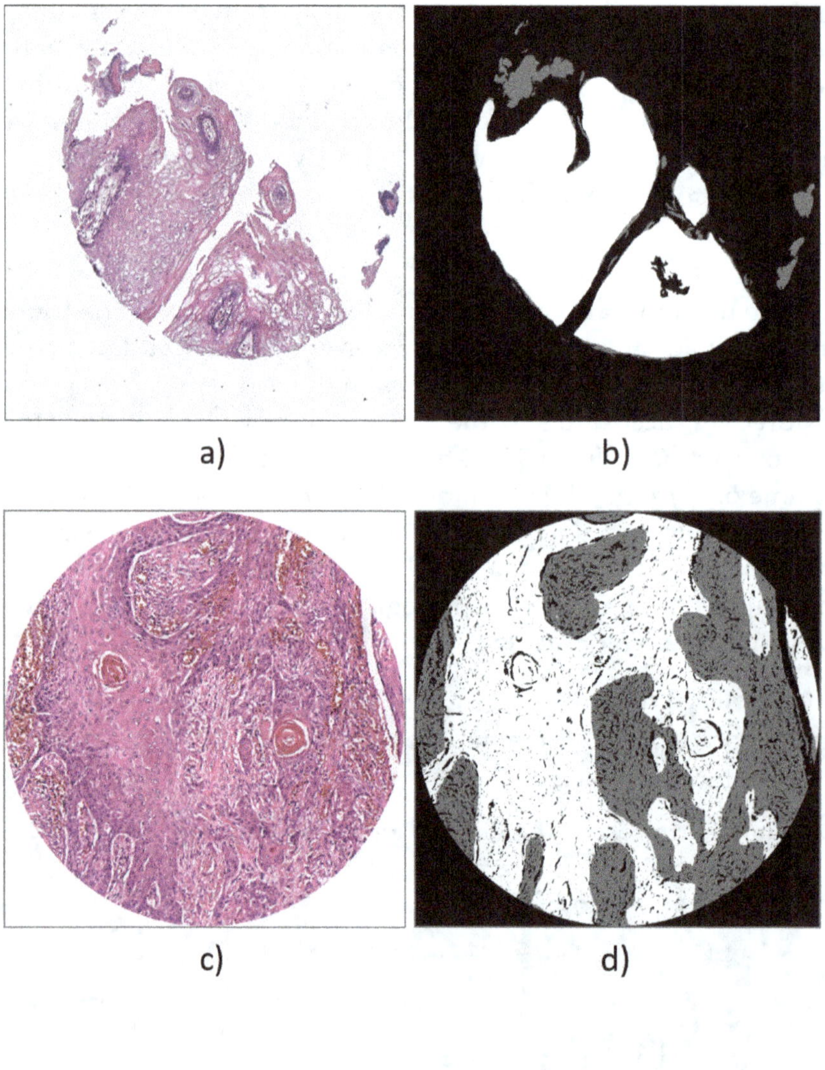

Figure 6. Top: Example of annotated data from the training dataset. (**a**) Original image. (**b**) Manually generated annotation mask. Bottom: Example of annotated data from the Oral Cancer Annotated (ORCA) dataset. (**c**) Original image. (**d**) Manually generated annotation mask.

3.2.2. ORCA Dataset

An important contribution of this work is the creation of a fully annotated dataset, called ORCA, consisting of couples of WSI samples plus corresponding annotation masks. An example of a couple <original image, annotated mask> from the ORCA dataset is shown on the bottom of Figure 6.

The original WSI samples belong to the Cancer Genome Atlas (TCGA), a landmark cancer genomics program, molecularly characterized over 20,000 primary cancer and matched normal samples spanning 33 cancer types [40]. TCGA data are publicly available for anyone in the research community to use. For each WSI included in the TCGA dataset, we defined one or two cores containing a representative tumor area. The dataset contains WSI scanned both at 20× and at 40×.

TCGA whole slide images were annotated using the Leica Aperio ImageScope software. For each image, a circular core region has been selected using the ImageScope ellipse tool, with a fixed size of 4500 × 4500 pixels in the case of the WSI scanned at 40× or 2250 × 2250 pixels in the case of WSI acquired at 20×. This allowed us to keep the same spatial dimension for all the selected cores. Then, the tumor contours have been drawn using a pen tool. The RGB images and the corresponding annotation masks were extracted using OpenCV and OpenSlide libraries.

All the couples of WSI samples plus corresponding annotation masks used in this work are available for downloading from the ORCA dataset web page at: https://sites.google.com/unibas.it/orca.

4. Experimental Results

In order to train and evaluate the networks, we split the image data into training, validation, and test sets. The training set consists of the 188 images from the Federico II Hospital plus a set of images obtained by applying a simple augmentation technique. This allows for augmenting the number of the available training samples. In particular, the data augmentation has been achieved by flipping the images vertically, horizontally, and in both ways. The final cardinality of the augmented training set is 756 images.

Each validation and test set includes 100 images from the ORCA data set. It is worth noticing that validation and test set are completely disjoint sets. In such a way, we tested the capability of the networks in generalizing the segmentation problem.

As stated above, we trained four different models:

- SegNet.
- U-Net.
- U-Net with VGG16 encoder.
- U-Net with ResNet50 encoder.

The source code of the used SegNet network is available at https://github.com/apennisi/segnet, while the source code for U-Net and its modifications is available at https://github.com/Mulham91/Deep-Learning-based-Pixel-wise-Lesion-Segmentationon-Oral-Squamous-Cell-Carcinoma-Images.

The four networks have been trained by using the Adam optimizer, with a learning rate of $1e-4$, without adopting any decay technique. The input image size has been set to 512 × 512 pixels.

For computing the loss, we used the Cross-Entropy function [41], which is a loss function widely used in deep learning. Cross entropy helps in speeding up the training for neural networks in comparison to the other losses [42]. The cross entropy for multi-class error computation is defined as follows:

$$s = -\sum_{c=1}^{M} y_{o,c} \log(p_{o,c}), \quad (1)$$

where c is the class id, o is the observation id, and p is the probability. Such a definition may also be called categorical cross entropy.

The training has been manually stopped after 60 epochs for all the considered network architectures because we noticed a trend of all the network in overfitting the training set.

We performed three kinds of experiments:

1. Using RGB images as input;
2. Taking into account the HSV color representation and concatenating the Hue channel with the Red channel from the RGB space;
3. Using the Red and Value channels.

An example of the different color models mentioned above is shown in Figure 7. The original RGB image is decomposed into single channels using the RGB and HSV color models. Then, some channels have been selected as input for the deep network. In particular, we used H + R and R + V.

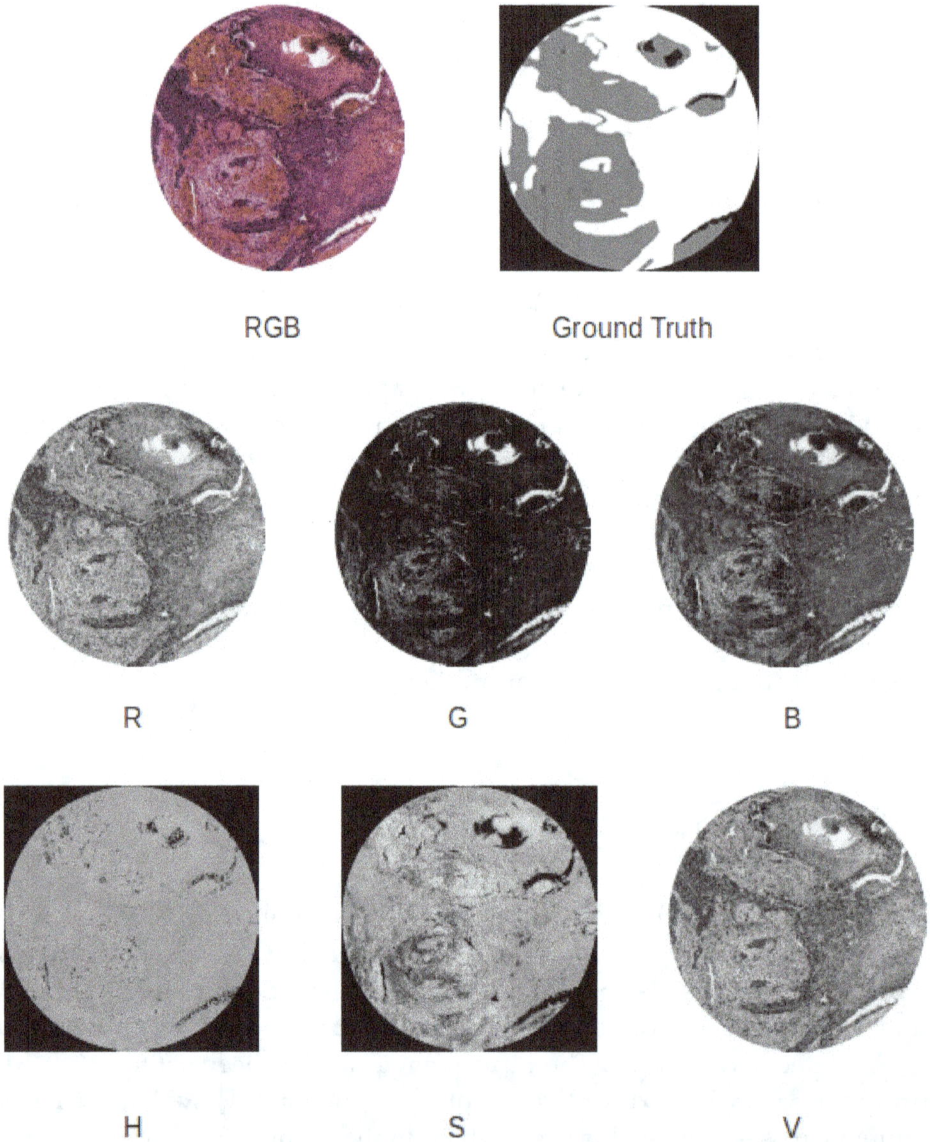

Figure 7. An example of the input images used for training the networks. First row: Original input and corresponding annotated mask. Second row: Red, Green, and Blue channels from the original RGB image. Third row: Hue, Saturation, and Value channels from the transformation of the original RGB image into Hue, Saturation, and Value (HSV).

The idea of using a multi-spectral input derives from the application of deep learning techniques in the area of precision farming, where multi-spectral inputs have denoted good performance on SSNs for the segmentation of crop and weed plants in images acquired from farming robots [43].

The prediction masks produced by the deep networks have been compared with the ground-truth annotation masks in order to measure the capability of our pipeline in generating accurate results. In particular, we have used the number of false-positive (FP), false-negative (FN), and true-positive (TP) carcinoma pixel detections as an indicator for the evaluation of the results. Figure 8 shows an example of how we computed FP, FN, and TP pixels to evaluate the predicted mask.

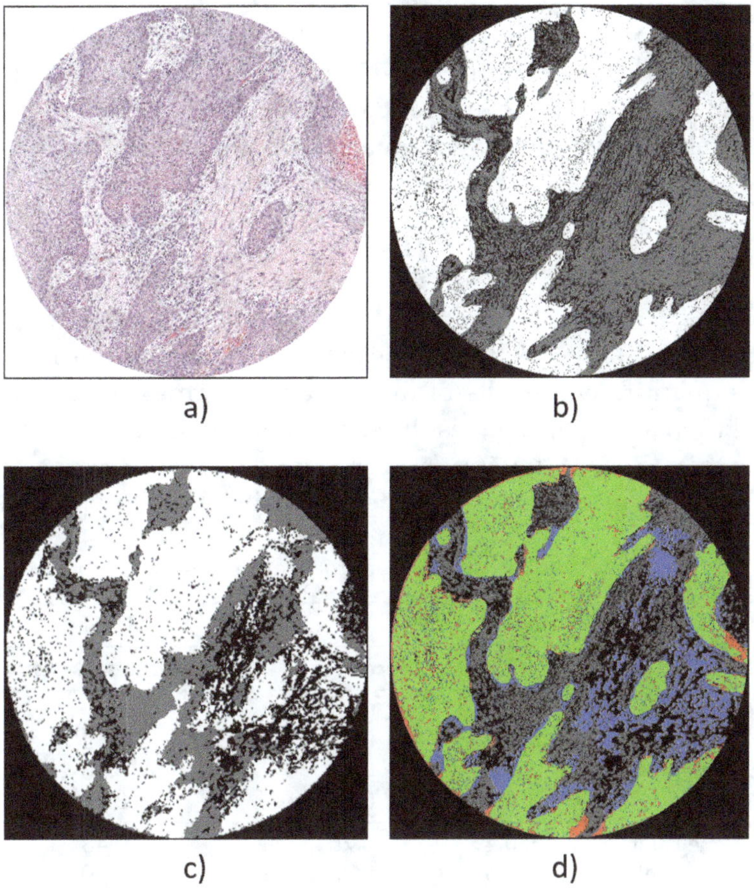

Figure 8. An example of error analysis for a test image. (**a**) The original image included in the test set. (**b**) The corresponding annotation mask, where carcinoma pixels are coloured in white. (**c**) The predicted mask generated from U-Net with ResNet50 encoder. (**d**) The coloured error mask, where green pixels are true-positive (TP) carcinoma pixels, blue are false-positives (FPs), and red are false-negatives (FNs).

4.1. Qualitative Evaluation

We evaluated the output of the trained network, in the first instance, by visual inspection. This allowed us to interpret the results and judge them in the light of the pathologist's experience and diagnostic reasoning in histopathology.

In most cases, we observed that the areas reported as false positives (blue pixels in Figure 8d) actually corresponded to small nests of stromal infiltration, located in correspondence with the tumor invasion front.

Vice versa, we observed that a portion of the pixels reported as false negatives actually referred to small areas of stroma within the tumor area.For example, by observing the colored mask in Figure 8d, it is visible that the stromal area within the tumor is considered as a set of false-negative pixels (coloured in red) even if they should be considered as true positives.

Given the discussion above, from a qualitative point of view, the algorithm has often reported pixels relating to areas of intense inflammatory infiltrate as false positives. However, single interspersed lymphocytes in the peritumor stroma were not per se a problem in the interpretation of the image.

Tumor grading was another determining factor in the efficiency of the algorithm. In fact, the trained network recognized with difficulty the highly differentiated tumor areas, with a prevalence of keratin pearls. This last factor could be attributable to the fact that the dataset used for the training was mainly composed of a series of high grade advanced squamous carcinomas.

4.2. Quantitative Results

To obtain a quantitative measure of the segmentation performance achieved by the four deep networks, we used the Mean Intersection-Over-Union (mIOU) metric. MIOU is one of the most common metrics for evaluating semantic image segmentation tasks. In particular, we first computed the IOU for each semantic class, namely carcinoma, tissue non-carcinoma, and non-tissue, and then computed the average over all classes. The $mIOU$ is defined as follows:

$$mIOU = \frac{1}{C}\sum_{i=1}^{C}\frac{TP_j}{TP_j + FP_j + FN_j}, \quad (2)$$

where TP is true-positive, FP is false-positive, FN is false-negative, and C is the total number of classes.

Table 1 shows the quantitative results of the semantic segmentation on three different inputs: RGB, (Red + Hue), and (Red + Value). The results show that the use of the combination (Red + Value) generates better results than (Red + Hue) input. Moreover, a deeper network, such as U-Net modified with ResNet50 as encoder, performs better than the original U-Net (having a more shallow encoder).

Table 1. Pixel-wise segmentation results.

Training Input	SSN Type	MIoU	IOU		
			Non-Tissue	Tissue Non-Carcinoma	Carcinoma
RGB	SegNet	0.51	0.74	0.49	0.30
	U-Net	0.58	0.79	0.52	0.45
	U-Net + VGG16	0.64	0.84	0.56	0.45
	U-Net + ResNet50	0.67	0.85	0.59	0.56
Red + Hue	SegNet	0.49	0.70	0.48	0.30
	U-Net	0.55	0.78	0.50	0.38
	U-Net + VGG16	0.33	0.22	0.28	0.53
	U-Net + ResNet50	0.57	0.80	0.48	0.43
Red + Value	SegNet	0.54	0.72	0.49	0.40
	U-Net	0.57	0.78	0.49	0.46
	U-Net + VGG16	0.62	0.79	0.50	0.55
	U-Net + ResNet50	0.63	0.80	0.52	0.56

4.3. Discussion

The histological evaluation of Hematoxylin Eosin stained slides from tumor samples, carried out by an experienced pathologist on an optical microscope, is a mandatory step in the diagnostic, prognostic and therapeutic pathway of patients suffering from squamous cell carcinoma of the oral cavity. To date, for the histological diagnosis of OSCCs, the gold standard is the visual analysis of histological preparations, stained with hematoxylin and eosin; tumor recognition basically takes place on the basis of the qualitative assessment of architectural characteristics of the neoplastic tissue, based on the wealth of knowledge pathologist's own. The qualitative assessment is subjective and can suffer from inter-individual variability, especially in borderline situations that are difficult to interpret. The use of a segmentation algorithm could minimize the interpretative variability and speed up the pathologists' work, providing they with a screening tool, particularly useful in those cases in which the histopathological diagnosis must be carried out on the extensive sampling of complex surgical samples that involve the generation of multiple blocks of formalin-fixed and paraffin-embedded tissue samples, from which numerous slides stained with hematoxylin and eosin are obtained.

Based on the presented results, our contribution is composed of: (i) a novel dataset, the ORCA set, which will allow us to conduct new studies on Oral Squamous Cell Carcinoma. Particularly, the dataset is composed of annotation from the TCGA dataset, a full comprehensive dataset enriched, as well as with diagnostic slide, with clinicopathological information and molecular biology data. This could facilitate the development of molecular characterization deep learning algorithms; (ii) our method relies on 2250×2250 and 4500×4500 images, without a tiling processing. Even though an improvement in its accuracy is mandatory for clinical practice, the utilization of so large images can hugely reduce time-demand for a WSI, making our approach easily scalable to clinical routine, when hundreds of slides need to be processed each day; (iii) after demanded improvements and a clinical trial, this kind of algorithm may be part of clinical practice via L.I.S. integration, fastening OSCC diagnosis and helping pathologists to identify OSCC areas on WSI. Indeed, we foresee to extend our method on lymphonodal metastasis, giving the pathologist an easy way to detect small tumor islands, and on distant metastasis, supporting the pathologist with cases of suspect metastasis of OSCC primary tumor.

We intend to propose this artificial intelligence algorithm as a Computer-Aided Diagnostic, aware that it cannot replace the pathologist in his routine activity, but that it will be able to provide they with valid help, especially for those who find themselves working in generalist diagnostic centres on the territory, not specialized in the diagnosis of an infrequent but extremely lethal disease.

5. Conclusions

In this work, we created a dataset called ORCA, containing annotated data from the TCGA dataset, to compare four different deep learning-based architectures for oral cancer segmentation, namely: SegNet, U-Net, U-Net with VGG16 encoder, and U-Net with ResNet50 encoder. The peculiarity of this work consists of the use of a training set completely different from the test data. In such a way, we tested the capability of the networks in generalizing the problem, providing promising segmentation results.

Despite the non-optimal results, to the best of our knowledge, this is the first attempt to use an automatic segmentation algorithm for oral squamous cell carcinoma and it represents an important novelty to this pathology. Furthermore, the publically-available ORCA dataset will facilitate the development of new algorithms and will boost the research on computational approaches to OSCC.

As future directions, we will aim at enlarging the training set and at making it publicly available. In this work, we considered color transformation by using a combination of HSV and RGB color models as a method for creating a multi-channel input. This was done because the group of pathologists that are authors of this work noticed that HSV color space contains a lot of visually distinguishing features about tumor cells. We did not use color modifications for augmenting the data. However, this is an interesting aspect that will be investigated in future work. Moreover, we foresee to improve our model to achieve a result that may be transferred to clinical practice.

Author Contributions: D.D.B., A.P. and F.M. (Francesco Merolla) conceived and designed the experiments; M.F. and F.M. (Francesco Martino) performed the experiments; F.M. (Francesco Merolla) and D.R. analyzed the data; G.I. contributed reagents/materials/analysis tools; S.S. and D.N. provide a critical review of the paper. All authors have read and agreed to the published version of the manuscript.

Acknowledgments: We thank Valerio Pellegrini for his contribution in the annotation of the dataset images.

References

1. Ettinger, K.S.; Ganry, L.; Fernandes, R.P. Oral Cavity Cancer. *Oral Maxillofac. Surg. Clin. N. Am.* **2019**, *31*, 13–29. [CrossRef]
2. The Global Cancer Observatory. Available online: https://gco.iarc.fr/ (accessed on 9 October 2020).

3. Bray, F.; Ferlay, J.; Soerjomataram, I.; Siegel, R.L.; Torre, L.A.; Jemal, A. Global cancer statistics 2018: GLOBOCAN estimates of incidence and mortality worldwide for 36 cancers in 185 countries. *CA Cancer J. Clin.* **2018**, *68*, 394–424. [CrossRef] [PubMed]
4. Pantanowitz, L.; Evans, A.; Pfeifer, J.; Collins, L.; Valenstein, P.; Kaplan, K.; Wilbur, D.; Colgan, T. Review of the current state of whole slide imaging in pathology. *J. Pathol. Inform.* **2011**, *2*, 36. [CrossRef] [PubMed]
5. Helin, H.; Tolonen, T.; Ylinen, O.; Tolonen, P.; Näpänkangas, J.; Isola, J. Optimized JPEG 2000 compression for efficient storage of histopathological whole-Slide images. *J. Pathol. Inform.* **2018**, *9*. [CrossRef]
6. Hanna, M.G.; Reuter, V.E.; Hameed, M.R.; Tan, L.K.; Chiang, S.; Sigel, C.; Hollmann, T.; Giri, D.; Samboy, J.; Moradel, C.; et al. Whole slide imaging equivalency and efficiency study: Experience at a large academic center. *Mod. Pathol.* **2019**, *32*, 916–928. [CrossRef]
7. Griffin, J.; Treanor, D. Digital pathology in clinical use: Where are we now and what is holding us back? *Histopathology* **2017**, *70*, 134–145. [CrossRef]
8. Dimitriou, N.; Arandjelović, O.; Caie, P.D. Deep Learning for Whole Slide Image Analysis: An Overview. *Front. Med.* **2019**, *6*, 264. [CrossRef]
9. Xu, H.; Park, S.; Hwang, T.H. Computerized Classification of Prostate Cancer Gleason Scores from Whole Slide Images. *IEEE/ACM Trans. Comput. Biol. Bioinform.* **2019**. [CrossRef]
10. Tian, K.; Rubadue, C.A.; Lin, D.I.; Veta, M.; Pyle, M.E.; Irshad, H.; Heng, Y.J. Automated clear cell renal carcinoma grade classification with prognostic significance. *PLoS ONE* **2019**, *14*. [CrossRef]
11. Jaber, M.I.; Song, B.; Taylor, C.; Vaske, C.J.; Benz, S.C.; Rabizadeh, S.; Soon-Shiong, P.; Szeto, C.W. A deep learning image-based intrinsic molecular subtype classifier of breast tumors reveals tumor heterogeneity that may affect survival. *Breast Cancer Res.* **2020**, *22*. [CrossRef]
12. Tang, Z.; Chuang, K.V.; DeCarli, C.; Jin, L.W.; Beckett, L.; Keiser, M.J.; Dugger, B.N. Interpretable classification of Alzheimer's disease pathologies with a convolutional neural network pipeline. *Nat. Commun.* **2019**, *10*. [CrossRef]
13. Guo, Z.; Liu, H.; Ni, H.; Wang, X.; Su, M.; Guo, W.; Wang, K.; Jiang, T.; Qian, Y. A Fast and Refined Cancer Regions Segmentation Framework in Whole-slide Breast Pathological Images. *Sci. Rep.* **2019**, *9*. [CrossRef]
14. Nielsen, F.S.; Pedersen, M.J.; Olsen, M.V.; Larsen, M.S.; Røge, R.; Jørgensen, A.S. Automatic Bone Marrow Cellularity Estimation in H&E Stained Whole Slide Images. *Cytom. Part A* **2019**, *95*, 1066–1074. [CrossRef]
15. Bueno, G.; Fernandez-Carrobles, M.M.; Gonzalez-Lopez, L.; Deniz, O. Glomerulosclerosis identification in whole slide images using semantic segmentation. *Comput. Methods Programs Biomed.* **2020**, *184*. [CrossRef]
16. Mahmood, H.; Shaban, M.; Indave, B.I.; Santos-Silva, A.R.; Rajpoot, N.; Khurram, S.A. Use of artificial intelligence in diagnosis of head and neck precancerous and cancerous lesions: A systematic review. *Oral Oncol.* **2020**, *110*, 104885. [CrossRef]
17. Sun, Y.N.; Wang, Y.Y.; Chang, S.C.; Wu, L.W.; Tsai, S.T. Color-based tumor tissue segmentation for the automated estimation of oral cancer parameters. *Microsc. Res. Tech.* **2009**, *73*. [CrossRef]
18. Rahman, T.Y.; Mahanta, L.B.; Chakraborty, C.; Das, A.K.; Sarma, J.D. Textural pattern classification for oral squamous cell carcinoma. *J. Microsc.* **2018**, *269*, 85–93. [CrossRef]
19. Fouad, S.; Randell, D.; Galton, A.; Mehanna, H.; Landini, G. Unsupervised morphological segmentation of tissue compartments in histopathological images. *PLoS ONE* **2017**, *12*, e0188717. [CrossRef]
20. Das, D.K.; Bose, S.; Maiti, A.K.; Mitra, B.; Mukherjee, G.; Dutta, P.K. Automatic identification of clinically relevant regions from oral tissue histological images for oral squamous cell carcinoma diagnosis. *Tissue Cell* **2018**, *53*, 111–119. [CrossRef]
21. Baik, J.; Ye, Q.; Zhang, L.; Poh, C.; Rosin, M.; MacAulay, C.; Guillaud, M. Automated classification of oral premalignant lesions using image cytometry and Random Forests-based algorithms. *Cell. Oncol.* **2014**, *37*. [CrossRef]
22. Krishnan, M.M.R.; Venkatraghavan, V.; Acharya, U.R.; Pal, M.; Paul, R.R.; Min, L.C.; Ray, A.K.; Chatterjee, J.; Chakraborty, C. Automated oral cancer identification using histopathological images: A hybrid feature extraction paradigm. *Micron* **2012**, *43*. [CrossRef]
23. Krishnan, M.M.R.; Shah, P.; Chakraborty, C.; Ray, A.K. Statistical analysis of textural features for improved classification of oral histopathological images. *J. Med. Syst.* **2012**, *36*, 865–881. [CrossRef]
24. Krishnan, M.M.R.; Choudhary, A.; Chakraborty, C.; Ray, A.K.; Paul, R.R. Texture based segmentation of epithelial layer from oral histological images. *Micron* **2011**, *42*. [CrossRef]

25. Krishnan, M.M.R.; Pal, M.; Bomminayuni, S.K.; Chakraborty, C.; Paul, R.R.; Chatterjee, J.; Ray, A.K. Automated classification of cells in sub-epithelial connective tissue of oral sub-mucous fibrosis-An SVM based approach. *Comput. Biol. Med.* **2009**, *39*, 1096–1104. [CrossRef]
26. Mookiah, M.R.K.; Shah, P.; Chakraborty, C.; Ray, A.K. Brownian motion curve-based textural classification and its application in cancer diagnosis. *Anal. Quant. Cytol. Histol.* **2011**, *33*, 158–168.
27. Martino, F.; Varricchio, S.; Russo, D.; Merolla, F.; Ilardi, G.; Mascolo, M.; Dell'aversana, G.O.; Califano, L.; Toscano, G.; Pietro, G.D.; et al. A machine-learning approach for the assessment of the proliferative compartment of solid tumors on hematoxylin-eosin-stained sections. *Cancers* **2020**, *12*, 1344. [CrossRef]
28. Graham, S.; Vu, Q.D.; Raza, S.E.; Azam, A.; Tsang, Y.W.; Kwak, J.T.; Rajpoot, N. Hover-Net: Simultaneous segmentation and classification of nuclei in multi-tissue histology images. *Med. Image Anal.* **2019**, *58*, 101563. [CrossRef]
29. Raza, S.E.; Cheung, L.; Shaban, M.; Graham, S.; Epstein, D.; Pelengaris, S.; Khan, M.; Rajpoot, N.M. Micro-Net: A unified model for segmentation of various objects in microscopy images. *Med. Image Anal.* **2019**, *52*, 160–173. [CrossRef]
30. Rahman, T.Y.; Mahanta, L.B.; Das, A.K.; Sarma, J.D. Automated oral squamous cell carcinoma identification using shape, texture and color features of whole image strips. *Tissue Cell* **2020**, *63*. [CrossRef]
31. Fraz, M.M.; Khurram, S.A.; Graham, S.; Shaban, M.; Hassan, M.; Loya, A.; Rajpoot, N.M. FABnet: Feature attention-based network for simultaneous segmentation of microvessels and nerves in routine histology images of oral cancer. *Neural Comput. Appl.* **2020**, *32*, 9915–9928. [CrossRef]
32. Shaban, M.; Khurram, S.A.; Fraz, M.M.; Alsubaie, N.; Masood, I.; Mushtaq, S.; Hassan, M.; Loya, A.; Rajpoot, N.M. A Novel Digital Score for Abundance of Tumour Infiltrating Lymphocytes Predicts Disease Free Survival in Oral Squamous Cell Carcinoma. *Sci. Rep.* **2019**, *9*, 1–13. [CrossRef]
33. Litjens, G.; Bandi, P.; Bejnordi, B.E.; Geessink, O.; Balkenhol, M.; Bult, P.; Halilovic, A.; Hermsen, M.; van de Loo, R.; Vogels, R.; et al. 1399 H&E-stained sentinel lymph node sections of breast cancer patients: The CAMELYON dataset. *GigaScience* **2018**, *7*, 1–8. [CrossRef]
34. The Cancer Genome Atlas (TCGA). Available online: https://www.cancer.gov/about-nci/organization/ccg/research/structural-genomics/tcga (accessed on 9 October 2020).
35. Weinstein, J.N.; The Cancer Genome Atlas Research Network; Collisson, E.A.; Mills, G.B.; Shaw, K.R.; Ozenberger, B.A.; Ellrott, K.; Shmulevich, I.; Sander, C.; Stuart, J.M. The cancer genome atlas pan-cancer analysis project. *Nat. Genet.* **2013**, *45*, 1113–1120. [CrossRef] [PubMed]
36. Badrinarayanan, V.; Kendall, A.; Cipolla, R. SegNet: A Deep Convolutional Encoder-Decoder Architecture for Image Segmentation. *IEEE Trans. Pattern Anal. Mach. Intell.* **2017**, *39*, 2481–2495.
37. Ronneberger, O.; Fischer, P.; Brox, T. U-Net: Convolutional Networks for Biomedical Image Segmentation. In Proceedings of the International Conference on Medical Image Computing and Computer-Assisted Intervention, Munich, Germany, 5–9 October 2015; pp. 234–241.
38. Simonyan, K.; Zisserman, A. Very Deep Convolutional Networks for Large-Scale Image Recognition. In Proceedings of the International Conference on Learning Representations, San Diego, CA, USA, 7–9 May 2015.
39. He, K.; Zhang, X.; Ren, S.; Sun, J. Deep Residual Learning for Image Recognition. In Proceedings of the IEEE Conference on Computer Vision and Pattern Recognition (CVPR), Las Vegas, NV, USA, 27–30 June 2016.
40. The National Cancer Institute (NCI). Available online: https://www.cancer.gov/ (accessed on 25 September 2020).
41. Janocha, K.; Czarnecki, W.M. On Loss Functions for Deep Neural Networks in Classification. *arXiv* **2017**, arXiv:1702.05659.
42. Sainath, T.N.; Kingsbury, B.; Soltau, H.; Ramabhadran, B. Optimization Techniques to Improve Training Speed of Deep Neural Networks for Large Speech Tasks. *IEEE Trans. Audio Speech Lang. Process.* **2013**, *21*, 2267–2276.
43. Fawakherji, M.; Potena, C.; Pretto, A.; Bloisi, D.D.; Nardi, D. Multi-Spectral Image Synthesis for Crop/Weed Segmentation in Precision Farming. *arXiv* **2020**, arXiv:2009.05750.

12

Classification Models for Skin Tumor Detection using Texture Analysis in Medical Images

Marcos A. M. Almeida [1,*] and Iury A. X. Santos [2]

[1] Departamento de Eletrônica e Sistemas, Centro de Tecnologia, Universidade Federal de Pernambuco, Recife-PE 50670-901, Brazil

[2] Departamento de Física, Universidade Federal Rural de Pernambuco, Recife-PE 52171-900, Brazil; iuryadones@gmail.com

* Correspondence: marcos.almeida@ufpe.br;

Abstract: Medical images have made a great contribution to early diagnosis. In this study, a new strategy is presented for analyzing medical images of skin with melanoma and nevus to model, classify and identify lesions on the skin. Machine learning applied to the data generated by first and second order statistics features, Gray Level Co-occurrence Matrix (GLCM), keypoints and color channel information—Red, Green, Blue and grayscale images of the skin were used to characterize decisive information for the classification of the images. This work proposes a strategy for the analysis of skin images, aiming to choose the best mathematical classifier model, for the identification of melanoma, with the objective of assisting the dermatologist in the identification of melanomas, especially towards an early diagnosis.

Keywords: texture analysis; melanoma; glcm matrix; machine learning; classifiers

---

1. Introduction

The skin cancer is among the most common types of cancer in the world [1]. Melanoma is the most dangerous type of skin cancer, caused by over production of melanin pigments that change the color and texture of skin, resulting as a dark area on the skin [2]. Data indicate that the incidence of melanoma, which is a type of cancer that metastasizes rapidly, has increased alarmingly [3].

However, visual analysis is limited by human visual ability, as well as human perception and sensitivity, in addition to the fact that not all melanomas have the same characteristics. The tumor is an exceptional expansion of human cells that reproduce in an unrestricted way and that can be identified by a variation of color and texture of the human tissue under study, making information contained in the images extremely valuable. Textures are visual patterns, which have brightness, color, slope, size and other attributes. When partitioned into sub-images by regions of interest, they are able to be properly classified.

Color is one of the significant features in the examination of skin lesion. The distribution of texture and color features presents significant information, as Figure 1 shows.

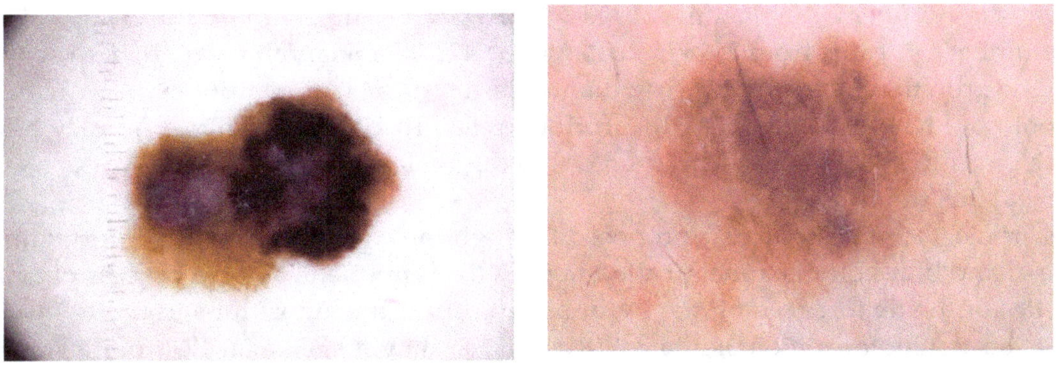

(a) (b)

Figure 1. Images of melanoma and nevus tissues: (**a**) Skin lesion from melanoma image; (**b**) Nevus Skin.

A technique of analysis that focuses on the extraction of intrinsic characteristics of the image such as—brightness and color, providing an idea of the roughness or smoothness, among other characteristics, is texture analysis. Digital image texture analysis refers to techniques that use image processing in order to extract representative features of the images studied which can have importance in the discrimination between images.

This makes it possible to accelerate decisions concerning diagnosis. In these cases, image quality is essential, relying on bandwidth, sensitivity, resolution and signal-to-noise ratio of the image systems. Artificial intelligence can be very useful in assisting oncologists and radiologists in making early diagnoses of tissue regions with melanoma [4].

In Figure 2 a graphical representation of nearly 300,000 cases predicted indicates melanoma was the 19th most-incident tumor in the world in 2018 and will continue rising, according to the World Health Organization's (WHO) International Agency for Research on Cancer (IARC) study Globocan [5].

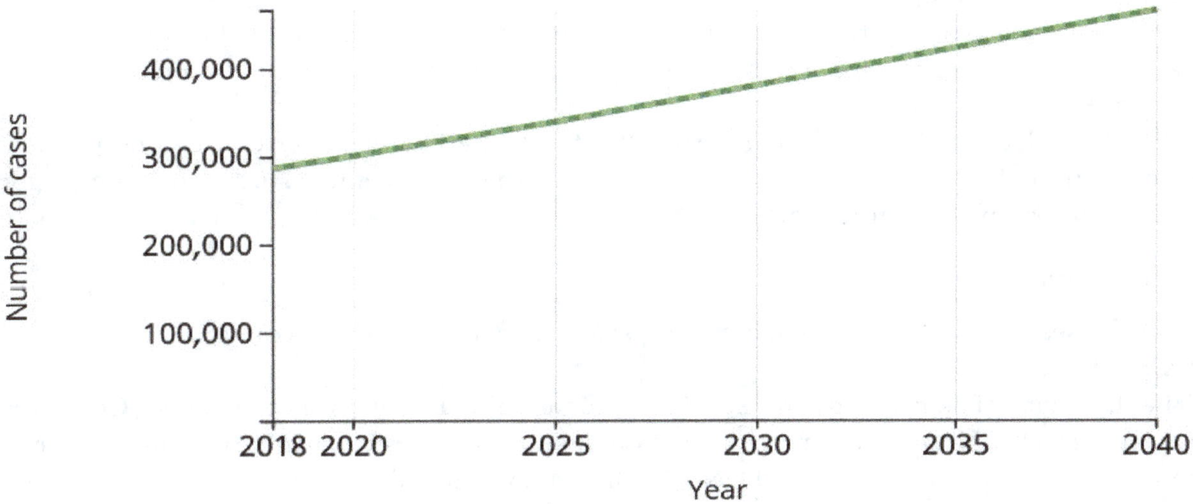

Figure 2. Estimated of incident cases from 2018 to 2040, melanoma of skin, both sexes, all ages. Source: International Agency for Research on Cancer of World Health Organization.

The estimate foresees that, this year, 2020, 1.81 million new cases of cancer and 9.5 million deaths due to neoplasia will occur. One in five men and one in six women are predicted to develop the disease over a lifetime. This is in contrast to the last survey published, in 2012, when the International Agency for Research on Cancer (IARC of WHO) predicted 14.1 million new cases and 8.2 million deaths.

According to the IARC, by 2020 there are expected to be 300,000 new cases of melanoma in the world.

In 2018, the number of melanoma cases was 287,723. The estimate for 2040 will be 466,914. Estimated number of deaths from 2018 to 2040 will be 42,208, melanoma of skin, both sexes, all ages.

Given the growth of demand for early diagnosis, a tool such as computer vision with a machine learning tool could help radiologists to produce relevant diagnoses more quickly and provide quantitative measures for regions suspected of having melanoma cancer. The works related to this research reveal this trend.

In this article, the new strategy is proposed through the addition of texture information, through the red, green and blue color channels, called here RGB components. In the process of acquiring the characteristics of the textures, using the Python syntax and the algorithms in the Python library to pinpoint the location of the region of interest (ROI) in the skin image, regardless of the image position.

Artificial intelligence when applied to the set of data representative of characteristic textures of the images, can assist oncologists and radiologists in identifying suspicious skin regions. Adequate experimental results have shown how this strategy can provide an accurate measure of quality that correspond to the subjective assessments by clinical experts [6].

The human eye, despite its perfection, is not able to capture certain details in an image or to distinguish small differences between certain micro-textures. Using Machine Learning, these differences can be measured, evaluated and compared to standard images and thus identify microtextural differences in medical examination images. Different parameters of texture reflect different properties within the image.

The purpose of resource extraction is to choose a data set representative of the original image measuring certain properties or resources that can distinguish a pattern between one sub-image and another.

This is a problem of binary classification, since the samples belonged to two classes—nevus tissue or melanoma, so the proposal for a solution for this new strategy for detecting melanoma is presented. All experimental simulations were implemented and executed using the Python language.

The paper is organized as follows—Section 2 presents the studies related to research, introducing the most common techniques used for the detection of tumors.

Section 3, deals with the theoretical framework in first and second order statistics.

Section 4 proposes strategies and solutions using a machine learning application for the detection of skin cancer.

Section 5 is dedicated to presenting the results of the experiments. Some discussions are presented in Section 6 and in Section 7 we make conclusions from the results of this study, with suggestions for new lines of research and future work.

2. Related Works

Some research works are related to our study because they use convergent techniques for texture analysis.

The diagnosis of skin lesions was studied by Zhang [7]. The analysis considered Convolutional Neural Networks (CNN) for automatic detection of skin cancer, comparing this with other research methods. The proposed method called CNN/WOA achieved an accuracy of 91.00%, with a sensitivity of 95.00% and specificity of 91.00%.

Pathan [8] reviewed the cutting-edge techniques declared in the literature, summarizing these state of art approaches. The steps included dermoscopic image pre-processing, segmentation, extraction and selection of peculiar characteristics and disposition of the skin lesions. The study also evaluated the consequences of the methodologies reported in the literature in addition to the results and future directions of research. The best result from the listed methods and algorithms was the Otsu threshold with Active Contour using a Sparse-Field level-set method, with a precision ability of 97.50% for the detection of melanomas.

Lee et al. [9] proposed the skin disease classification solution using Fine-tuned Neural Networks. The model achieved an accuracy of 89.90% and 78.50% in the validation set and the test set, respectively.

Using the technique of aggregating robust convolutional neural networks (CNNs) into a structure, Harangi [10] achieved classification results in three classes of injuries. The experimental results concluded that the average area under the receiver operating characteristic curve (AUC) was 89.10% for the task of categorizing the 3 classes.

Li [11] proposed two deep learning methods to address three main tasks emerging in the area of skin lesion image processing, that is, lesion segmentation (task 1), lesion dermoscopic feature extraction (task 2) and lesion classification (task 3). The proposed deep learning frameworks were evaluated on the ISIC 2017 dataset. Experimental results show the promising accuracies of these frameworks, that is, 75.30% for task 1, 84.80% for task 2 and 91.20% for task 3 were achieved.

A method proposed by Abbadi [12], takes into account the techniques known as ABCD—Asymmetry, Edge, Color and Diameter. For the detection of melanoma, the metric TDS (Total Dermoscopy Score) was calculated to perform the classification. The accuracy found in the results was 95.45%.

Fernandez [3] proposed in his research the extraction of characteristics that appear in the image of the lesion and treated with the Gray Level Co-occurrence Matrix (GLCM) method. Then, during the detection phase, a set of classifiers determined the occurrence of a malignant tumor. The experiments were carried out on images obtained from the ISIC repository. The proposed system provides skin cancer detection accuracy above 88.00%.

Ansari [13] proposed a skin cancer detection framework using SVM for early detection of skin cancer. The dermoscopic image of skin cancer was obtained and submitted to different pre-processing strategies using filtering images. The GLCM system was used to select specific highlights on the image which were then used to help establish the classifier. The classification determined whether the image was of a cancerous or non-cancerous tissue. The accuracy of the proposed structure is 95.00%.

The following are references from other authors with their respective works and applications, using similar techniques for extracting characteristics in medical images.

The diagnosis of breast cancer subtypes using image texture analysis was studied by Waugh [14]. The analysis considered the distribution of the pixel intensities in the magnetic resonance images. The entropy parameters of the GLCM matrix resulted in significant contributions to image classification, which can be useful in the treatment and monitoring of breast cancer therapeutics.

Recently, Vamvakas [15] proposed the solution of a challenge in the diagnosis of magnetic resonance images, using advanced techniques such as Diffusion Tensor Imaging—distinguishing ambiguous images in the appearance of Glioblastoma Multiforme and solitary metastasis, using 3D textural resources with GLCM.

Jennitta [16] using GLCM and Local Standard Descriptor parameters, applied to magnetic resonance images of the brain, showed a promising approach to medical diagnosis.

Hiba Asri [17], with the objective of diagnosing breast cancer, used machine learning techniques, such as—Support Vector Machine (SVM), Decision Tree, Naive Bayes and K closest neighbors, in the Wisconsin Breast Cancer database. The results proved that the SVM had the best accuracy—97.13%.

In a recent study on lung cancer, Yoon et al. [18], selected parameters for texture analysis in magnetic resonance images. Correlation between tumor area and size was calculated by linear regression. The injection of contrast material was used to check the MRI images and improvements were recorded in the selected texture parameters, in a time window between 120–180 s.

A predictive and two probabilistic model for detecting cancer in the human liver using computed tomography images was shown by Seal [19]. Haralick [20] calculated parameters in the GLCM of images of the liver with injury and without injury, as made available with several classification models such as—Logistic Regression (LR), Linear Discriminant Analysis (LDA) and a predictive model using Multilayer Perceptron (MLP), to estimate the likelihood of a patient having liver cancer or not. It was proved that logistic regression (96.67%) obtained the best accuracy when compared to LDA (95.00%) and MLP (94.40%).

Harshavardhan [21] used the SVM (Support Vector Machine) to classify data extracted from brain images to characterize benign or malignant tumors. To evaluate the performance of these resources, several texture methods were used, such as the histogram, Gray Level Co-occurrence Matrix (GLCM), gray level execution length matrix (GRLM), all analyzed separately. Performance results ranged from 82.97% to 92.83%.

Bahadure [22] demonstrated an efficient proposal to identify normal and abnormal tissues from MRI images of the brain. The experimental results identified one classified with an accuracy of 96.51%, specificity of 94.20% and sensitivity of 97.72%. Machine learning techniques were used, with data on texture, color, contrast and GLCM of the studied images.

Abdel-Nasser et al. [23] proposed a method that generates a set of compact representations of infrared breast images, with competitive results (AUC = 0.989), able to differentiate between normal and cancerous cases.

3. Materials and Methods

There follows a general description of the statistical parameters used in the proposal of this work, for the extraction of characteristics from the images. These characteristics make up the co-occurrence matrix (GLCM) and are part of the keypoints, applied to each image.

Let f (x, y) be a function of two discrete variables x and y, $x = 0, 1, \ldots, N-1$ and $y = 0, 1, \ldots, M-1$. The discrete function f (x, y) can assume values for $i = 0, 1, \ldots$, L − 1, where L is the number of grayscale levels. The intensity-level histogram is a function showing (for each intensity level) the number of pixels in the whole image, which have this intensity:

$$h(i) = \sum_{x=0}^{N-1} \sum_{y=0}^{M-1} \delta(f(x,y), j), \tag{1}$$

where $\delta(i, j)$ is the Kronecker delta function

$$\delta(i,j) = \begin{cases} 1. & i = j \\ 0. & i \neq j \end{cases}. \tag{2}$$

The probability of occurrence of each pixel in the image that will appear in the histogram is given by:

$$p(i) = \frac{h(i)}{M}, \qquad i = 0,\ 1,\ \ldots,\ L-1. \tag{3}$$

These resources are determined automatically, constituting the first order statistics (Equations (4)–(7)) and used at keypoints. The average intensity of the grayscale is calculated by:

$$\mu = \sum_{i=0}^{L-1} ip(i). \tag{4}$$

The variance shows the degree of variability around the average grayscale distribution:

$$\sigma^2 = \sum_{i=0}^{L-1} (i-\mu)^2 p(i). \tag{5}$$

Skewness measures the asymmetry of the histogram:

$$\mu_3 = \sigma^{-3} \sum_{i=0}^{L-1} (i-\mu)^3 p(i). \tag{6}$$

Kurtosis is a measure of whether the data are heavy-tailed or light-tailed relative to the normal distribution. The kurtosis is a measure of flatness of the histogram.

$$\mu_4 = \sigma^{-4}\sum_{i=0}^{L-1}(i-\mu)^4 p(i) - 3. \tag{7}$$

The second-order histogram is defined as that Gray-Level Co-occurrence Matrix, that is a square matrix is formed by elements that indicate the probability of occurrence for a pair of pixels with intensities that depend on the distance d and the angle θ. Equations (8) through (14) make up the second-order statistics set.

$$\mathrm{p(i,j,d,}\ \theta) = \{((x_1, y_1), (x_2, y_2)) : h(x_1, y_1) = i\ ,\ h(x_2, y_2) = j\}, \tag{8}$$

where

$$(x_2,\ y_2) = (x_1\ ,\ y_1) + (dcos\theta, dsen\theta). \tag{9}$$

In this study, the distances considered were d = 1, 2, . . . , 5, with angles $\theta = 0°, 45°, 90°$ and 135°.

Energy derived from the second angular momentum measures the local uniformity of the shades of gray.

$$E = \sum_i\sum_j [p(i,j)]^2. \tag{10}$$

Entropy measures the degree of clutter between the image pixels:

$$H = -\sum_i\sum_j p(i,j)log_2[p(i,j)]. \tag{11}$$

Correlation is a measure of how a pixel is associated with its neighbor across the image and assumes values ranging from ±1.

$$\rho = \sum_{i=0}^{L-1}\sum_{j=0}^{L-1} p(i,j)\frac{(i-\mu_X)(j-\mu_Y)}{\sigma_X\sigma_Y}. \tag{12}$$

Contrast is a difference moment of the GLCM and measures the amount of local variations in an image:

$$C = \sum_{i=0}^{L-1}\sum_{j=0}^{L-1}(i-j)^2 p(i,j). \tag{13}$$

Haralick [20] proposed a set of scalar quantities for summarizing the information contained in a GLCM. Originally these comprised a total of 14 features namely, angular second moment, contrast, correlation, sum of variance, inverse difference moment, sum average, sum variance, sum entropy, entropy, difference variance, difference entropy, information measures of correlation and maximal correlation coefficient. In order to obtain texture features, the normalized GLCM was computed for each of four orientations (0°, 45°, 90° and 135°).

GLCM expresses the texture feature according to the calculation of the conditional probability of the pixel pair of the gray intensities, for the different spatial positions [24].

$$p(i,j|\mathrm{d},\theta) = \frac{p(i,j,\mathrm{d},\ \theta)}{\sum_i\sum_j p(i,j|d,\theta)}. \tag{14}$$

The next step was to format a proposal, containing the extraction of characteristics from medical images to build a classification based on several state-of-the-art classifiers.

4. Proposed Strategy

The present study investigates the best strategy for aiding in the diagnosis of the presence or absence of melanoma through skin imaging. In the proposed strategy, what differentiates it from other methods of texture analysis is the inclusion of RGB components, adding texture information to the keypoints.

The developed strategy involves the following steps:

1. Random selection of a set of images with melanoma and nevus.
2. Generation of keypoints containing:
   a. first order statistics information;
   b. second order statistics parameters;
   c. RGB component information.
3. Extraction of characteristics from all training images.
4. Classification phase with the modeling using the training database.
5. Application of the selected model to a test image database.
6. Result of the model applied to the test database.

In addition, the algorithm used to read the keypoints does not depend on the image position, when capturing information in the region of interest—ROI.

The block diagram in Figure 3 shows the proposed strategy.

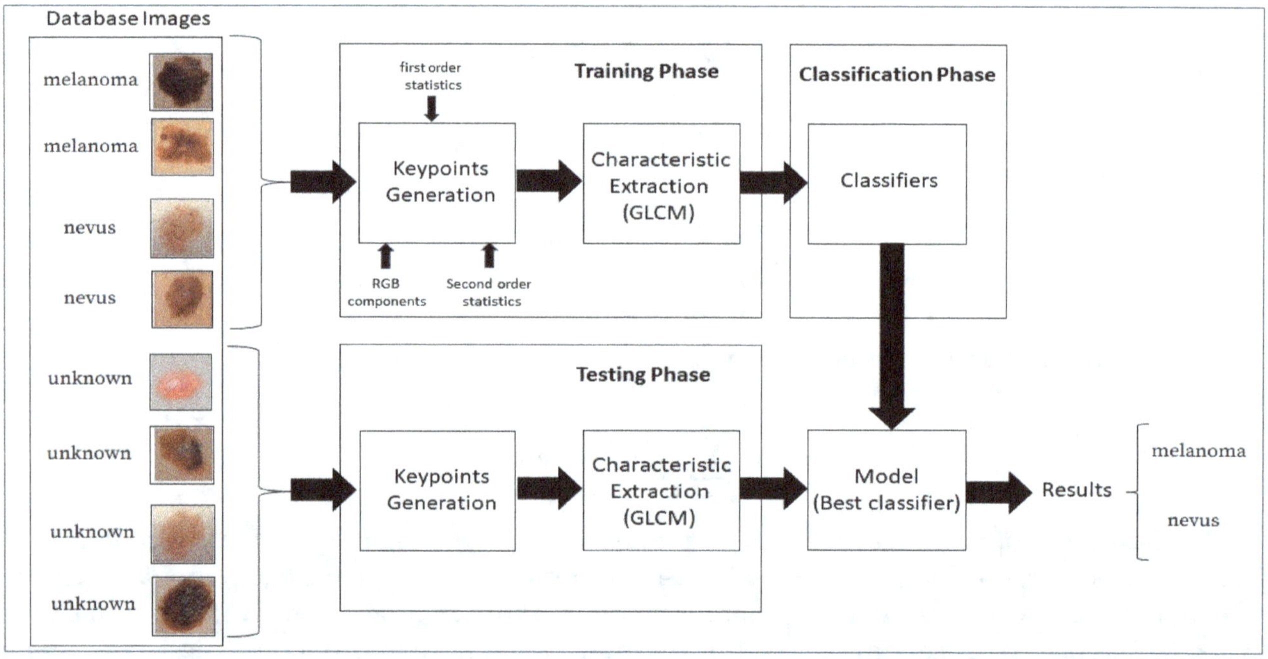

Figure 3. Block Diagram of the proposed strategy.

All data sets used are available in the Skin Lesion Analysis Towards Melanoma—International Skin Imaging Collaboration (ISIC) 2019 [25].

The database was formed by 2000 jpeg skin images, selected at random. The learning process was performed on 75% of the database, as in this research, 10 samples were used per image, the learning process analyzed a total of 15,000 samples. In the testing process, the remaining 25% of the images in the database were used, making a total of 5000 samples in the testing phase. Each sample had a dimension of 6 pixels × 6 pixels.

To increase the efficiency in extracting characteristics for differentiation of the tissues, it was necessary to add parameters as first and second order statistics into keypoints, such as—mean, variance, kurtosis, skewness, contrast, correlation, entropy, energy, maximum and minimum value, as well as RGB components.

After extracting the characteristics of the images, modeling was performed through training the database, using the best-known classifiers and their variations, as found in the academic literature:

- Stochastic Gradient Classifier. The basic idea of this classifier method is straightforward—iteratively adjust the parameters θ in the direction where the gradient of the cost function is large and negative. In this way, the training procedure ensures the parameters flow towards a local minimum of the cost function.
- Naïve Bayes Classifier. A Naive Bayes classifier is a simple probabilistic classifier based on applying Bayes' theorem (from Bayesian statistics) with strong (naive) independence assumptions. This classifier is among those common learning methods grouped by similarities which makes use of Bayes' theorem of probability to build ML models, especially those related to disease prediction and document classification.
- Decision Tree Classifier. A decision tree is a decision support tool that uses a tree-like graph and its possible results. It is a way to display the algorithm.
- Random Forest Classifier. Random forests are an ensemble learning method for classification, regression and other tasks, that operate by constructing a multitude of decision trees at training time. As a result, the classes (classification) or average forecast (regression) of these individually generated trees are grouped. This method aims at averaging many approximately unbiased but noisy trees to obtain low variances results. Is a collection of decisions tress, which, together, forms a forest.
- KNN Classifier. Classification is achieved by identifying the nearest neighbors to a query example and using those neighbors to determine the class of the query.
- Support Vector Machine Classifier. The objective of the SVM classifier is to find the hyperplane that separates the points of classes C_1 and C_2 with a maximum margin, linearly penalizing points within the margin through a regularization parameter selected by the user. Support vector machines bring a new option to the pattern recognition problem with clear connections in statistical learning theory. They differ radically from other methods, for example, neural networks—the training of an SVM always finds a global minimum and its simple geometric interpretation provides much scope for deeper investigations.
- Model Logistic Regression Classifier. Logistic regression classifies by using the log-ratios between the probability of groups given the data. For the groups g_1 and g_2:

$$log\frac{P(G = g_1|X = x)}{P(G = g_2|X = x)} = \beta_0 + x\,\beta_x = 0. \tag{15}$$

The decision boundary is the value where the probability of the group given the data is equal. To find it, the likelihood function of β is maximized:

$$L(\beta) = \sum_{i=1}^{N} logPg_i(x|\beta). \tag{16}$$

In machine learning, the classification identifies to which Class a set of observed data belongs. Classification is an example of pattern recognition. Some variants of the classifiers cited and available in the library of the Python environment were used, to increase the set of classifiers tested:

1. sklearn.linear_model.SGDClassifier;
2. sklearn.naive_bayes.GaussianNB;
3. sklearn.naive_bayes.BernoulliNB;

4. sklearn.naive_bayes.MultinomialNB;
5. sklearn.tree.DecisionTreeClassifier;
6. sklearn.ensemble.ExtraTreesClassifier;
7. sklearn.ensemble.RandomForestClassifier;
8. sklearn.ensemble.GradientBoostingClassifier;
9. sklearn.neighbors.KNeighborsClassifier;
10. sklearn.svm.LinearSVC;
11. sklearn.svm.SVC;
12. sklearn.linear_model.LogisticRegression.

After the computational effort using the twelve classifiers, the five best ones were selected, based on the area under the Receiver Operating Characteristics:

1. Linear Model Logistic Regression.
2. Gradient Boosting (Stochastic Gradient Boosting).
3. SVM Linear SVC (Support Vector Machine Linear—Support Vector Classification).
4. Linear Model Stochastic Gradient Descendent (Linear Model SGD).
5. SVM SVC (Support Vector Machine—Support Vector Clustering).

The results of the database simulation are provided in detail in the following sections.

5. Results

First-order statistics concern the distribution of gray levels in an image, where the first-order histogram is used as the basis for extracting its characteristics, such as—mean, standard deviation, kurtosis and skewness, as shown in Table 1. These are not sufficient, however, for decision making between what is melanoma tissue and what is healthy tissue. The Mann-Whitney U test applied to the parameters in Table 1 show that ($p < 0.05$), therefore, the null hypothesis is rejected. Meaning that the distributions of both samples (melanoma and nevus) are not the same.

Table 1. First-order statistics.

Parameters	Nevus Tissue	Melanoma Tissue	*p*-Value
Mean Intensity	0.4514 ± 0.14340	0.4204 ± 0.1543	0.000
Kurtosis	3.0953 ± 5.4136	3.6476 ± 6.7590	0.003
Skewness	0.1935 ± 1.7280	0.2479 ± 1.8501	0.022

The boxplot in Figure 4 shows that it is not possible to differentiate nevus tissue from tissue with melanoma by only observing the average intensity values.

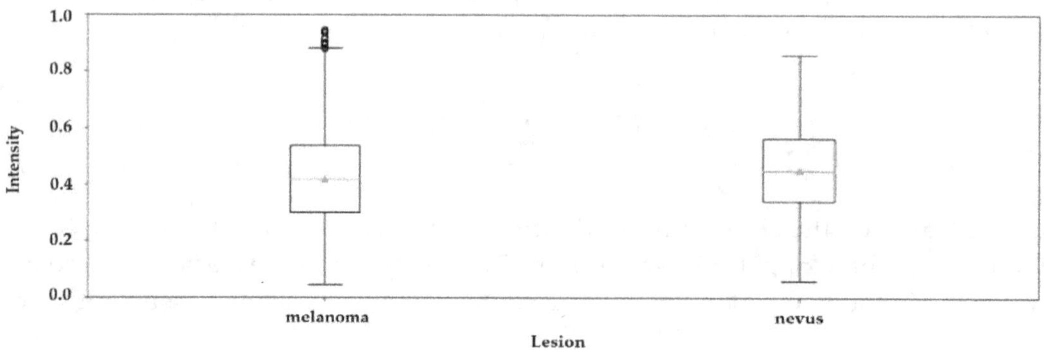

Figure 4. Boxplot with average intensities of grayscale images with melanoma and nevus.

Performance Metrics for Classifiers

In academic medical literature, instances are designated as positive, indicating the existence of the disease and negative, indicating the absence of the disease; thus, four possibilities arise when medical images are submitted to the classifiers:

- TP-True Positive: correctly classified positive cases.
- TN-True Negative: correctly classified negative cases.
- FP-False Positive: incorrectly classified negative cases.
- FN-False Negative: incorrectly classified positive cases.

The metrics that were considered to evaluate the classifiers for these were:

1. Accuracy is the ratio of the number of instances correctly classified to the number of all instances in the test suite.

$$Accuracy = \frac{TP + TN}{TP + TN + FP + FN} \tag{17}$$

2. Sensitivity, also known as recall, is the ratio of positives predicted correctly relative to the actual number of positives in the test set.

$$Sensitivity = \frac{TP}{TP + FN} \tag{18}$$

3. Specificity is the version of the sensitivity for negatives and indicates the proportion of negatives correctly predicted relative to the actual number of negatives.

$$Specificity = \frac{TN}{TP + FP} \tag{19}$$

4. The F score is a metric that considers both precision and sensitivity by taking their harmonic mean.

$$F - score = 2 * \frac{recall * precision}{recall + precision} \tag{20}$$

The ideal limit for all metrics is to reach the unit value.

Table 2 shows the five best classifiers in descending order by Area Under the Receiver Operating Characteristics (AUC); these presented the best performance, of the twelve tested.

In this study, considering the test database, the AUC of this set of classifiers, reached levels between 95.04% and 97.46%. All experiments were conducted under the same Python software setup.

Having a unique metric evaluation facilitates the decision-making process for selection of the best classifier from a set of the top five. This metric is the AUC. It provides a clear classification of preferences among all of them and therefore a clear choice of direction. Thus, the best classifier was the Linear Logistic Regression Model.

Table 2. Classifiers ordered by Area Under the Receiver Operating Characteristics (AUC).

	Classifiers	AUC	Precision	Recall	F1-Score	Support
1.	Logistic Regression	0.9746				
	Melanoma		0.98	0.97	0.98	269
	Nevus		0.96	0.98	0.97	231
	Accuracy				0.97	
	Weighted average		0.97	0.98	0.97	500
2.	Gradient Boosting	0.9699				
	Melanoma		0.97	0.97	0.97	269
	Nevus		0.97	0.97	0.97	231
	Accuracy				0.97	
	Weighted average		0.97	0.97	0.97	500
3.	SVM Linear SVC	0.9659				
	Melanoma		0.99	0.94	0.97	269
	Nevus		0.93	0.99	0.96	231
	Accuracy				0.96	
	Weighted average		0.96	0.97	0.96	500
4.	Linear Model SGD	0.9551				
	Melanoma		0.95	0.97	0.96	269
	Nevus		0.96	0.94	0.95	231
	Accuracy				0.96	
	Weighted average		0.96	0.96	0.96	500
5.	SVM SVC	0.9504				
	Melanoma		0.94	0.97	0.96	269
	Nevus		0.96	0.93	0.95	231
	Accuracy				0.95	
	Weighted average		0.95	0.95	0.95	500

[1] Linear Model Logistic Regression. [2] Stochastic Gradient Boosting. [3] Support Vector Machine Linear—Support Vector Classification. [4] Linear Model Stochastic Gradient Descendent. [5] Support Vector Machine—Support Vector Clustering.

The receiver operating curve (ROC) in Figure 5 is another common tool used with the binary classifier. It clarifies resource selection and the accuracy of the logistic regression classifier. The blue dotted line represents the ROC curve of a purely random classifier. A good classifier stays as far away from that line as possible, as here, in the upper left corner.

A suitable overall measure for the curve is the area under the curve (AUC).

The confusion matrix of the Logistic Regression method that describes the complete performance of the model is shown in Figure 6. This generates a sensitivity and specificity of 0.97.

The accuracy of a classification can be evaluated by computing the number of correctly recognized class examples (true positives), the number of correctly recognized examples that do not belong to the class (true negatives) and examples that either were incorrectly assigned to the class (false positives) or that were not recognized as class examples (false negatives) [26].

In the Linear Logistic Regression model, the recall for identification of melanoma was 97%. So, of the 500 medical images in the test database, 269 images were of melanoma and the classifier was 97% correct, that is, it identified TP = 261 images correctly, wrongly classifying FN = 8 of the images as nevus.

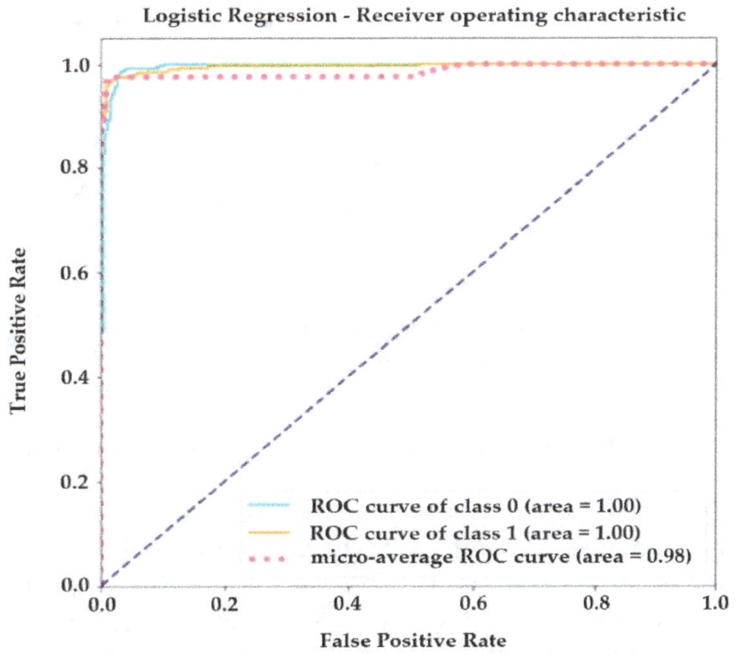

Figure 5. Receiver operating curve (ROC) curve of logistic regression.

Similarly, the recall for nevus identification was 98.00%. The classifier recognized TN = 226 images as nevus, classifying FP = 5 images as melanoma, for a total of 231 nevus medical images.

The same reasoning can be made for the other classifiers listed in Table 2.

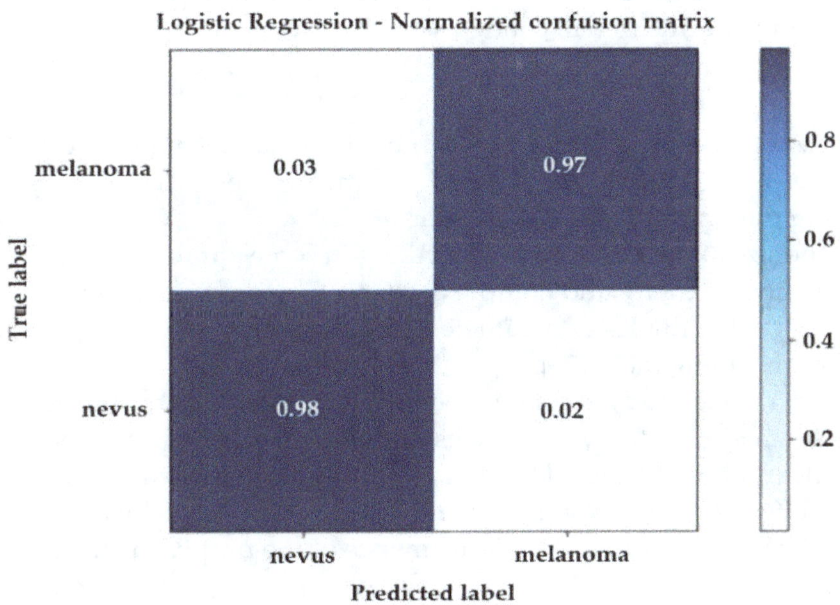

Figure 6. Confusion Matrix considering the Logistic Regression Model.

For the best performance model, the probability curve is shown through the sigmoid curve showed in Figure 7.

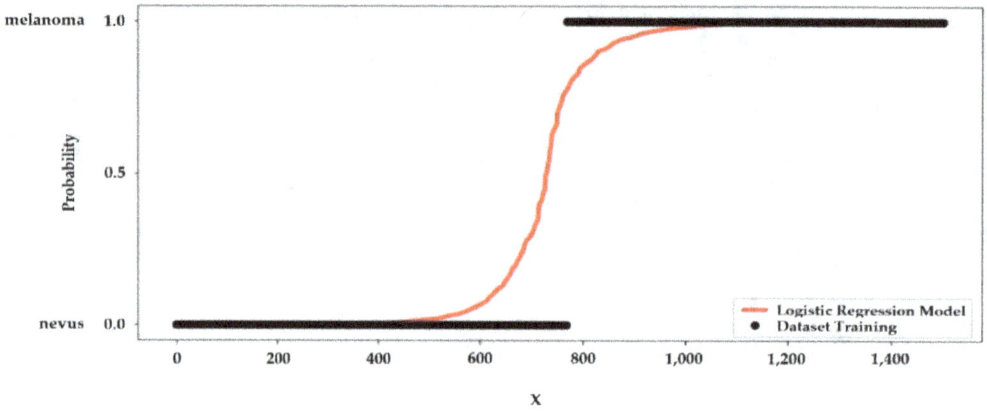

Figure 7. Logistic Regression Model of the Proposed Strategy.

Just as linear regression uses the least common square method to minimize error and to attain the best possible solution, logistic regression achieves the best results using the maximum likelihood method, plotting the probability curve as a function of the number of samples tested. The steeper this curve, the smaller the sample range that leads to the probability curve $0 < p < 1$, for diagnosis detection, $p > 0.5$ probably the tissue will be melanoma, if $p < 0.5$ the tissue will be nevus.

A ROC curve is a graphical tool used to understand the performance of a classification model. For a logistic regression model, a prediction can either be positive or negative. Also, this prediction can either be correct or incorrect.

$$False\ Positive\ Rate = \frac{FP}{TN + FP} = 1 - Specificity. = 84.01\%. \tag{21}$$

The Specificity is 15.99%. The number of positive and negative outcomes change as we change the threshold of probability values to classify a probability value as a positive or negative outcome. Thus, the Sensitivity and Specificity will change as well [27].

6. Discussion

Although the results were satisfactory with the use of statistical techniques, for future studies, it should be noted that when second order GLCM parameters were used, it is necessary to take some precautions regarding the size of the region of interest.

In some cases, the size of the ROI can change values in some parameters. For example, parameters describing the image homogeneity and complexity (angular second moment, entropy, sum entropy and difference entropy) are examples of parameters that depend on the ROI size, especially with small ROI sizes that approach a limit value [28].

The AUC found in this study, as shown in Table 2, considering the test database, reached levels between 95.04% and 97.46%, which corresponds to an accuracy between 95.00% and 97.00%, respectively. The Linear Model Logistic Regression classifiers were the most accurate.

This shows the effectiveness of second-order statistics and the inclusion of RGB components in the composition of keypoints in improving performance of the proposed strategy.

7. Conclusions

The proposed mechanism of identifying and classifying skin tissue is general; in future work it can be applied to other medical images to verify the results, since the strategy analyzes the texture of the images and reveals their differences according to the parameters set, enabling the image classification.

Texture analysis utilizes the changes in the grey value of image pixels and their distribution pattern, which can reflect microscopic pathological changes that are not visible to the human eye and can be used in the analysis of various images. Thus, texture analysis in medical imaging can be a substantial support for the clinical decision-making process in the diagnosis and classification of tumors. This methodology is expected to become more accurate than the human eye in detecting minute deviations in cell and tissue structures.

Statistical methods using GLCM features, associated with red, green and blue color information to perform micro-texture analyzes of human tissues and image classification for tumor detection showed great efficiency in the results presented.

The results show that for the detection of melanoma in human tissues, the logistic regression model was the best model with 97.00% of accuracy and precision on benchmark dataset and also a sensitivity and specificity of 97.00%.

The second-best method of classifying the data of the evaluated medical images was the Classification of the Gradient Boosting.

Author Contributions: M.A.M.A. and I.A.X.S. contributed in equal proportion to the development of the algorithm presented in this paper, which was written by the first author. I.A.X.S. was responsible for the Python implementation of the proposed algorithm. All authors have read and agreed to the published version of the manuscript.

Acknowledgments: We would like to thank the International Skin Imaging Collaboration (ISIC), sponsored by the International Society for Digital Skin Imaging (ISDIS) for making publicly available databases on the ISIC Archive containing the largest publicly available collection of quality controlled dermoscopic images of skin lesions.

References

1. World Cancer Research Fund—American Institute for Cancer Research. Available online: https://www.wcrf.org/dietandcancer/cancer-trends/skin-cancer-statistics (accessed on 1 June 2020).
2. Karabulut, E.M.; Ibrikci, T. Texture Analysis of Melanoma Images for Computer-aided Diagnosis. In Proceedings of the Annual Int'l Conference on Intelligent Computing, Computer Science and Information Systems (ICCSIS-16), Pattaya, Thailand, 28–29 April 2016; Volume 1, pp. 26–29.
3. Fernandez, H.C.; Ortega, O.L. Félix Castro-Espinozaa and Volodymyr Ponomaryov. An Intelligent System for the Diagnosis of Skin Cancer on Digital Images taken with Dermoscopy. *Acta Polytech. Hung.* **2017**, *14*, 169–185.
4. Almeida, M.A.M. Use of Statistical Techniques to Analyze Textures in Medical Images for Tumor Detection and Evaluation. *Adv. Mol. Imaging Interv. Radiol.* **2018**, *1*, 1–6.
5. World Health Organization's (WHO); International Agency for Research on Cancer (IARC). Available online: https://www.iarc.fr (accessed on 2 May 2020).
6. Singh, P.; Mukundan, R.; De Ryke, R. Texture Based Quality Analysis of Simulated Synthetic Ultrasound Images Using Local Binary Patterns. *J. Imaging* **2017**, *4*, 3. [CrossRef]
7. Zhang, L.; Gao, H.J.; Zhang, J.; Badami, B. Optimization of the Convolutional Neural Networks for Automatic Detection of Skin Cancer. *Open Med.* **2020**, *15*, 27–37. [CrossRef] [PubMed]
8. Pathan, S.; Prabhu, G.; Siddalingaswamy, P. Techniques and algorithms for computer aided diagnosis of pigmented skin lesions—A review. *Biomed. Signal Process. Control.* **2018**, *39*, 237–262. [CrossRef]
9. Lee, Y.C.; Jung, S.H.; Won, H.H. WonDerM: Skin Lesion Classification with Fine-tuned Neural Netwporks. In *ISIC 2018 Lesion Analysis Towards Melanoma Detection*; Cornell University: Ithaca, NY, USA, 2018; pp. 1–4.
10. Harangi, B. Skin lesion classification with ensembles of deep convolutional neural networks. *J. Biomed. Inform.* **2018**, *86*, 25–32. [CrossRef]
11. Li, Y.; Shen, L. Skin Lesion Analysis towards Melanoma Detection Using Deep Learning Network. *Sensors* **2018**, *18*, 556. [CrossRef]
12. Abbadi, N.K.; Faisal, Z. Detection and Analysis of Skin Cancer from Skin Lesions. *Int. J. Appl. Eng. Res.* **2017**, *12*, 9046–9052.
13. Ansari, U.B. Skin Cancer Detection Using Image Processing. *Int. Res. J. Eng. Technol.* **2017**, *4*, 2875–2881.
14. Waugh, S.; Purdie, C.; Jordan, L.B.; Vinnicombe, S.; Lerski, R.A.; Martin, P.; Thompson, A.M. Magnetic resonance imaging texture analysis classification of primary breast cancer. *Eur. Radiol.* **2015**, *26*, 322–330. [CrossRef]

15. Vamvakas, A.; Tsougos, I.; Arikidis, N.; Kapsalaki, E.; Fountas, K.; Fezoulidis, I.; Costaridou, L. Exploiting morphology and texture of 3D tumor models in DTI for differentiating glioblastoma multiforme from solitary metastasis. *Biomed. Signal Process. Control.* **2018**, *43*, 159–173. [CrossRef]
16. Jenitta, A.; Ravindran, R.S. Image Retrieval Based on Local Mesh Vector Co-occurrence Pattern for Medical Diagnosis from MRI Brain Images. *J. Med Syst.* **2017**, *41*, 1–10. [CrossRef] [PubMed]
17. Asri, H.; Mousannif, H.; Al Moatassime, H.; Noel, T. Using Machine Learning Algorithms for Breast Cancer Risk Prediction and Diagnosis. *Procedia Comput. Sci.* **2016**, *83*, 1064–1069. [CrossRef]
18. Yoon, S.H.; Park, C.M.; Park, S.J.; Yoon, J.-H.; Hahn, S.; Goo, J.M. Tumor Heterogeneity in Lung Cancer: Assessment with Dynamic Contrast-enhanced MR Imaging. *Radiol.* **2016**, *280*, 940–948. [CrossRef] [PubMed]
19. Seal, A.; Bhattacharjee, D.; Nasipuri, M. Predictive and probabilistic model for cancer detection using computer tomography images. *Multimedia Tools Appl.* **2017**, *77*, 3991–4010. [CrossRef]
20. Haralick, R.M. Statistical and structural approaches to texture. *Proc. IEEE* **1979**, *67*, 786–804. [CrossRef]
21. Harshavardhan, A.; Babu, S.; Venugopal, T. Analysis of Feature Extraction Methods for the Classification of Brain Tumor Detection. *Int. J. of Pure Appl. Math.* **2017**, *117*, 147–154.
22. Bahadure, N.; Ray, A.K.; Thethi, H.P. Image Analysis for MRI Based Brain Tumor Detection and Feature Extraction Using Biologically Inspired BWT and SVM. *Int. J. Biomed. Imaging* **2017**, *2017*, 1–12. [CrossRef]
23. Abdel-Nasser, M.; Moreno, A.; Puig, D. Breast Cancer Detection in Thermal Infrared Images Using Representation Learning and Texture Analysis Methods. *Electron.* **2019**, *8*, 100. [CrossRef]
24. Ayyachamy, S. Registration Based Retrieval using Texture Measures. *Appl. Med Inform.* **2015**, *37*, 1–10.
25. International Skin Imaging Collaboration. Available online: https://challenge2019.isic-archive.com/ (accessed on 2 December 2019).
26. Ashish, K. *Learning Predictive Analytics with Phyton*; Packet Publishing—Open Source: Birmingham, UK, 2016; pp. 346–352.
27. Sokolova, M.; Lapalme, G. A systematic analysis of performance measures for classification tasks. *Inf. Process. Manag.* **2009**, *45*, 427–437. [CrossRef]
28. Sikiö, M.; Holli-Helenius, K.K.; Ryymin, P.; Dastidar, P.; Eskola, H.; Harrison, L. The effect of region of interest size on textural parameters. In Proceedings of the 2015 9th International Symposium on Image and Signal Processing and Analysis (ISPA), Zagreb, Croatia, 7–9 September 2015; Institute of Electrical and Electronics Engineers (IEEE): Piscataway, NJ, USA, 2015; pp. 149–153.

13

Deep Learning in Selected Cancers' Image Analysis

Taye Girma Debelee [1,2,*], Samuel Rahimeto Kebede [1,3], Friedhelm Schwenker [4] and Zemene Matewos Shewarega [1]

1 Artificial Intelligence Center, 40782 Addis Ababa, Ethiopia; samuelrahimeto@dbu.edu.et (S.R.K.); zemene.matewos@aic.et (Z.M.S.)
2 College of Electrical and Mechanical Engineering, Addis Ababa Science and Technology University, 120611 Addis Ababa, Ethiopia
3 Department of Electrical and Computer Engineering, Debreberhan University, 445 Debre Berhan, Ethiopia
4 Institute of Neural Information Processing, University of Ulm, 89081 Ulm, Germany; friedhelm.schwenker@uni-ulm.de
* Correspondence: tayegirma@gmail.com

Abstract: Deep learning algorithms have become the first choice as an approach to medical image analysis, face recognition, and emotion recognition. In this survey, several deep-learning-based approaches applied to breast cancer, cervical cancer, brain tumor, colon and lung cancers are studied and reviewed. Deep learning has been applied in almost all of the imaging modalities used for cervical and breast cancers and MRIs for the brain tumor. The result of the review process indicated that deep learning methods have achieved state-of-the-art in tumor detection, segmentation, feature extraction and classification. As presented in this paper, the deep learning approaches were used in three different modes that include training from scratch, transfer learning through freezing some layers of the deep learning network and modifying the architecture to reduce the number of parameters existing in the network. Moreover, the application of deep learning to imaging devices for the detection of various cancer cases has been studied by researchers affiliated to academic and medical institutes in economically developed countries; while, the study has not had much attention in Africa despite the dramatic soar of cancer risks in the continent.

Keywords: deep learning; medical image analysis; breast cancer; brain tumor; cervical cancer; colon cancer; lung cancer

1. Introduction

Over the last decades, three different approaches have been practiced to deal with medical images. The first is creating awareness among the community for a regular check-up and it was not be practiced among communities. The second approach is using medical imaging technologies for screening and it is witnessed over the last decades. However, the benefits of medical imaging technology depend on the experience of the image interpreting experts or radiologists. Then, applying a computer-aided detection (CAD) approach using machine learning techniques has brought a promising result along with the imaging technologies. Machine learning techniques have evolved rapidly in recent years to solve complex problems.

The architecture of deep convolutional neural networks (DCNNs) is composed of convolutional layers, pooling layers and fully connected layers to perform feature extraction (see Figure 1), features down sampling (see Figure 2) and classification, respectively during the process of optimization [1].

In convolutional layers, local features such as colors, end-points, corners and oriented-edges are collected in the shallow layers. These local features in the shallow layers are integrated into larger structural features like circles, ellipses, specific shapes or patterns when the layer goes deeper. Afterwards, these features of structures or patterns constitute the high-level semantic representations that describe feature abstraction for each category. In pooling layers, feature down sampling is performed either using average pooling or max-pooling layers to reduce the dimensionality of the features extracted using convolutional layers [2]. On the other hand, in fully connected layers, it takes the extracted features from the convolutional layers as inputs and works as a classifier, well known as multilayer perceptron (MLP). These fully connected layers encode the spatial correspondences of those semantic features and convey the co-occurrence properties between patterns or objects.

There have been many survey papers produced on the application of deep learning on medical image analysis and few among many produced in 2017 are considered in this survey paper. Suzuki [3] in his survey paper claimed that machine learning in deep learning form has emerged in computer vision and paved the way for many researchers to work on medical image analysis using deep learning approach. The popularity of deep learning started after the AlexNet model won the competition in 2012. Suzuki has produced an interesting survey paper that aimed to address four major points: the machine learning techniques used in the computer vision field, changes observed in machine learning after the introduction of deep learning, available machine learning models in deep learning and the impact of deep learning for medical image analysis. As claimed by Litjens et al. [4], convolutional neural network-based deep learning has become a method for medical image analysis. In their survey paper, they considered papers that were related to medical image analysis, specifically for image classification, object detection, segmentation, registration and other tasks. In addition, the areas of application of deep learning were neuro, retinal, pulmonary, digital pathology, breast, cardiac, abdominal and musculoskeletal.

Dinggang Shen et al. [5] claimed that deep learning has helped many researchers in the area of computer vision to identify, classify and quantify patterns in medical images. They specifically argued that deep learning is useful in exploiting hierarchical features from data itself than feature engineering using handcrafting using human effort. Suzuki [6] in his survey paper overviewed the area of deep learning and its application in medical imaging analysis to assess what was changed before and after the introduction of deep learning in machine learning, identifying the reasons that make deep learning powerful and their applications to medical image analysis.

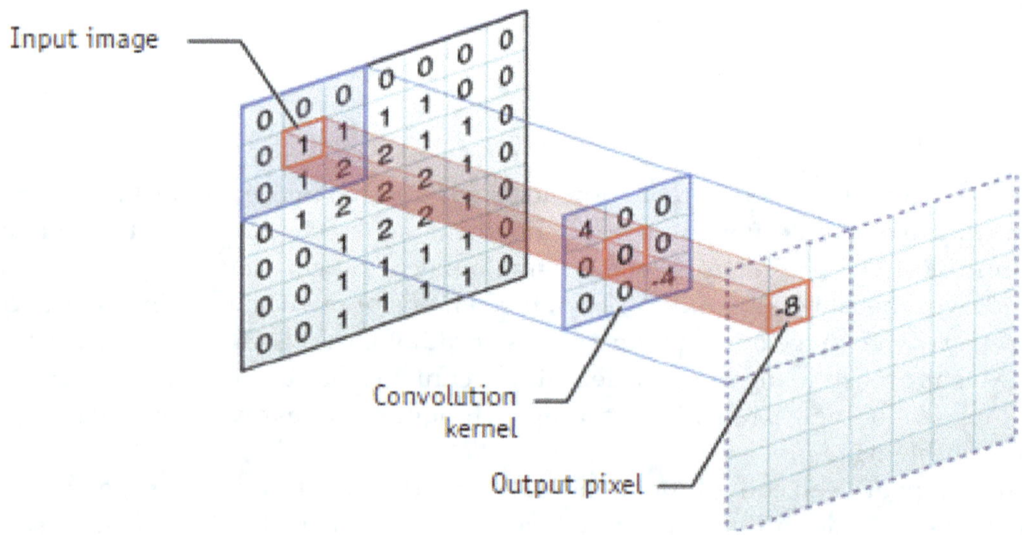

Figure 1. Example of convolution operation from [7].

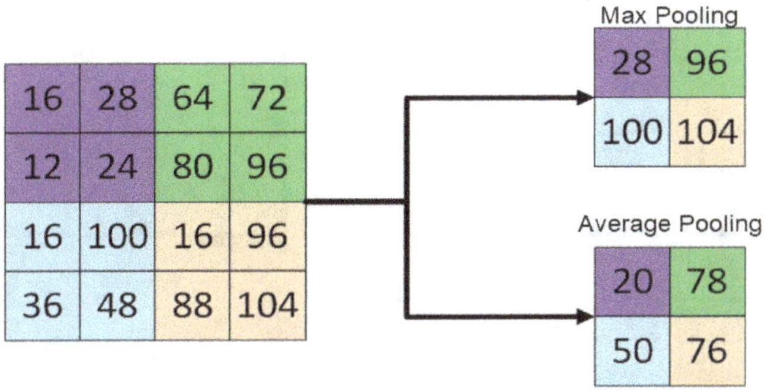

Figure 2. Example of down sampling operation using max-pooling and average-pooling.

In this survey paper, we briefly describe the breast cancer, cervical cancer, brain tumor, colon cancer and lung cancer along with their respective screening methods. Finally, we reviewed the application of deep learning for each cancer type in terms of deep learning application types like feature extraction, detection, segmentation, prediction and classification. The motivation behind selecting the cancer type for the survey was based on the cancer statistics reported in 2018 by the World Health Organization as presented in Table 1.

Table 1. World Health Organization 2018 statistical report through the global cancer observatory.

Cancer Type	New Cases (%)	Death Rate (%)
Breast Cancer	11.6	6.6
Colon Cancer	10.2	9.2
Brain Tumor	3.5	2.8
Cervical Cancer	3.2	2.5
Stomach Cancer	5.7	8.2
Liver Cancer	4.7	8.2
Lung Cancer	11.6	18.4

2. Methods

Published papers from 2016 to 2020 were considered and reviewed to (1) assess the application of deep learning for breast cancer, (2) assess the application of deep learning for cervical cancer, (3) assess the application of deep learning for a brain tumor and (4) assess the application of deep learning for colon cancer. We first defined a search criterion for the selected search databases. Our general search criteria for this survey paper are ((“colon” OR “colorectal”) AND (“cancer” OR “polyp”) AND (“deep learning”) AND (“Image”) AND (“detection” OR “classification” OR “segmentation” OR “Localization”)) OR ((“breast”) AND (“cancer” OR “mass”) AND (“deep learning”) AND (“Image”) AND (“detection” OR “classification” OR “segmentation” OR “Localization”)) OR ((“Brain”) AND (“Tumor”) AND (“deep learning”)AND (“MRI”) AND (“detection” OR “classification” OR “segmentation” OR “Localization”)) OR (“Cervix” OR “Cervical”) AND (“Deep Learning”) AND (“Classification” OR “segmentation”). The searches were carried out from four databases: (1) PubMed, (2) Science Direct, (3) IEEE Xplore Digital Library and (4) Google Scholar. The search framework of the survey paper is presented in Figure 3 and the major performance metrics used to evaluate deep learning approach applied to the selected medical images are presented in Section 2.1.

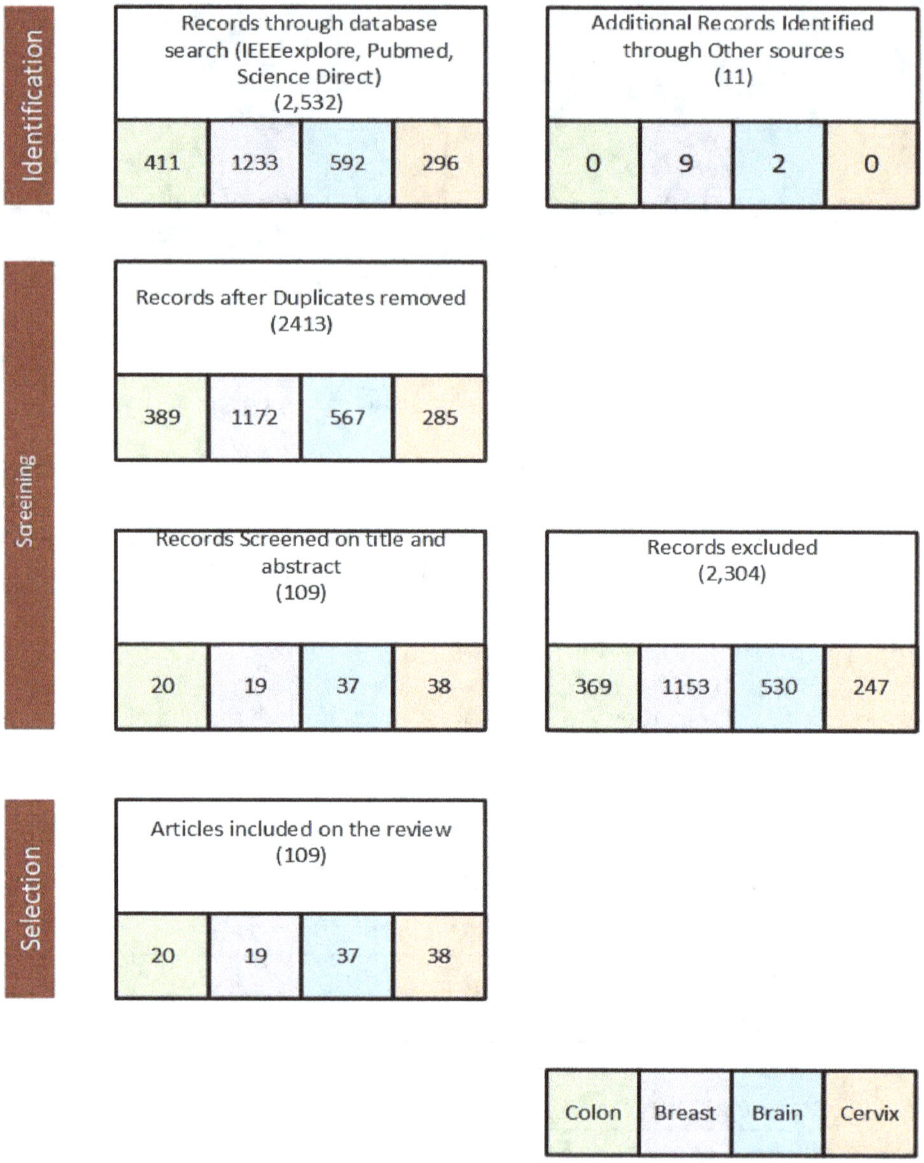

Figure 3. Search criteria framework used for IEEExplore, PubMed, Google Scholar and Science Direct engines to select papers for review.

2.1. Segmentation and Classification Performance Metrics

Most of the performance metrics encountered in the review include area under curve (AUC), sensitivity (Sn), specificity (Sp), accuracy (Acc), precision (P), recall (R), positive predictive values (PPV), Matthews correlation coefficient (MCC), geometric mean (G-Mean), which are usually successful in describing the classification performance [8,9]. Performance measures including Dice similarity coefficient (DSC) or Zijdenbos similarity index (ZSI) or F1-score, Hausdorff distance (H) and intersection over union (IoU) are the most effective metrics for measuring system's segmentation performance [10]. Here, the true positives for the segmentation are the correctly labeled pixel while it is correctly labeled class for classification case.

3. Deep Learning in Tumor Detection, Segmentation and Classification

Region-based segmentation technique was in use in medical image analysis until the deep learning approach evolved in the field of computer vision [8]. However, Lee et al. [7] in their survey paper indicated that the existence of deep learning in the research community has become a reason to use object recognition in an image. In addition to object detection, deep learning has been applied for feature extraction, abnormality detection, cancer/tumor segmentation and classification [11].

3.1. Breast Cancer

Breast cancer occurs when there is uncontrolled growth of cells in the breast [12]. It is the most widely diagnosed type of cancer in women and the first prevalent cancer type in Ethiopia [11,13]. There are four types of breast cancer manifestation that include: mass, calcification, architectural distortion and bilateral asymmetry [11].

3.1.1. Screening Methods

As presented in Debelee et al. [11], breast cancer image analysis and breast abnormality detection start with breast cancer screening. Breast cancer screening methods include screen film mammography (SFM), digital mammography (DM), ultrasound (US), magnetic resonance imaging (MRI), digital breast tomosynthesis (DBT) and combinations of the screening methods.

3.1.2. Datasets

There are many datasets prepared for medical image analysis based on the different imaging modalities. The most common and available dataset for the breast cancer is of mammography and histopathology datasets. Some of the most common datasets are discussed in Table 2.

Table 2. Image datasets for breast cancer image analysis.

Dataset	Size	#Classes/Targets	Format	Type	Author/Repository, Year
MIAS	322	2	pgm	Mammography	Suckling, J. et al. [14]
DDSM	55,890		npy	Mammography	Scuccimarra [15]
InBreast		410	XML	Mammography	Moreira et al. [16]
Breast Cancer Wisconsin	568	3	csv	Mammography	Dua, D. and Graff, C. [17]
BreakHis	7909	2	png	Histology	Bukun [18]
BACH/ICIAR2018	400	4	tiff	Histology	G.Aresta [19]

3.1.3. Deep Learning for Detection of Breast Cancer Through Diagnostic Medical Imaging Techniques

Li Shen et al. [2] proposed a deep learning-based breast cancer detection algorithm using end-to-end training approach using mammographic images from the Digital Database for Screening Mammography (DDSM) and INbreast databases. The deep learning architectures used in their paper were ResNet-50 and VGGNet-16. The proposed approach was evaluated in terms of AUC at single model and four-model (ResNet-ResNet, ResNet-VGGNet, VGGNet-VGGNet and VGGNet-ResNet) averaging level. For the DDSM dataset, the best single model achieved a per-image AUC of 0.88, and four-model averaging improved the AUC to 0.91 with sensitivity of 86.1% and specificity of 80.1%. For INbreast database, the best single model achieved per-image AUC of 0.95, and four-model averaging achieved a better AUC value of 0.98 with sensitivity of 86.7% and specificity of 96.1%.

Wu et al. [20] proposed a DCNN architecture based on four columns of ResNet-22 to classify breast cancer screening exams using mammography. There was a total of 200,000 exams which incorporated over 1,000,000 images to train and evaluate the proposed DCNN model. The performance of their network achieved an AUC of 0.895 in predicting whether there is a cancer in the breast, when tested on the screening population and the result was compared to 14 radiologists reading results.

Alzubaidi et al. [21] transfer learning approach on their proposed 74 layer CNN. Their model was pre-trained on one same domain image dataset (erythrocytesIDB dataset, which has images of peripheral blood smears samples taken from patients with Sickle Cell Disease). They divided the original microscopy image into 12 patches and used majority voting for the classification, where the most frequent patch label is chosen to be the image label. The model achieved a patch level accuracy of 90.5% and image-level accuracy of 97.4%. The majority voting they employed seemed not a correct way since if the cells are the majority of normals and if it still has cancerous cells, the system might classify them as normal, which is not good.

Zhu et al. [22] proposed two deep learning approach to predict the occurrence of invasive cancer on MRI images. The first approach was based on transfer learning using GoogleNet pre-trained model to predict the presence of invasive cancer. As a second approach, the authors extracted features from the natural images and used SVM to predict the invasive disease. The best classification result gained in terms of AUC was 0.53 for transfer learning approach and 0.70 for extracted features.

Li et al. [23] explored the abilities of digital breast tomosynthesis (DBT) and full-field digital mammography (FFDM) in mass classification using deep neural networks equipped with or without transfer learning. They also explored an eligible combination strategy of DBT and FFDM in enhancing classification performance. They applied a 16-layer VGG network (VGG-16) and 11-layer deep convolutional neural network (DCNN) for the 2D images and extend the 11-layer DCNN to accommodate the extra dimension in 3D DBT images. The best performer from these methods, a 2D-DCNN which was trained by combining the DBT and FFDM, achieved the highest performance with average AUC, accuracy, sensitivity and specificity of 0.95, 92.13%, 83% and 93.84%, respectively on three class classification (benign, malignant, normal).

Zeiser et al. [24] explored the application of the U-Net model with different depths with or without data augmentation for the segmentation of masses on mammograms. The U-Net model trained with depth of 5 and with data augmentation was the best performer with sensitivity of 92.32%, specificity of 80.47%, accuracy of 85.95%, Dice index of 79.39% and AUC of 86.40% on the DDSM dataset.

Shen et al. [2] applied an ensemble of four best performing deep learning models which were designed based on Resnet50 and VGG16 as patch classifiers and Resnet and VGG blocks as top layer for breast cancer classification. The ensemble of these classifiers achieved the best AUC of 0.91 (sensitivity: 86.1%, specificity: 80.1%) on the detection of benign and malignant masses and classifications on the DDSM dataset.

Zhang et al. [25] used U-net architecture for the segmentation and extraction of fat tissue, fibroglandular tissue (FGT) inside the breast, and all nonbreast tissues outside the breast in breast MRI. They achieved mean DSC of 0.95 for breast and 0.91 for FGT; and mean accuracy of 0.98 for breast and 0.97 for FGT.

Zhou et al. [26] applied 3D deep convolutional neural network (CNN) based on 3D DenseNet [27] architecture with 37 layers for diagnosing breast cancer and localizing the lesions at dynamic contrast enhanced (DCE) MRI data in a weakly supervised manner. The proposed algorithm performance for breast cancer diagnosis showed 83.7% accuracy, 90.8% sensitivity, 69.3% specificity, 0.859 AUC and 0.501 Dice distance.

Summary of the performance of the above reviewed work can be summarized in Table 3.

3.1.4. Deep Learning for Breast Histopathology Image Analysis

Breast histopathology helps to confirm the presence of cancerous sales detected by other imaging modalities. Since histology slides may contain millions of cells and identifying the cancerous sales from the slides is time consuming and tedious job. Hence there are many varieties of research done in this area.

Table 3. Summary of scientific papers on detection of breast cancer using diagnostic medical imaging techniques.

Author and Citation	Dataset	AUC	Sn (%)	Sp (%)	Acc (%)	Target
	Siemens and Hologic	0.933	-	-	-	Detection
Wu et al. [20]	Personal	0.895	-	-	-	Classification/Prediction
Shen et al. [2] (Single-Model)	DDSM INbreast	0.88 0.95	- -	- -	- -	Detection Detection
Shen et al. [2] (Four-Models Average)	DDSM INbreast	0.91 0.98	86.1 86.7	80.1 96.1	- -	Detection Detection
Zhu et al. [22] (Transfer learning)	-	0.53	-	-	-	Prediction
Zhu et al. [22] (SVM)	-	0.7	-	-	-	Prediction
Li et al. [23]	-	0.95	83	93.84	92.13	Classification
Zeiser et al. [24]	DDSM	0.86	92.32	80.47	85.95	Segmentation
Zhang et al. [28]	-	-	-	-	97.5	Detection
Zhou et al. [26]	-	0.86	90.8	69.3	83.7	Classification

Sheikh et al. [29] proposed a multi-scale input and multi-feature CNN network for the classification of histopathological images. They concatenate four scales ($1\times$, $0.5\times$, $0.33\times$ and $0.25\times$) of the original normalized image to accommodate the scale variant property of the cells and used it as an input to the CNN network. They trained their proposed model on ICIAR2018 and BreakHits datasets. The model achieved a satisfactory max accuracy of 0.83 for the ICIAR2018 dataset and 0.98 for the BreakHis dataset for binary classification. For the multiclass classification, the proposed model's accuracy was rather unsatisfactory reaching as low as 60% for the ICIAR2018 dataset.

Li et al. [30] modified the Densenet-121 architecture by removing the pooling layers of the 4th Dense-block and feeding the extracted feature maps from each Dense-block to the squeeze-and-excitation (SENet) module for breast histopathology images. The used SENet for receiving more channel-wise information. After concatenating each SENet output, they used a fully-connected layer for the classification purpose. They used a pre-trained Densenet model for their architecture using the transfer-learning approach. Using the publicly available BreakHis dataset, their algorithm achieved an average accuracy of 88% over different magnification levels for binary classification.

Yan et al. [31] used the transfer-learning approach by using Google's Inception-V3 model as patch-wise feature extraction and image-wise long short-term memory (LSTM) for classifying breast histopathological images into four classes, namely normal, benign, in situ and invasive. They fine-tuned the Inception-V3 model. Their proposed model achieved an average accuracy of 91% on the ICIAR2018 dataset.

Sharma et al. [32] studied the use of pre-trained deep learning networks as feature extractor from breast cancer histopathology images. They used transfer learning on the pre-existing networks (VGG16, VGG19 and ResNet50) for using them as feature extractor. The extracted features were then classified using SVM classifier. The VGG16 network with linear SVM achieved the highest accuracy (93.97% for $40\times$, 92.92% for $100\times$, 91.23% for $200\times$ and 91.79% for $400\times$ magnifications).

Vang et al. [33] proposed ensemble classifier and reinforcement backed deep learning approach using inception-V3 for multiclass (normal, benign, in situ and invasive) classification. The ensemble fusion approach for image level prediction involved majority voting, gradient boosting machine (GBM) and logistic regression. Their approach performed low in terms of sensitivity for the two classes (benign and normal). The sensitivity of the normal and benign predicted classes was improved by adding a dual path network (DPN) to use it as feature extractor. However, the extracted features were further sent to the next layer of ensemble prediction fusion using GBM, logistic regression and support vector machine (SVM) to refine predictions. This approach was evaluated in terms of accuracy and scored an accuracy of 87.5%.

Alzubaidi et al. [21] transfer learning approach onto their proposed 74 layer CNN. They pre-trained their model on one same domain image dataset (erythrocytesIDB dataset, which has images of peripheral blood smears samples taken from patients with Sickle Cell Disease). They divided the original microscopy image into 12 patches and used majority voting for the classification, where the most frequent patch label is chosen to be the image label. The model training was don on the ICIAR 2018 dataset. The model achieved patch level accuracy of 90.5% and image level accuracy of 97.4%. The majority voting they employed seemed not a correct way since if the cells are majority of normal and if it still has cancerous cells the system might classify them as normal, which is not good.

The summary of papers explored in classification of breast histological slides can be summarized in Table 4. From the literature reviews the algorithm proposed by Yan et al. [31] seems the best method for histopathological breast cancer detection.

Table 4. Summary of scientific papers on classification of breast cancer using histopathological images.

Author and Citation	Dataset	Acc	Sn (%)	Sp (%)
	Siemens and Hologic	0.933	-	-
Vang et al. [33]	ICIAR2018 (H & E)	87.5	-	-
Sharma and Mehra [32]	BreakHis	93.97	-	-
Sheikh et al. [29]	ICIAR2018 and BreakHis	83 98	-	-
Li et al. [30]	ICIAR2018	88	-	-
Yan et al. [31]	ICIAR2018	91	-	-
Alzubaidi et al. [21]	ICIAR 2018	97.4	-	

3.1.5. Summary

As presented in Tables 5 and 6, the deep learning architecture involved in the recently published, from 2016 to 2020, breast cancer we considered in this survey paper were ResNet, VGGNet, AlexNet, Inception V3, U-Net and DenseNet.

Table 5. Summary of breast cancer scientific papers in terms of convolutional neurla network (CNN) architecture and type of environment used in the selected papers.

Authors	Network	Pre-Training	Transfer Learning	Environment
Wu et al. [20]	ResNet-22	Yes	No	TensorFlow
Shen et al. [2]	ResNet-50, VGGNet-16	Yes	Yes	-
Vang et al. [33]	Inception V3	Yes	No	TensorFlow
Zhu et al. [22]	GoogleNet	Yes	Yes	Caffe
Li et al. [23]	VGGNet-16	Yes	Yes	-
Sharma and Mehra [32]	VGGNet-16, VGGNet-19, ResNet50	Yes	Yes	Keras, TensorFlow
Zeiser et al. [24]	U-net	No	No	-
Zhang et al. [28]	U-net	No	No	TensorFlow
Zhou et al. [26]	3D DensNet	No	No	-
Sheikh et al. [29]	MSI-MFNet	No	No	Keras
Li et al. [30]	IDSNet	Yes	Yes	Tensorflow
Yan et al. [31]	Inception-V3	Yes	Yes	Tensorflow
Alzubaidi et al. [21]	ResNet	Yes	Yes	-

Table 6. Summary of breast cancer scientific papers in terms of publication year, name of journal/conference for the selected papers and its impact factor with year of impact factor.

Authors	Publication Year	Journal/Conf.	Impact Factor	Year of Impact Factor
Wu et al. [20]	2020	ITMI	6.85	2020
Shen et al. [2]	2019	Scientific Reports	3.998	2019
Vang et al. [33]	2018	CBM	5.4	2019
Zhu et al. [22]	2019	CBM	3.434	2020
Li et al. [23]	2019	European Radiology	4.101	2019
Sharma and Mehra [32]	2020	Journal of Digital Imaging	2.99	2018
Zeiser et al. [24]	2020	Journal of Digital Imaging	2.99	2018
Zhang et al. [28]	2018	Academic Radiology	2.50	2020
Dembrower et al. [34]	2020	Radiology	7.608	2018
Zhou et al. [26]	2019	Journal of Magnetic Resonance Imaging	2.112	2018
Sheikh et al. [29]	2020	MDPI, Cancers	6.126	2019
Li et al. [30]	2020	Plos One	2.74	2019
Yan et al. [31]	2020	Elsevier, Methods	3.812	2019
Alzubaidi et al. [21]	2020	MDPI, electronics	2.412	2019

As indicated in Table 7, the result of almost all papers in this survey paper were not compared with the domain specialists and performance of the traditional machine learning algorithms.

Table 7. Summary of breast cancer scientific papers in terms of comparison to specialists and/or traditional techniques.

Author and Citation	Comparison to Specialists	Comparison to Traditional Technique (Yes/No)
Hagos et al. [35]	No	No
Wu et al. [20]	Yes	No
Shen et al. [2]	No	No
Vang et al. [33]	No	No
Zhu et al. [22]	No	No
Li et al. [23]	No	No
Sharma and Mehra [32]	No	Yes
Zeiser et al. [24]	No	Yes
Zhang et al. [28]	No	No
Zhou et al. [26]	Yes	Yes
Sheikh et al. [29]	No	Yes
Li et al. [30]	No	Yes
Yan et al. [31]	No	Yes
Alzubaidi et al. [21]	No	yes

3.2. *Cervical Cancer*

Cervical cancer is one of the most common cancers among women worldwide, especially in developing nations, and it has a relatively high incidence and mortality rates [36]. Cervical cancer usually develops slowly over time. When cervical cancer begins in the cervix, cervical cells go through changes called dysplasia, in which cells that are not normal begin to appear in the cervical tissue. In its later stage, cancer cells start to multiply and proliferate more deeply into the cervix and to surrounding areas. Fortunately, cervical cancer is mostly preventable with active screening and detection techniques.

For example, preventive screening and early detection can decrease the morbidity of cervical cancer by about 70% in the United States [37].

3.2.1. Screening Methods

Nowadays, there are a few frequently-used cervical cancer screening techniques, such as high-risk human papillomavirus (HPV) testing, Pap smear cytology testing, colposcopy and visual inspection of the cervix with acetic acid (VIA), each of which has its advantages and disadvantages.

- **Bimanual pelvic examination.** This is a visual and physical inspection by the physician. It consists of both visual inspections using a device called a speculum and physical inspection by using fingers. This test is not enough on its own and the Pap test is usually performed next.
- **Cervical cytopathology** Papanicolaou Smear (Pap smear) or liquid-based cytology is a process of gently scraping cervical cells and inspection of those cells under a microscope. It can also be analyzed digitally using computers.
- **HPV typing test.** Cervical cancer usually occurs from persistent infection of the cervix with some carcinogenic types of human papillomavirus (HPV) such as HPV16 and HPV18 [38]. It is usually performed along with a Pap test or after Pap test results show abnormal changes to the cervix. The occurrence of HPV does not confirm cancer.
- **Colposcopy.** Colposcopy is a visual inspection of the cervix using a special instrument called a colposcope. The device magnifies the cervix area under inspection like a microscope. It can be used for pregnant women.

Other types of tests were also used for cervical cancer screening such as X-ray, CT scan, MRI and PET scan but they are more expensive and used to detect advanced stages of cancer.

Cervical cytology (Pap test) is the most common test used to look for early changes in cells that can lead to cervical cancer [39]. It has been widely used for the screening of cervical cancer in developed countries and is effective in reducing the number of deaths. It is still unavailable for population-wide screening in the developing countries. This is because screening using cervical cytology is difficult, tedious, time-consuming, expensive and subjected to errors because each slide contains around three million cells with large shape and appearance variation between cells, the poor contrast of cytoplasm boundaries and the overlap between cells [40]. In developed countries like the United Kingdom, cervical cancer screening is performed every 3 years for women aged 25 to 49 years and every 5 years aged 50 to 64 years [41]. Over the past few decades, many types of research were performed in developing a computer-assisted cervical cancer screening method. Most of these researches tried to automatically identify the various stages of cancer or abnormality types by classifying cells on the Pap-smear slides. Most of these classifications consist of cell or nuclei segmentation, feature extraction and classification steps [42].

3.2.2. Datasets for Cervical Cancer

Most of the research regarding the detection and segmentation of cervical cancer used the Herlev dataset. The pap-smear benchmark database provides data for comparing classification methods. The data consists of 917 images of pap-smear cells, classified carefully by cyto-technicians and doctors [43]. The dataset is distributed unevenly into seven classes, namely superficial squamous, squamous intermediate, columnar, moderate dysplasia, moderate dysplasia, severe dysplasia and carcinoma in situ. Each image in the Herlev dataset contains only a single cell. Each slide contains many cells and cells might also overlap. Hussien [44] prepared a more realistic dataset for the classification of cervical cells. Summary of the publicly available datasets for classification and segmentation of cervical cells and cervix is given in Table 8.

Table 8. Image datasets for cervical cancer.

Dataset	Size	#Classes/Targets	Format	Type	Author, Year
Herlev	917	187	Bit Map(BMP)	Histology	Dr J. Jantzen [43]
DANS-KNAW	963	4	jpg	Histology	Hussien [44]
CRIC	400	6	png and csv	Histology	M.T. Rezende et al. [45]
Zenodo	962	4	jpg	Histology	Franco et al. [46]
ALTS	938	2	jpg	Colposcopy	Alts Group [47]
MobileODT	1448	3	jpg	Colposcopy	MobileODT [48]

3.2.3. Deep Learning for Segmentation of Cervical Cells

Traditional cytological criteria for classifying cervical cell abnormalities are based on the changes in the nucleus to cytoplasm ratio, nuclear size, irregularity of nuclear shape and membrane. In normal cells, the cytoplasm appears much larger than the nucleus with the regular shaped nuclei. Therefore numerous works are focusing on the segmentation of cell or cell components (nuclei, cytoplasm) [41]. Deep learning has been applied for the segmentation of cervical cell nuclei and the whole cell itself. The successful segmentation of each cervical cell from the slides gives a better performance for cancerous cells. Nuclei detection is only maybe helpful and is easier than segmentation of the whole cell and may be enough for the detection of cancer or help for the segmentation of the whole cell.

Song et al. [49] tried to improve cervical cell segmentation by using learning-based segmentation when overlapping cells are encountered. They include high-level shape information to guide the segmentation algorithm which is done by the convolutional neural network algorithm. They evaluated their algorithm in nuclei detection and cervical cell segmentation. By using the datasets ISBI 2015 challenge dataset, and SZU dataset they achieved a Dice similarity coefficient (DSC) of 0.95 and 0.89, respectively.

Zhao et al. [50] proposed an algorithm called Progressive Growing of U-net + (PGU-net +) for Automated Cervical Nuclei Segmentation, which tried to modify the original U-net algorithm [51], which augmented the limited medical dataset for use of deep learning. They claimed these augmentations mix the information of different scales that affect each other; hence, it limits the segmentation accuracy of the model. they proposed a progressive growing U-net (PGU-net +) model, which extracts image features at each scale independently and passing residual information with the next scale. They achieved a segmentation accuracy of 0.925 on the Herlev dataset, with precision 0.901 ± 0.13, recall 0.968 ± 0.04 and ZSI of 0.925 ± 0.09.

Sompawong et al. [52] applied a pre-trained Mask R-CNN for cervical cancer nuclei detection, segmentation and classification into normal and abnormal ones. They used liquid-based histological slides obtained from Thammasat University (TU) Hospital and obtained mean average precision (mAP) of 57.8%, the accuracy of 91.7%, the sensitivity of 91.7% and specificity of 91.7% per image. They used DeepPap as a benchmark to evaluate their algorithm. Since DeepPap used the Herlev dataset (containing images of single cells) for training and testing. It needs to be modified and retrained on the TU dataset. They showed the proposed algorithm performs better than the modified DeepPap on the TU dataset. They did not evaluate the Mask R-CNN algorithm on the Herlev dataset.

Liu et al. [53] proposed a cervical nucleus segmentation method in which pixel-level prior information was utilized to provide the supervisory information for the training of a mask regional convolutional neural network (Mask R-CNN). They added a local fully-connected conditional random field (LFCCRF) to refine the segmentation. Using the Herlev Pap smear dataset, the proposed method achieved 0.96 in both precision and recall and 0.95 in the Zijdenbos similarity index.

Liang et al. [42] used a comparison based detection which combines the decision of two CNN architectures. First reference, samples were obtained by using the ResNet50 with Feature Pyramid Network (FPN) architecture from each cell image from the dataset. At the same time features from the whole slide image, which contains many cells, were extracted through ResNet50 with FPN and region proposal network (RPN). They replaced the original parameter classifier from their baseline network, Faster R-CNN with FPN with their comparison classifier. Their proposed algorithm can detect 11 different cell types from the whole slide. The performance of the proposed algorithm achieved mean average precision (mAP) of 26.3% and average recall (AR) of 35.7%. They argue these performance measurements do not reflect how good the algorithm was since the proposed algorithm groups multiple neighboring cells with the same category into one result.

Kurnianingsih et al. [54] used deep learning methods to segment cervical cells and classify them. For the segmentation purpose, transfer learning was applied on Mask R-CNN weights trained using the COCO dataset. The pre-trained model was trained to segment cervical cell area consisting of both nuclei and cytoplasm. In the segmentation phase, when Mask R-CNN is applied to the whole cell, it outperforms the previous segmentation method in precision (0.92 $\pm$ 0.06), recall (0.91 $\pm$ 0.05) and ZSI (0.91 $\pm$ 0.04).

Deep learning-based segmentation into nuclei segmentation and cell segmentation can be summarized (see Tables 9 and 10).

Table 9. Summary of selected papers on nuclei segmentation.

Authors	Method	Dataset	Acc	P	R	F1	Sp	Sn	ZSI
Zhao et al. [50]	Progressive Growing of U-net+(PGU-net+)	Herlev	0.925	0.901	0.968				0.925
Liu et al. [53]	Mask-RCNN with LFCCRF	Herlev		0.96	0.96				0.95
Sompawong et al. [52]	Mask-RCNN	TU	89.8%				94.3%	72.5%	

Table 10. Summary of selected papers on cervical cell segmentation.

Authors	Method	Dataset	Acc	P	R	ZSI	DSC
Kurnianingsih et al. [54]	Mask R-CNN	Herlev		0.92	0.91	0.91	
Song et al. [49]	CNN with Shape information	Herlev					0.92
Liang et al. [42]	comparison based Faster R-CNN	local		26.3	35.7		

3.2.4. Deep Learning for Cervical Cell Classification

Zhang et al. [55] tried to directly classify cervical cells—without prior segmentation—based on deep features, using convolutional neural networks (ConvNets). In their algorithm (DeepPap), a pre-trained ConvNets was trained on a cervical cell dataset consisting of adaptively re-sampled image patches coarsely centered on the nuclei. Then they applied aggregation to average the prediction scores of a similar set of image patches. The proposed algorithm achieved classification accuracy (98.3%), area under the curve (AUC) (0.99) values and specificity (98.3%) on the Herlev dataset.

Hyeon et al. [56] proposed a CNN-based pre-trained model, VGGNet-16 for feature extraction, and use different classifiers namely: logistic regression, random forests, AdaBoost and SVM for classification of the pap-test images into normal and abnormal. From these classifiers, the highest scoring one is the SVM classifier with an F1-score of 0.7817 on a dataset collected locally.

LIN et al. [57] applied the transfer learning approach to fine-tune different CNN models (AlexNet, GoogLeNet, ResNet and DenseNet) which were pre-trained on ImageNet dataset [58]. The pre-trained models were fine-tuned on the Herlev cervical dataset with additional cytoplasm and nucleus morphological masks. They achieved classification accuracies of 94.5%, 71.3% and 64.5%, for two-class (abnormal versus normal), four-class (normal, low-grade squamous intraepithelial lesion (LSIL), high-grade squamous intraepithelial lesion (HSIL) and carcinoma-in-situ (CIS) [59]) and seven-class ("World Health Organization classification system") classification tasks, respectively.

Chen et al. [60] tried to combine features extracted from different types of tests. They proposed a Faster R-CNN, which is based on Faster R-CNN for fusing acetic and iodine images of the cervix.

They fuse non-image features extracted from the cervix transformation zone type, pap test, HPV test and age after they non-linearly compression of the fused image features to 29D by using one fully connected (FC) layer. They did not mention which classifier they used for normal–abnormal classification but achieved an accuracy of 87.4% (88.6% sensitivity and 86.1% specificity) on a locally collected dataset.

Kurnianingsih et al. [54] trained a compact VGG network based on their Mask R-CNN based segmentation algorithm. For the classification, a compact VGG Net classifier yields a sensitivity score of more than 96% with a low standard deviation (± 2.8%) for the binary classification problem and yields a higher result of more than 95% with low standard deviation (maximum 4.2%) for the 7-class problem.

Performance comparison of different pre-trained deep learning models on Pap smear classification was done by Promworn et al. [61]. They compared the performance of CNN models namely resnet101, densenet161, AlexNet, vgg19_bn and squeeznet1_1, which are the top five models based on accuracy in ImageNet. The models are retrained on the Herlev dataset. Based on accuracy, densenet161 was the best performer on both binary classification (94.38%) and multiclass classification (68.54). Based on sensitivity, AlexNet and resnet have achieved 100% on binary classification. Whereas densenet161 was the best performer on multiclass classification with 68.18%. Again, based on specificity, densenet161 was superior with values 82.61% for binary and 69.57% for multiclass classification.

Yutao Ma et al. [62] developed a CADx system by using a convolutional neural network (CNN) for feature extraction and support vector machines (SVM) for classifying the optical coherence microscopy (OCM) images into five classes namely normal, ectropion, low-grade and high-grade squamous intraepithelial lesions (LSIL and HSIL) and cancer. They also used HPV test results for the classification in conjunction with features extracted from the OCM images by the CNN. An 88.3 ± 4.9% classification accuracy was achieved for all five classes. In the binary classification task (low-risk (normal, ectropion and LSIL) vs. high-risk (HSIL and cancer)), the CADx method achieved an area under the curve (AUC) value of 0.959 with 86.7 ± 11.4% sensitivity and 93.5 ± 3.8% specificity.

Ahmed et al. [63] proposed transfer learning-based approaches for the classification of cervical cells. They explored six different methods for the classification of cervical cells by combining three pre-trained models as features, shallow CNN, which consisted of only two convolutional layers and two max-pooling layers, VGG-16 Net and CaffeNet as a feature extraction technique and two classifiers, extreme learning machine (ELM) and auto encoder (AE) for the classification purpose. They used the Herlev dataset for training and testing their system. The best performer from these combinations is the CaffeNet+ELM which achieved a binary classification accuracy of 99.7 and 97.2 for the 7 class classification.

Dong et al. [64] used artificially extracted features such as color, texture and morphology along with the Inception-V3 model for the classification of cervical cells. They used features extracted manually since the features extracted from the CNN architecture since the knowledge of cervical cells is lacking there. Nine artificial features were combined with features extracted from the Inception-V3 architecture joined on the fully connected layer and used the Softmax function for the classification. They keep the aspect ratio of the cells when resizing for the Inception-V3 network will harm the morphological features. The proposed algorithm achieved an overall accuracy of 98.2%, the sensitivity of 99.4% and specificity of 96.73% for normal abnormal classification on the Herlev dataset.

Martinez-Mias et al. [65] tried to improve and make it realistic the cervical classification from PAP smears using a cell merger approach. They used CNN for PAP smear image classification, and optimize and integrate the cell fusion approach since most PAP smear slides contain overlapping cells. They used a local PAP smear dataset collected from ten patients and labeled using biopsy results. Hence, it was used as a gold standard. They trained the CaffeNet model using data prepared using a cell merger to reflect the reality of the PAP smear examination. For classifying the cervical cells into four classes the CaffeNet with the cell merger dataset achieved an average accuracy of just 55.6% with the performance as low as just 16.7% for LSIL class. For the normal/abnormal classification, their proposed algorithm achieved an accuracy, sensitivity and specificity of 88.8%, 0.92 and 0.83, respectively. This performance is satisfactory considering the classification was done on overlapping cell regions.

Xiang et al. [66] used YOLOv3 as a cell detector and Inception-V3-based classifier for cervical cell classification into ten classes that could be present on the slide namely, normal cells (NORMAL), atypical squamous cells-undetermined significance (ASC-US), atypical squamous cells-cannot exclude HSIL(ASC-H), low-grade squamous intraepithelial lesion (LSIL), high-grade squamous intraepithelial lesion (HSIL), atypical glandular cells (AGC), adenocarcinoma (ADE), vaginalis trichomoniasis (VAG), monilia (MON) and dysbacteriosis (DYS). The model achieves 97.5% sensitivity (Sens) and 67.8% specificity (Spec) on cervical cell image-level screening.

The cervical cell classification algorithms can be categorized into two categories, binary and multiclass. In the binary classification cervical cells are classified into normal and abnormal cells (see Table 11). Multiclass classification describing the severity of the cancer including the normal ones (see Table 12).

Table 11. Summary of selected papers on cervical cell binary classification.

Authors	Method	Dataset	Acc(%)	Sn(%)	Sp(%)	AUC	F1	P	R
Zhang et al. [55]	DeepPap	Herlev	98.3	-	98.3	0.99	-	-	-
Hyeon et al. [56]	VGG16	SVM	local	-	-	-	0.78	0.78	0.78
Lin et al. [57]	GoogleNet5C	Herlev	94.5	-	-	-	-	-	-
Chen et al. [60]	Mask R-CNN 7 class	local-	87.4	88.6	86.1	-	-	-	-
Kurnianingsih et al. [54]	Mask R-CNN	Herlev	98.1	96.7	98.6	96.5	-	-	-
Promworn et al. [61]	densenet161	Herlev	94.38	100	-	-	-	-	-
Yutao Ma et al. [62]	CNN and SVM	OCM image	-	86.7	93.5	0.96	-	-	-
Ahmed et al. [63]	CaffNet+ELM	Herlev	99.5	-	-	-	-	-	-
Dong et al. [64]	Inception-V3	Herlev	98.23	99.4	96.7	-	-	-	-
Martinez-Mias et al. [65]	CaffeNet	Local	88.8	92	83	-	-	-	-

Table 12. Summary of selected papers on cervical cell multiclass classification.

Authors	Method	Dataset	Acc	Sn	Sp	Others
	regressor 7 classes					
Yutao Ma et al. [62]	CNN and SVM 5 classes	OCM image	88.3			
Lin et al. [57]	GoogleNet5C 4 classes	Herlev Dataset	71.3			
Lin et al. [57]	GoogleNet5C seven classes	Herlev Dataset	64.5			
Kurnianingsih et al. [54]	Mask R-CNN 7 class	Herlev	95.9	96.2	99.3	
Promworn et al. [61]	densenet161 7 classes	Herlev dataset	68.54	68.18	69.57	
Ahmed et al. [63]	CaffNet+ELM	Herlev	91.2	-	-	-
Martinez-Mias et al. [65]	CaffeNet	Local	55.6	-	-	-
Xiang et al. [66]	YOLOv3+InceptionV3	local	89.3	97.5	67.8	-

3.2.5. Deep Learning for Cervix Classification

Colposcopic images are also used for cervical cancer detection using deep learning methods. A colposcopy helps to observe the cervix at up to $\times 10$ magnification [67]. Cervical intraepithelial lesions are easily recognized when treated with acetic acid solutions using colposcopy.

Cervix type classification from smartphone camera was tried in [68] using capsule networks which achieves an accuracy of 94%. A more advanced approach called CervixNet [69] which is designed based on a novel hierarchical convolutional mixture of experts (HCME) method achieved an accuracy of 96.77%.

M. Arora et al. [70] used the transfer learning approach from a pre-trained CNN, Inception V3 model [71] by modifying the output layer. The output layer was replaced by a pooling layer and a fully connected layer for the classification of the cervix based on its image. A cervical image dataset from Kaggle was used here, which has three types of cervix based on the location of the transformation layer. The type of cervix will help the physician whether further tests are needed or not. They obtained an average accuracy of just 54.54%.

Guo et al. [72] explored the application of two versions of regions with convolutional neural networks (R-CNN), Mask R-CNN and $Mask^X$ R-CNN, on three different dataset for cervix classification for automatic segmentation of cervix region. Mask R-CNN is effective on datasets with annotations having the exact boundaries. The $Mask^X$ R-CNN can also trained the bounding box annotation. The highest performance was achieved using Mask R-CNN with Dice and IoU of 0.947 and 0.901, respectively. $Mask^X$ R-CNN also achieved a very good performance with Dice and IoU of 0.92 and 0.86 respectively. These colposcopy images suffer from presense of many distractors such as pubic hair, intra-uterine devices (IUDs), the speculum and even parts of human hand. The main problem in cervix classification from cervix photos is the presence of out of focus images [73].

Guo et al. [74] used an ensemble of three deep learning architectures, RetinaNet, Deep SVDD and a customized CNN for the detection of cervix on smarthphone captured images. They achieved an average accuracy and F1-score of 91.6% and 0.890, respectively.

3.2.6. Summary

Screening through a Pap test for cervical cancer can take days for the final analysis to complete since the pathologist needs to go through millions of cells. A deep learning-based system can detect those cells in minutes if it is accurate enough to be trusted. One of the main challenges of deep learning methods is the presence of other types of cells and other materials present in the image and the overlapping between two adjacent cervical cells. To solve these problems, a large and carefully annotated dataset needs to be built for the algorithms to learn. Building this many datasets for medical images is very difficult. The most commonly used dataset for cervical cancer screening is the Herlev dataset as shown in Table 10.

Deep learning has been applied for cervical cancer screening in many of its screening methods. Most of the successful deep learning-based cervical cancer detection methods were based on a dataset using pap smear histology images. Colposcopic images are also taking more attention since they are easy to take and not invasive. Their accuracies on the detection of cervical cancers is not as good as that of the histology images. Cervical cancer detection using the deep learning methods based on the colposcopic images are becoming common since a large dataset can be collected and annotated easily. Colposcopic screening could be applied for mass screening purposes with the aid of deep learning, since taking samples are easy. As we can see from Tables 9–12, the Herlev dataset is the most used dataset for cervical cell classification and segmentation works. Most of the coloscopic datasets used for cervix classifications are locally collected. We can also see that the deep learning methods for nuclei segmentation are more accurate than that of cell segmentations since cell boundaries might overlap between adjacent cells. For the classification case, binary classifiers are more accurate than that of multiclass classifiers which can detect the type of abnormalities in the cells.

From Tables 11–13, we can see those deep learning methods with pre-trained networks and those with transfer learning mechanisms are more accurate than networks trained from scratch with TensorFlow the widely used software.

Most of the reviewed papers on the application of deep learning on cervical cancer screening were published in 2019 with an average impact factor of 3.4 (see Table 14). And, as shown in Table 15, only one of the papers compares the algorithm performance with that of the specialist.

Table 13. Summary of cervical cancer scientific papers in terms of CNN architecture, and type of environment used in the selected papers.

Author and Citation	Network	Pre-Training	Transfer Learning	Environment
Zhao et al. [50]	U-Net	No	No	-
Liu Y. et al. [53]	Mask-RCNN	Yes	No	Tensorflow
Sompawong et al. [52]	Mask-RCNN	Yes	Yes	-
Kurnianingsih et al. [54]	Mask-RCNN and VGGNet	Yes	Yes	-
Song et al. [49]	CNN-Custom	No	No	-
Lianget al. [42]	ResNet50	Yes	Yes	Tensorflow
Zhang et al. [55]	ConvNet	Yes	Yes	Caffe
Hyeon et al. [56]	CNN	Yes	Yes	-
Yutao Ma et al. [62]	VGG-16	Yes	Yes	Tensorflow
Lin et al. [57]	GoogLeNet	Yes	Yes	Caffe
Promworn et al. [61]	DenseNet161	No	No	PytTorch
Wimpy and Suyanto [68]	Capsule Network	Yes	No	Tensorflow
Gorantla et al. [69]	ResNet101	yes	Yes	-
Arora et al. [70]	CNN-Custom	No	No	-
Ahmed et al. [63]	CaffeNet	yes	yes	Caffe
Martinez-Mias et al. [65]	CaffeNet	yes	yes	Caffe

Table 14. Summary of cervical cancer scientific papers in terms of article publication year, name of the journal for the selected papers and its impact factor with year of impact factor.

Author and Citation	Publication Year	Journal/Conference	Impact Factor	Impact Assigned Year
Zhao et al. [50]	2019	MMMI 2019	-	-
Liu Y. et al. [53]	2018	IEEE Access	4.098	2018
Sompawong et al. [52]	2019	Conference ACEMBS	0.54	2019
Kurnianingsih et al. [54]	2019	IEEE Access	4.098	2018
Song et al. [49]	2016	Conference ISBI	1.51	2019
Liang et al. [42]	2019	Neurocomputing	3.317	2016
Zhang et al. [55]	2017	JBHI	5.223	2020
Hyeon etal. [56]	2017	Conference ICMDM	-	-
Yutao Ma et al. [62]	2019	IEEE Transaction on Biomedical Engineering	4.78	2019
Lin et al. [57]	2019	IEEE Access	4.098	2018
Promworn et al. [61]	2019	Conference ICNEMS	0.312	2019
Wimpy and S. Suyanto [68]	2019	Conference ISRITI	-	-
Gorantla et al. [69]	2019	BIBE	0.392	2012
Arora et al. [70]	2018	Conference ICSCCC	0.91	2019
Ahmed et al. [63]	2019	Future Generation computer systems	6.125	2019
Dong et al. [64]	2020	ASCJ	5.5	2020
Martinez-Mias et al. [65]	2020	ESWA	5.45	2020

Table 15. Summary of cervical cancer scientific papers in terms of comparison to specialists and/or traditional techniques.

Author and Citation	Comparison to Specialists	Comparison to Traditional Technique (Yes/No)
Zhao et al. [50]	No	Yes
Liu Y. et al. [53]	No	Yes
Sompawong et al. [52]	No	Yes
Kurnianingsih et al. [54]	No	Yes
Song et al. [49]	No	Yes
Lianget al. [42]	No	Yes
Zhang et al. [55]	Yes	No
Hyeon et al. [56]	No	No
Yutao Ma et al. [62]	Yes	No
Lin et al. [57]	No	Yes
Promworn et al. [61]	No	Yes
Wimpy and S. Suyanto [68]	No	Yes
Gorantla et al. [69]	No	Yes
Arora et al. [70]	No	No
Ahmed et al. [63]	No	Yes
Dong et al. [64]	No	Yes
Martinez-Mias et al. [65]	No	No

3.3. Brain Tumor

Brain tumor is a group of abnormal cells around or inside the brain due to the uncontrolled division of cells with a serious effect of deterring the normal functionality of the brain activity and destroying the healthy cells[75].

Brain tumor is classified into benign or low-grade (grade I and II) and malignant or high-grade (grade III and IV). Benign is a non-cancerous tumor that does not exhibit any progression and cannot spread to other parts of the body; it started in the brain with a very low growth rate. On the other hand, a malignant tumor is cancerous with an attribute of growing rapidly and spreading to other parts of the body. Malignant tumors can further be categorized as primary and secondary. Primary malignant tumor originates in the brain itself; whereas, the secondary type begins from somewhere else in the body and spreads to the brain. Cancerous cells that spread to the brain commonly originate from the lung, kidney, breast, skin and colon. A metastatic brain tumor is another expression for this type of brain tumor. Glioblastoma multiform (GBM) is the most common type of primary brain tumor that grows fast from glial cells. An intense clinical treatment plan is required for high-grade gliomas (HGG) as they have a higher spreading rate than the low-grade gliomas (LCG) [76]. It is evidenced that patients with GBMs decease in less than a year. Early detection helps a therapeutic plan of patients and improves the overall survival rate [77]. The most prevalent brain cancer is high-grade glioma with 85% of new cases of malignant primary tumor diagnosed every year [78].

3.3.1. Screening Methods

Magnetic resonance imaging is the most common brain tumor diagnosis and has a great role in treatment planning strategies [79]. These images have an important contribution towards an automatic medical image analysis field as they provide quite a lot of information about the brain structure and abnormalities [80].

This is the reason why MRI images have a great impact on the automatic medical image analysis field. There are various steps taken in the course of brain tumor treatment. The first step is determining if the tumor does exist in the brain or not. Then, the infected region in the brain tissues must be extracted from an MRI image in a process called segmentation [81]. Segmentation is not an easy task as MRI images may not help human readers easily discern regions of concern for various technical reasons. However, segmentation is a very important task in properly conducting the diagnosis, treatment and appraisal of treatment outcomes. A great number of automatic segmentation methods with varying degrees of accuracy have been developed as applications of the computational science for utilization of imaging devices advance.

There are different modalities of the MRI including T1-weighted (T1), T2-weighted contrast-enhanced (T1c), T2-weighted (T2) and T2-weighted fluid attenuated inversion recovery (FLAIR) for segmenting the brain tumor [82]. Moreover, features of the MRI like textures, local histograms and structure tensor eigenvalues have been used in brain tumor segmentation [83]. Deep learning-based methods have become state-of-the-art as they score superior performance in image analysis fields [84].

3.3.2. Datasets

Most of the researchers have applied publicly available brain tumor image datasets to test their methods. Summary of publicly available datasets for brain tumor segmentation and classification is summarized in Table 16.

Table 16. Image datasets for brain tumor (N—normal, AB—abnormal).

Dataset	Size	#Classes	Format/Targets	Type	Author, Year
LBPA40	288	2	html	MRI	Shattuck et al. [85]
BRATS 2015	43,708	2	.mha	MRI	Menze et al. [86]
BRATS2013	1799	2	.mha	MRI	Menze et al. [86]
RIDER_NEURO_MRI	29	2	.tcia	MRI	Barboriak et al. [87]
SUH	49	2	-	MRI	Fabelo et al. [88]
HMS	66	2	.gif	MRI	Keith A. Johnson
FBT	3064	2	.mat	MRI	C. Jun [89]
NHTM	3064	2	.png	MRI	C. Jun [89]
GCE	150	2	.png	MRI	Jun Cheng [90]

3.3.3. Deep Learning in Brain Tumor Segmentation

Alkassar et al. [91] proposed transfer learning and fully convolution network (FCN) to achieve robust tumor segmentation using VGG-16 networks. The proposed method achieved a global accuracy of 0.97785 and a 0.89 Dice score in terms of whole tumor segmentation on MRI images from the BRATS2015 dataset.

Amiri et al. [92] proposed a simple and reliable brain segmentation method in MRI images through recursively and deeply transferring a learned random forest (RF) to guide an SVM classifier for segmenting tumor lesions while capturing the complex characteristics of brain tumor appearance. They tested this method on 20 patients with high-grade gliomas from the Brain Tumor Image Segmentation Challenge (BRATS) dataset. Their method outperforms both SVM and RF with a high statistical significance using paired t-test; i.e., a mean Dice index of 72% compared to SVM (59%) and RF (63%).

Chahal et al. [93] proposed a novel approach using deep learning which utilizes both global and local brain image datasets for precise segmentation. Their proposed deep learning model combines two-pathway and cascade architectures to analyze and implement brain segmentation. The results are evaluated over Input Cascade and the outcomes showed better performance—that is, a metrics of Dice score for high grade and low-grade image with values 0.943 and 0.950, respectively—than existing MFC cascade.

Ding et al. [94] proposed deep residual dilate network with middle supervision (RDM-Net) which combines the residual network with dilated convolution. By evaluating their framework on the BRATS 2015 challenge, their framework proved to achieve better performance than other state-of-the-art methods incomplete tumor (Dice score of 0.86) and core tumor segmentation (Dice score of 0.78). However, the Dice score for enhancing tumors only achieves 0.63 which is not as good as the other counterpart methods. The reason for this could be the focus on the 2D slices segmentation by the proposed framework which pays less attention to the context information within slices by comparing with 3D segmentation. The loss of context information may lead to worse performance on the enhancing tumor segmentation.

Mallick et al. [95] have used a deep wavelet autoencoder (DWA) for an image compression technique which blends the basic feature reduction property of autoencoder along with image decomposition property of wavelet transform for further classification task by using DNN. The performance of the DWA-DNN classifier was compared with other existing classifiers like autoencoder-DNN or DNN and the proposed method surpasses them all with an overall accuracy of 96% where that of AE-DNN is 93% and DNN is 91%.

Ramirez et al. [96] proposed a new variational model for saliency detection in images and its application to brain tumor segmentation. The model works by incorporating a saliency term to a classical total variation-based restoration functional and hence discriminates what is relevant (salient) from the background. They have, therefore, introduced a deep learning framework for using available knowledge from a specific application to optimize the parameters of the energy functional. The proposed framework achieved a Dice score of 0.857, precision 0.845 and recall 0.882.

Sajid et al. [97] proposed a deep learning-based method that uses different modalities of MRI for the segmentation of brain tumors. The proposed hybrid convolutional neural network architecture uses a patch-based approach and deals with the over-fitting problems by utilizing dropout regularize alongside batch normalization, whereas the data imbalance problem is dealt with by using a two-phase training procedure. The proposed method contains a preprocessing step, in which images are normalized and bias field corrected, a feed-forward pass through a CNN and a post-processing step as a means of removing remnant false positives in the skull portion. The proposed method is validated on the BRATS 2013 dataset, where it achieves scores of 0.86, 0.86 and 0.91 in terms of Dice score, sensitivity and specificity for whole tumor region, improving results compared to existing state-of-the-art techniques.

Wang et al. [98] proposed an automatic method named residual and pyramid pool network (WRN-PPNet) to segment brain tumor by first obtaining 2D slices from 3D MRI brain tumor images and then normalizing the 2D slices and putting them in the model. The model will output the tumor segmentation results. The experimental results show that the proposed method is simple and robust compared to the other state-of-the-art methods with an average Dice, sensitivity and PPV values on randomly selected datasets 0.94, 0.92 and 0.97, respectively.

Zhao et al. [99] proposed a new method for brain segmentation which is an integration of fully convolutional neural networks (FCNNs) and conditional random fields (CRFs) in a unified framework. The result helps to obtain segmentation results with the appearance and spatial consistency. The following steps are taken to for training the deep learning model using 2D image patches and image slices: (1) training FCNNs using image patches; (2) training CRFs as recurrent neural networks (CTF-RNN) using image slices with parameters of FCNNs fixed; and (3) fine-tuning the FCNNs and the CRF-RNN using image slices. In the model, 3 segmentation models are particularly trained using 2D image patches and slices obtained in axial, coronal, and sagittal views respectively are combined to segment brain tumors using a voting-based fusion strategy. The method used BRTS 2013, BRATS 2015 and BRATS 2016 with an experimental result of a competitive score. The method achieved a promising performance on the BRATS 2013 and BRATS 2015 testing dataset. The method could also achieve competitive performance with only 3 imaging modalities (FLAIR, T1c and T2) rather than 4(FLAIR, T1, T1c and T2). In BRATS 2016, the method ranked first on its multi-temporal evaluation.

Kuzina et al. [100] proposed a knowledge transfer method between diseases via the generative Bayesian prior network to mitigate the common challenge of obtaining large image datasets for automatic segmentation. They have applied deep weight prior; hence the name UNet-DWP for their method, to incorporate information about the structure of previously learned convolutional filters during the training of a new model. A comparison between a pre-trained approach and random initialization to this approach proves that this method yields the best results in terms of the Dice similarity coefficient metric on a small subset of the BRATS2018 dataset. The performance of the model was rated by taking subsets containing 5, 10, 15 or 20 randomly selected images from the dataset and comparing them with the fixed test sample size of 50 images. They have also used a blend of binary cross-entropy and Dice losses to train U-Net in the non-Bayesian setting. The results indicate that the model outperforms both pre-trained and randomly initialized U-Nets for all the training sizes.

Zeineldin et al. [101] proposed a new generic deep learning architecture named DeepSeg to address the challenge of distinguishing tumor boundaries from healthy cells in the brain tumor diagnosis. This method helps to wholly automate detection and segmentation of the brain lesion using FLAIR MRI data. The developed system is a decoupling framework interacting encoding and decoding relationship where the encoder part performs spatial information using a convolutional neural network and the decoder provides the full-resolution probability map from the resulting semantic map. The study has employed different CNN models such as residual neural network (ResNet), dense convolutional network (DenseNet) and NASNet using modified U-Net architecture. The proposed architecture has been tested on MRI datasets of brain tumor segmentation (BRATS2019) challenge which includes s336 cases as training data and 125 cases for validation data yielding Dice and Hausdorff distance scored of about 0.81 to 0.84 and 9.8 to 19.7, respectively. The proposed DeepSeg is open source and freely available at https://github.com/razeineldin/DeepSeg/.

Fabelo et al. [102] suggested a deep learning-based hyperspectral image (HSI) processing modality to be used as a reliable support in real-time neurosurgical procedure for carrying out accurate resection of the tumor without affecting much of the normal brain tissue. The study employed a number of deep learning techniques for the detection of brain tumors using HSI. The HS image database was obtained during the course of operation and the system employed a highly sophisticated and specialized visible and near-infrared (VNIR) push broom camera. Classification methods with 2D-CNN and pixel-wise classification with 1D-DNN have been found to yield a very good result. Despite the challenge in obtaining sufficient number of training samples and the anomalies incurred due to brain movement during scanning, the overall average accuracy for the proposed method was 80%. The method has also achieved a very high specificity for both binary and multiclass classification schemes with values of 100% and 90%, respectively.

The summary of researches on deep learning methods for brain tumor segmentation is presented in Table 17.

3.3.4. Deep Learning in Brain Tumor Classification

Like in the segmentation, deep learning-based methods have performed fairly well in image classification of brain tumors. Yet, variation in the shape, size, location and contrast of tumor tissue cells is the major factor that impacts the accurate classification of brain tumors from MRI images [103].

Deep learning techniques involving different enhancement methods are used to classify different types of brain tumors—glioma, meningioma and pituitary. The classification is further categorized into axial, coronal and sagittal planes that are used by various algorithms to minimize the error rate of neural networks in identifying the brain tumor [104].

Mohsen et al. [80] employed a DNN classifier where a 7-fold cross-validation technique was applied for building and training the DNN of 7-hidden layers structure for classifying a dataset of brain MRIs into four classes, i.e., normal, glioblastoma, sarcoma and metastatic bronchogenic carcinoma.

They have combined the classifier with the discrete wavelet transform (DWT)—a powerful feature extraction tool—and principal components analysis (PCA). They achieved a classification rate of 96.97%, recall 0.97, precision 0.97, F-measure 0.97 and AUC (ROC) 0.984.

Table 17. Summary of selected papers on brain tumor segmentation.

Authors	Method Learning	Dataset	Acc.	P	R	F	Sp	Sn	Dice	PPV
Alkassar et al. [91]	DNN+FCN+VGG-16	BRATS2015	0.98						0.89	
Amiri et al. [92]	RF-SVM	BRATS							0.72	
Chahal et al. [93]	CNN	BRATS2013		0.96				0.93	0.95	
Ding et al. [94]	RDM-Net	BRATS2015							0.86	
Mallick et al. [95]	DWA-DNN	RIDER_NEURO_MRI	0.93			0.93	0.92	0.94		
Ramirez et al. [96]	CNN+TVS	Flair-MRI Brats2015		0.84	0.88				0.86	
Sajid et al.[97]	hybrid CNN	BRATS 2013					0.91	0.86	0.86	
Wang et al. [98]	WRN-PPNet	BRATS2015						0.92	0.94	0.97
Zhao et al. [99]	FCNNs and CRF-RNN	BRATS 2013–16						0.82	0.84	0.89
Kuzina et al. [100]	UNet-DWP	BRATS2018							0.76	
Zeineldin et al. [101]	DeepSeg	BRATS 2019							0.81–0.84	
Fabelo et al. [102]	HSI+2D-CNN	SUH	80					80–100		

Alqudah et al. [105] used a convolutional neural network (CNN) for classifying a dataset of 3064 T1 weighted contrast-enhanced brain MR images for grading the brain tumors into three classes called glioma, meningioma and pituitary. The research has used T1-weighted contrast-enhanced brain MR images for classifying brain tumor grades. They have used a free online available dataset at [90] which contains images having the above-mentioned attributes. A total of 18 layers in the proposed CNN architecture would enable the classifier to rate the brain tumor effectively. In their work they proved that the proposed CNN classifier is a powerful tool with an accuracy of 98.93% and sensitivity 98.18% for cropped lesions; for the uncropped lesions, they have obtained an accuracy of 99% and 98.52% sensitivity; for segmented lesion images, the result is 97.62 accuracy and 97.40% sensitivity.

Ucuzal et al. [106] developed a deep learning free web-based software that can be utilized in the detection and diagnosis of the three types of brain tumors (glioma/meningioma/pituitary) on T1-weighted magnetic resonance imaging. In the research, 3064 T1-weighted MR image scans for the three types of brain tumors have been used. Out of which, 2599 instances were used in the training phase; whereas, the remaining 465 were used in the testing phase. A python programming language library called Auto Keras was used in image pre-processing (image rotation, changing width and length, truncating images, rescaling, etc). Furthermore, a Bayesian optimization technique was used to tune the hyperparameters of the model. With this, they have verified that all the calculated performance metrics—i.e., accuracy, precision, sensitivity, specificity, F1-score, MCC, G-Mean of the experimental results are higher than 98% for classifying the types of brain tumors on the testing dataset obtained from Nanfang Hospital and Tianjin Medical University General Hospital which is an open-source dataset downloaded from [107]. This data set consists of 3064 T1-weighted contrast-enhanced MR images from 233 patients: 708 meningiomas, 1426 glioma and 930 pituitary tumors. The developed web-based software can be publicly available at [108].

Selvy et al. [109] developed a model that makes use of an image processing technique and artificial neural network for successful detection of the brain tumor. To enhance the contrast of the original image in its analysis and manipulation, they have used histogram equalization (HE) technique where gray level co-occurrence matrix (GLCM) would be used on the feature extraction. A probabilistic neural network (PNN) classifier is applied to the obtained feature to accurately determine tumor location in brain MRI images. The PNN classifier has produced an accuracy of 90.9%, specificity of 100% and sensitivity 85.75%.

Sultan et al. [110] proposed a deep learning (DL) model to classify different brain tumor types. The model which bases a convolutional neural network has employed two publicly available datasets acquired from Nanfang Hospital and General Hospital, Tianjing Medical University, China from 2005 to 2010. The two datasets entail 233 and 73 patients with a total of 3064 and 516 images on T1-weighted contrast-enhanced images, respectively. The overall accuracy of the proposed network is 96.13% for the first and 98.7% for the second dataset. The result inferred that the model has the ability to perform brain tumor multi-classification. The network training and performance computations are finally presented. The system parameters used to train the neural network structure are Intel i7-7700HQ CPU (2.8 GHz), NVIDIA GTX 1060 (6 GB) GPU, 16GB RAM, Matlab 2018b and Python 3. The network is constructed from 16 layers where the input layer holds the pre-processed images passing through the convolution layers and their activation functions (3 convolution, 3 ReLU, normalization and 3 max-pooling layers). Additionally, two dropout layers are used to prevent overfitting followed by a fully connected layer and a softmax layer to predict the output and finally a classification layer that produces the predicted class. Although the dataset is relatively not big (due to the variety of imaging views), data augmentation helped well to show better results and hence, overcome this problem.

Badža and Barjaktarovic [111] presented a new CNN architecture for Brain Tumor Image Segmentation and classification for three tumor types. The study has employed an image database that contains 3064 T1-weighted contrast-enhanced MRI images acquired from Nanfang Hospital and General Hospital, Tianjin Medical University, China from 2005 to 2010. The input layer of the proposed network was represented by MRI images of the database after being normalized to 256 × 256 pixels. The network architecture having consisted of input, two main blocks, classification block and output was employed to perform tumor classification. The blocks consist of the rectified linear unit (ReLU) activation layer, the dropout layer and the max-pooling layer engaged in fine-tuning and resizing the images. A CNN developed in Matlab R2018a (The MathWorks) was employed for the tumor classification. The evaluation of the network was assessed using four approaches: combinations of two 10-fold cross-validation methods and the two databases mentioned above. The generalization capability of the network was tested with one of the 10-fold methods, subject-wise cross-validation, and the improvement was tested by using an augmented image database. The best result for the 10-fold cross-validation method was obtained for the record-wise cross-validation for the augmented data set, and, in that case, the accuracy was 96.56%. With good generalization capability and good execution speed, the new developed CNN architecture could be used as an effective decision-support tool for radiologists in medical diagnostics.

The summary of the papers reviewed is presented in Table 18.

Table 18. Summary of selected papers on brain tumor classification.

Authors	Method	Dataset	Acc.	P	R	F	Sp	Sn	MCC	G-Mean
Mohsen et al. [80]	DWT-DNN	Harvard		0.97	0.97	0.97				
Alqudah et al. [105]	CNN	Online	98.40	98.19			99.19	98.18		
Ucuzal et al. [106]	CNN Multiclass	NHTM	99.74	99.58		99.59	99.81	99.60	99.39	99.70
Selvy et al. [109]	PNN	GCE	90			100	85.75			
Sultan et al. [110]	CNN	NHTM	96.13–98.7							
Badža and Barjaktarovic [111]	CNN	NHTM	96.56							

3.3.5. Summary

As shown in Table 19, papers from 2016,2018, 2019, and 2020 were reviewed here. Unlike other cancer type papers, reviewed papers on brain tumors consist of a significant number of papers that compared the performance of their model with that of the domain expert(see Table 20).

As indicated in Tables 17 and 18, Brain Tumor Image Segmentation Challenge (BRATS) of various versions is the most widely used dataset among the researchers and appeared in ten out of the seventeen papers reviewed.

From Table 21 it was found that a Tensor flow-based framework run by a high-speed core processor or a GPU was widely used, seven out of seventeen, followed by PyTorch, two out of seventeen, to implement the experiments and conducting the deep learning training. However, the rest of the papers have not explicitly indicated which software platform they have applied. On the other hand, VGGNet is the most frequently applied network to achieve robust tumor segmentation 52.9% of the papers have made a comparison with domain experts; on the other hand, 94.1% of the paper has made a comparison with the traditional method.

Table 19. Summary of brain tumor scientific papers in terms of article publication year, name of journal for the selected papers and its impact factor with year of impact factor.

Author and Citation	Publication Year	Journal	Impact Factor	Impact Assigned Year
Alkassar et al. [91]	2019	ICECCPCE19 Conference	0.627	2019
Amiri et al. [92]	2016	ATSIP 2016 Conference	0.17	2019
Chahal et al. [93]	2019	RDCAPE Conference	-	-
Ding et al. [94]	2019	IEEE Access	3.745	2019
Mallick et al. [95]	2019	IEEE Access	3.745	2019
Ramirez et al. [96]	2018	ISBI Conference	1.51	2019
Sajid et al.[97]	2019	Arabian Journal for Science and Engineering	0.33	2019
Wang et al. [98]	2019	IJCNN Conference	0.37	2019
Zhao et al. [99]	2018	Medical Image Analysis	3.88	2019
Kuzina et al. [100]	2019	Frontiers in Neuroscince	3.7	2020
Mohsen et al. [80]	2018	Future Computing and Informatics	3.88	2019
Alqudah et al. [105]	2019	IJATCSE	0.2	2019
Ucuzal et al. [106]	2019	ISMSIT	0.84	2019
Zeineldin et al. [101]	2020	IJCARS	1.961	2017
Fabelo et al. [102]	2019	MDPI	3.275	2019
Selvy et al. [109]	2019	IJSRCSEIT	1.638	2016
Sultan et al. [110]	2019	IEEE Access	3.745	2019
Badža and Barjaktarovic [111]	2020	MDPI	2.474	2019

Table 20. Summary of brain tumor scientific papers in terms of comparison to specialists and/or traditional techniques.

Author and Citation	Comparison to Specialists (Yes/No)	Comparison to Traditional Technique (Yes/No)
Alkassar et al. [91]	Yes	Yes
Amiri et al. [92]	No	Yes
Chahal et al. [93]	No	Yes
Ding et al. [94]	No	Yes
Mallick et al. [95]	No	Yes
Ramirez et al. [96]	Yes	Yes
Sajid et al.[97]	No	Yes
Wang et al. [98]	Yes	Yes
Zhao et al. [99]	Yes	Yes
Kuzina et al. [100]	No	Yes
Mohsen et al. [80]	No	Yes
Alqudah et al. [105]	No	Yes
Ucuzal et al. [106]	Yes	No
Zeineldin et al. [101]	Yes	Yes
Fabelo et al. [102]	Yes	Yes
Selvy et al. [109]	No	No
Sultan et al. [110]	Yes	Yes
Badža and Barjaktarovic [111]	No	Yes

Table 21. Summary of brain tumor scientific papers in terms of CNN architecture, and type of environment used in the selected papers.

Author and Citation	Network	Pre-Training	Transfer Learning	Environment
Alkassar et al. [91]	VGGNet-16	Yes	Yes	
Amiri et al. [92]	RF+SVM	Yes	Yes	
Chahal et al. [93]	CNN	Yes	Yes	
Ding et al. [94]	RDM-Net	Yes	Yes	
Mallick et al. [95]	DWA-DNN	Yes	Yes	Tensor flow
Ramirez et al. [96]	CNN+TVS	Yes	Yes	Tensor flow
Sajid et al.[97]	hybrid CNN	Yes	Yes	Tensor Flow
Wang et al. [98]	WRN-PPNet	Yes	Yes	Tensor flow
Zhao et al. [99]	FCNNs and CRF-RNN	Yes	Yes	Tensor flow
Kuzina et al. [100]	UNet-DWP	Yes	Yes	
Mohsen et al. [80]	DWT-DNN	Yes	Yes	
Alqudah et al. [105]	VGGNet-19	Yes	Yes	
Ucuzal et al. [106]	UNet-DWP	Yes	Yes	Tensor flow and Keras
Zeineldin et al. [101]	ResNet+DenseNet+NasNet	Yes	Yes	Keras, Tensor Flow
Fabelo et al. [102]	UNet	Yes	Yes	Tensor Flow
Selvy et al. [109]	GLCM+PNN	Yes	Yes	
Sultan et al. [110]	CNN	Yes	Yes	Matlab 2018b and Python
Badža and Barjaktarovic [111]	CNN	Yes	Yes	Matlab 2018b

3.4. *Colorectal Cancer (CRC)*

Worldwide in 2018, more than 1,849,518 (which accounts for 10.2% of overall cancer cases) new cases of colorectal cancer (CRC) are diagnosed and nearly 880,792 people died which is 9.2% of all cancer-related deaths [112]. It is the third most common cancer worldwide and the second most deadly [112]. Since colorectal cancer takes a long time before it becomes invasive, it is often curable if found early. Hence, casual screening for colorectal cancer can substantially reduce its mortality. Approximately 95% of all colorectal cancers are adenocarcinomas [113]. Colorectal adenocarcinomas develop in the lining of the colon or rectum and are characterized by glandular formation.

3.4.1. Screening Methods

There are three common screening methods for colorectal cancer: fecal occult blood test (FOBt), flexible sigmoidoscopy (FS) and total colonoscopy (TC) [114]. FOBt reveals traces of blood in stool samples which is an early sign of colorectal cancer. FS involves visual inspection of the distal bowel for polyps and cancers. TC visualizes the entire bowel and therefore is a more invasive examination. The advancement of whole slide imaging (WSI) scanners has opened new opportunities in automating pathology image analysis by digitizing the slides [115]. Histological examination of the glands, most frequently with the hematoxylin & eosin (H & E) stain, is routine practice for assessing the differentiation of cancer within colorectal adenocarcinoma [113]. Pathologists use the degree of glandular formation as an important factor in deciding the grade of the tumor. Accurate segmentation of structures of the glandular formations such as glands and nuclei have crucial importance, because their morphological properties can assist the pathologist in screening the malignancy [113].

3.4.2. Datasets

In Table 22, we present some of the publicly available and widely used datasets for colorectal cancer detection and segmentation.

Table 22. Publicly available datasets for colorectal cancer (CRC), UMCM—University Medical Center Mannheim, CVC—computer vision center.

Dataset	Size	#Classes/Targets	Format	Type	Author, Year
CVC-EndoSceneStill	912	4	bmp	Colonoscopy	Vázquez et al. [116], 2017
CVC-ColonDB	300	4	bmp	Colonoscopy	J. Bernal et al. [117], 2012
CVC-ClinicDB	612	4	tiff	Colonoscopy	J. Bernal et al. [118], 2015
UMCM	500	8	mat	histology	Kather et al. [119], 2016

3.4.3. Deep Learning for Cell Detection and Classification on Histological Slides

Kainz et al. [120] applied deep learning methods to segment and classify colon glands into benign and malignant types for GlaS@MICCAI2015 challenge. They first pre-processed the stained RGB by taking the Red channel and ignoring the others. Then contrast enhancement was performed using contrast limited adaptive histogram equalization (CLAHE) technique. Two CNN classifiers were trained: Object-Net, Separator-Net. Object-Net is for the detection of benign and malignant glands from their respective backgrounds. Separator-Net is for classifying gland-separating structures since the Object-Net architecture segment two neighboring glands as one. These to classifiers are then regularized using a figure-ground segmentation based on weighted total variation to produce the final segmentation result. They have achieved 96% average accuracy on the two tests provided by the challenge.

Sirinukunwattana et al. [121] proposed a spatially constrained convolutional neural network (SC-CNN) that includes parameter estimation layer and spatially constrained layer for spatial regression to predict the probability of a pixel being the center of a nucleus in hematoxylin and eosin (H & E) stained histopathology images. For classifying the detected nuclei they combine neighboring ensemble predictor (NEP) with a standard softmax CNN (s-CNN). For the nuclei detection using SC-CNN, they achieved 0.77 precision, 0.82 recall, and 0.8 F1-score. The NEP&s-CNN classifier achieved an F1-score of 0.784 and the overall nuclei detection and classification (SC-CNN+NEP&s-CNN) achieved an F1-score of 0.69.

Graham et al. [113] used a fully convolutional neural network that counters the loss of information caused by the max-pooling layer by introducing original down-sampled image into the residual unit using the minimal information loss (MIL) units. They applied atrous spatial pyramid pooling for multi-level aggregation and preserving the resolution. They achieved an F1-score of 0.92 for gland segmentation using the GlaS challenge dataset.

Chamanzar et al. [122] develop a deep learning method that can detect and segment a single cell using only point labeled dataset. They combined Voronoi transformation, Local pixel clustering and Repel encoding methods with U net with Resnet encoder by feeding them to a multi-task scheduler for training the system. They achieved an accuracy of 93% for cell segmentation and 94.1% for detection of adenocarcinoma.

Sari et al. [123] proposed a novel approach for feature extraction, which defines the features by considering only the salient subregions of the image. The salient subregions were detected by the detection of nuclear and non-nuclear pixels using an algorithm presented in [124]. Then a deep belief network of restricted Boltzmann machines (RBMs) re-characterizes these regions and extract features. These features are clustered using the k-means clustering algorithm and SVM classifier for categorizing those regions. They achieved an average precision, recall, and F1-score of 82.3%, 89.9% and 85.1, respectively at the detection of colon adenocarcinoma.

Shapcott et al. [125] proposed a deep learning-based cell identification on histological images of the colon with a systematic random sampling of the WSI slides. Their proposed system consists of two CNNs in series in which the first one detects cells on the WSI slide while the second one classifies those cells into epithelial, inflammatory, a fibroblast or "other". The training was performed on a local dataset and Evaluated using the "The Cancer Genome Atlas (TCGA)" dataset. Using five patients' slides, they achieved an average accuracy of 65% in the detection of cells and 76% in the classification.

Tang et al. [126] proposed Segnet based gland segmentation on the histology image of the colon. Augmented MICCAI2015 challenge dataset was used to train the SegNet network which is a CNN with encode-decoder architecture for pixel-wise segmentation. SegNet achieved an average Dice similarity index of 0.872 and Hausdorff distance of 104.61.

Vuong et al. [127] proposed an algorithm based on DenseNet121 that can perform both classification and regression tasks on WSI images, for improving the overall performance of the system. They designed this multi-task deep learning model by adding two fully connected layers, one for classification and one for regression, after the DenseNet121 network. The classifier classifies the tissue image into four distinctive pathologies and the regressor considers these four pathological categories as continuous values. They achieved 85.1% accuracy in classifying colon tissues into four categories.

Sabol et al. [128] proposed a semantically explainable fuzzy classifier called cumulative fuzzy class membership criterion (CFCMC) for classifying WSI of colorectal cancer tissue into eight different tissue types. They compared many CNN architectures as feature extraction for the CFCMC classifier with the Xception architecture performance being the best feature extractor for the CFCMC. The explainability of the system is its ability to provide a degree of confidence for each of its predictions. The proposed method achieved an accuracy of 92.78% for the classification of the different tissue samples. The explainability was evaluated by pathologists based on its objectivity, level of details, reliability and quality. Based on these measures, they confirmed that the explainability of the system is better than the traditional CNN architectures.

3.4.4. Deep Learning for Classification of Polyps on Endoscopic Images

Colorectal polyps are abnormalities in the colon tissues that can develop into colorectal cancer. The survival rate for patients is higher when the disease is detected at an early stage and polyps can be removed before they develop into malignant tumors. These tests are usually performed using endoscopic analysis of the colon. During this study, the endoscopist explores the colon cavity looking for abnormal growths of tissue, polyps. However, polyp detection is a challenging problem given its high variation in appearance, size, shape and in many cases its high similarity with the surrounding tissue.

The application of CTs for the screening of colorectal cancer suffers from false positives due to the similarity between polyps and colorectal tubes on the CT image. Approaches in [129] can help to distinguish between colorectal tubes and polyps in CT scans of the colon area using a three dimensional massive-training artificial neural network (3D-MTANN). The proposed model manages to reduce false positives by 33% while keeping a sensitivity of 96%.

Ornela Bardhi et al. [130] used CNNs with auto-encoders for the automatic detection of colon polyp. They used the SegNet architecture from the TensorFlow to build the model and train it from scratch using three datasets: CVC-ColonDB, CVC-ClinicDB and ETIS-LaribPolypDB. They achieved a maximum accuracy of 96.7% on the EITS dataset for the detection of colon polyps.

Bour et al. [131] trained different architectures: ResNet50, ResNet101, Xception, VGG19 and Inception V3 for classification of polyps. ResNet50 achieved the highest accuracy of 87.1 % with precision 87.1%, recall 87.1%, F1-score 87.1% and specificity 93%.

Liu et al. [132] used a deep learning network, faster_rcnn_inception_resnet_v2 model for localization and classification of endoscopic images of the colon. They achieved 90.645% mean average precision and 0.5 for the intersection over union (IoU).

Ozawa et al. [133] used deep convolutional neural network (CNN) architecture called single shot multibox detector (SSD) for the detection of colorectal polyps. All layers were fine-tuned using stochastic gradient descent with a global learning rate of 0.0001. The trained SSD detected the trained CNN detected 1246 colorectal polyps from a dataset collected at Tada Tomohiro Institute of Gastroenterology and Proctology with a sensitivity of 92% and a positive predictive value (PPV) of 86%.

Nadimi et al. [134] used a modified version of ZF-net, a CNN architecture proposed by Matthew D. Zeiler and Rob Fergus [135], as the basis for a Faster R-CNN to localize regions of images containing colorectal polyps. They trained their architectures using a locally collected dataset labeled as colorectal polyps (N = 4800) and normal mucosa (N = 6500). The proposed architecture achieved an accuracy, sensitivity and specificity of 98.0%, 98.1% and 96.3%, respectively. The proposed approach produces the bounding box annotation of the polyp.

3.4.5. Summary

The most common colorectal cancer screening methods use endoscopic images to find abnormal colon tissues, polyps and locating cancerous cells or glands on WSI images. Hence most of the application of deep learning for detecting colorectal cancer is either finding adenocarcinoma on WSI or detection of polyps on colonoscopic images. Most of the research shows promising results in both polyp detection and adenocarcinoma or glands detection as seen in Tables 23 and 24.

Table 23. Summary of selected papers on detection and classification for colorectal cancer histological slides.

Authors	Method	Dataset	Acc	P	R	F1	DSC	H
Kainz et al. [120]	Separator-Net and Object-Net	MICCAI2015	96	59	74	62	-	-
Graham et al. [113]	MILD-Net	$GlaS^{+}$	-	-	-	87	88	142
Chamanzar et al. [122]	WSMTL	local	93	-	-	79.1	78.4	-
Sari et al. [123]	DeepFeature	local	-	82.3	89.9	85.1	-	-
Shapcott et al. [125]	CNNs	local and TCGA	65	-	-	-	-	-
Sirinukunwattana et al. [121]	SC-CNN+NEP & s-CNN	MICCAI2015	-	-	-	-	69	-
Tang et al. [126]	Segnet	MICCAI2015	-	-	-	-	87.2	104.61
Vuong et al. [127]	Multitask DensNet121	local	85.1	-	-	-	-	-
Sabol et al. [128]	CFSCMC	UMCM	92.78	-	-	-	-	-

The main challenge for the analysis of colposcopic images is most of the dataset suffers from out of focus problems. Detection of polyps from endoscopic images presents a big opportunity for deep learning methods to shine since most of the physicians may miss smaller polyps. Still, challenges are there due to low-quality samples and the operator might miss some areas.

Papers who used pre-trained models and applied transfer learning approaches discuss their findings in detail and are from reputable journals (see Tables 25 and 26). From Table 27, only two of the papers measure the performance of their proposed model against expert physicians.

Table 24. Summary of selected papers on colorectal cancer polyp detection.

Authors	Method	Dataset	Acc	P	R	F1	Sp	Sn	PPV
Ornela Bardhi et al. [130]	SegNet	EITs	96.7	-	-	-	-	-	-
Bour et al. [131]	Resnet50	local	87.1	87.1	87.1	87.1	93	-	-
Liu et al. [132]	faster_rcnn_inception_resnet_v2	local	90.6	-	-	-	-	-	-
Ozawa et al. [133]	SSD	local	-	-	-	-	-	92	86
Nadimi et al. [134]	mZF-net+ResNet	local	98	-	-	-	98.1	96	-

Table 25. Summary of colorectal cancer in terms of article publication year, name of journal for the selected papers and its impact factor with year impact factor has been assigned.

Author and Citation	Publication Year	Journal/Conference	Impact Factor	Impact Assigned Year
Kainz et al. [120]	2017	PeerJ	2.38	2019
Graham et al. [113]	2018	Medical Image Analysis	8.79	2018
Chamanzar et al. [122]	2020	ISBI conference	2.283	2019
Sari et al. [123]	2019	IEEE Transactions on Medical Imaging	9.71	2019
Shapcott et al. [125]	2019	Frontiers in bioengineering and biotechnology	3.644	2020
Sirinukunwattana et al. [121]	2016	IEEE transactions on medical imaging	9.71	2019
Tang et al. [126]	2018	Conference YAC	1.461	2019
Vuong et al. [127]	2020	Conference ICEIC	0.76	2019
Ornela Bardhi et al. [130]	2017	Conference ISSPIT	1.393	2019
Bour et al. [131]	2017	Conference ISSPIT	1.393	2019
Liu et al. [132]	2019	Conference ISNE	0.152	2019
Ozawa et al. [133]	2020	Therapeutic advances in gastroenterology	4.08	2020
Nadimi et al. [134]	2020	CEE	2.663	2020
Sabol et al. [128]	2020	YJBIN	3.526	2020

Table 26. Summary of colorectal cancer in terms of CNN architecture and type of environment used in the selected papers.

Author and Citation	Network	Pre-Training	Transfer Learning	Environment
Kainz et al. [120]	Object-Net and SeparatorNet—custom	No	No	Matlab
Graham et al. [113]	MILD-Net—custom	No	No	Tensorflow
Chamanzar et al. [122]	U-net and Resnet	Yes	Yes	PyTorch
Sari et al. [123]	DeepBelief	Yes	Yes	-
Shapcott et al. [125]	-	No	No	Tensorflow
Sirinukunwattana et al. [121]	-	No	No	Matlab
Tang et al. [126]	SegNet	No	No	Caffe
Vuong et al. [127]	DensNet121	No	No	PyTorch
Ornela Bardhi et al. [130]	SegNet	No	No	Tensorflow
Bour et al. [131]	ResNet50	Yes	Yes	Tensorflow
Liu et al. [132]	faster_rcnn_inception_resnet_v2	No	No	Tensorflow
Ozawa et al. [133]	Single Shot MultiBox Detector (SSD)	No	No	Caffe
Nadimi et al. [134]	mZF-Net+ResNet	Yes	Yes	Matlab 2018a
Sabol et al. [128]	Xception+CFCMC	Yes	Yes	-

Table 27. Summary of colorectal cancer papers in terms of comparison to specialists and/or traditional techniques.

Author and Citation	Comparison to Specialists	Comparison to Traditional Technique (Yes/No)
Kainz et al. [120]	No	No
Graham et al. [113]	No	Yes
Chamanzar et al. [122]	No	Yes
Sari et al. [123]	No	No
Shapcott et al. [125]	No	No
Sirinukunwattana et al. [121]	No	Yes
Tang et al. [126]	No	Yes
Vuong et al. [127]	No	No
Ornela Bardhi et al. [130]	No	No
Bour et al. [131]	Yes (Approval)	No
Liu et al. [132]	No	Yes
Ozawa et al. [133]	No	No
Nadimi et al. [134]	No	No
Sabol et al. [128]	Yes	Yes

3.5. Lung Cancer

Lung cancer is the deadliest cancer worldwide with the highest incidence rate [112]. The death rate is so high because the majority of the cases are discovered at an advanced stage, where curative treatment is no longer feasible. Hence, screening for early detection is significant enough for decreasing mortality.

3.5.1. Screening Methods

The recommended screening test for lung cancer is low-dose computed tomography (LDCT), which uses a low dose of X-ray radiation to get detailed images of the lungs. Physicians will study different slices of the LDCT to determine the presence of an abnormal area called lung nodule (or mass) [136]. Other approaches also exist like chest X-ray(the usual X-ray image), sputum cytology (microscopic analysis of mucus from the lungs). According to a study performed in [136], these approaches do not seem to decrease the mortality rate.

3.5.2. Datasets

In Table 28, some of the publicly available and widely used datasets for lung cancer detection and segmentation are listed.

Table 28. Publicly available datasets for CRC, UMCM—University Medical Center Mannheim, CVC—computer vision center.

Dataset	Size	#Classes/Targets	Format	Type	Author, Year
UCI ML repository	32	3		CSV	Hong and Yang [137], 1991
SPIE-AAPM-NCI	22489	2	dicom	CT	Armato et al. [138], 2015
Lung Nodule Malignancy	6690	2	hdf5	CT	Scott Mader [139], 2017
LUNA2016	888	2	mhd.zip	CT	Consortium for Open Medical Image Computing [119], 2016

3.5.3. Deep Learning for Lung Nodules Detection

Before the introduction of convolution-based deep learning methods, Suzuki [140] uses massive training artificial neural networks (MTANN) for the detection and decreasing false positives in lobules detection using extracted subregions from LDCT images. MTANNs are designed based on the concepts of artificial neural network filters, where MTANN will classify each subregion (kernel) independently. Hence, the convolution process is external. They used Multiple MTANNs in parallel to distinguish between nodules and non-nodules by training each MTANN with the same nodules but different types of non-nodules. multi-MTANN was applied to differentiate between benign and malignant nodules from LDCT images in [141].

Tajbakhsh and Suzuki [142] compared the performances of the two widely studied deep learning models, CNNs and MTANNs, for the detection and classification of lung nodules. The proposed MTANN-based architecture outperforms the best performing CNN (AlexNet in their experiment) insensitivity and false-positive rates achieving 100% sensitivity and 2.7 false positives per patient. In the classifications of the nodules into benign and malignant the MTANNs achieved an AUC of 0.88.

Gu et al. [143] proposed a novel CAD system for the detection of lung nodules using a 3D-CNN. They implemented a multiscale approach for making the system more efficient at the detection of various sizes of nodules. The proposed CAD system considers the preprocessing step, which is usually essential in building a standalone CAD system. It has a volume segmentation step for generating ROI cubes for the 3D-CNN to classify them. After the classification, DBSCAN was used to merge neighboring regions into one since they might be different parts of the same nodule. Using the LUNA16 dataset, they found out that small scale cubes are efficient in the detection of smaller nodules (92% sensitivity and four false positives per patient), but larger ones have lower sensitivity (88%), but with an average of one false positive per patient.

Sahu et al. [144] proposed a multiple view sampling-based multi-section CNN model for nodule classification and malignancy estimation from CT scans. Their proposed model is computationally lighter than the widely used and relatively efficient 3D-CNNs. They used sample slices extracted at different orientations, with spherical sampling performing the best, and a pre-trained MobileNet network to build their system. On the classification task, the proposed model achieved a sensitivity of 96% and AUC of 98% on the LUNA2016 dataset. They measure the severity of malignancy by training the logistic regression model to estimate the class probability of malignancy. It achieved an accuracy of 93.79% on malignancy estimation. Since it is a lightweight model, the model can work on smaller devices such as smart-phones, tablets, etc.

Ozdemir et al. [145] proposed an efficient end-to-end CAD system by coupling nodule detection with malignancy ranking step. They called the nodule detection system as CAD_e (detection) whose output is an input for malignancy ranking step, CAD_x (diagnosis) step in the complete CAD system. Training and evaluation were performed on the LUNA16 and Kaggle Bowl datasets [146]. The proposed model includes model uncertainty in its decision, making it relatively trustworthy in a real-world application. The proposed CAD_e system achieved a sensitivity of 96.5%+ and 19.7 false positives per patient without using false positive reduction techniques. The CAD_x system also achieves an AUC of 98%. The combination of the two systems was further tuned to build the full CAD system.

Bansal et al. [147] proposed Deep3DSCan for lung cancer segmentation and classification. They used a deep 3D segmentation algorithm to extract a 3D volume of interest from CTs. A combination of features extracted using a deep fine-tuned residual network and morphological features were used to train the ResNet based model. Training and testing used the publicly available LUNA16 dataset. The proposed architecture achieved an accuracy of 88% in segmentation and classification tasks with an F1-score of 0.88.

3.5.4. Summary

Many of the papers discussed here studied the detection and classification of lung nodules from the LDCT images. The end-to-end papers covered in these reviews ([142,145,147]) can help to build an effective CAD system to assist the radiologist.Bansal et al. [147] seems to work better than the other works reviewed here since its performance covers both the detection and classification tasks (see Table 29). We must also consider MTANN-based papers since they deliver a satisfactory result with smaller data sizes. Papers reviewed here can be summarized in Tables 30 and 31. Here we did not consider to create a table for domain expert approval since none was participated in the papers we reviewed.

Table 29. Summary of selected papers on lung cancer detection and classification.

Authors	Method	Dataset	Acc	FPR	Sp	Sn	AUC
Tajbakhsh and Suzuki [142]	MTANN, detection	local	-	2.7	-	100	
Tajbakhsh and Suzuki [142]	MTANN, classification	local	-	-	-	-	0.88
Gu et al. [143]	3D-CNN, detection	LUNA16	-	2.5	-	90	
Sahu et al. [144]	multi-section MobileNet	LUNA16	93.8	-	-	96	0.98
Ozdemir et al. [145]	V-Net, classification	LUNA16	-	19	-	96.5	0.98
Bansal et al. [147]	ResNet	LUNA16	88	-	89.7	87	0.88

Table 30. Summary of lung cancer in terms of article publication year, name of journal for the selected papers and its impact factor with the year impact factor has been assigned.

Author and Citation	Publication Year	Journal/Conference	Impact Factor	Impact Assigned Year
Tajbakhsh and Suzuki [142]	2017	Pattern Recognition	7.196	2019
Gu et al. [143]	2018	CBM	3.43	2019
Sahu et al. [144]	2019	IEEE-JBHI	5.180	2020
Ozdemir et al. [145]	2020	IEEE Transactions on Medical Imaging	9.71	2020
Bansal et al. [147]	2020	IET Image Processing	2.61	2020

Table 31. Summary of Colorectal cancer in terms of CNN architecture and type of environment used in the selected papers.

Author and Citation	Network	Pre-Training	Transfer Learning	Environment
Tajbakhsh and Suzuki [142]	MTANN	-	-	Caffe
Gu et al. [143]	3D-CNN	-	-	Keras
Sahu et al. [144]	Mobile-Net	Yes	Yes	Keras
Ozdemir et al. [145]	Vnet	-	-	-
Bansal et al. [147]	Resnet	-	-	Pythorch

3.5.5. Deep Learning for Other Cancer Detection and Segmentation

In this sub-section, we included the application of deep learning on skin, liver and stomach cancer detection. Melanoma is skin cancer which is the deadliest cancer in its nature. In a normal diagnosis distinguishing melanoma lesions from nonmelanoma, lesions are very challenging [148]. For such difficulties, researchers have introduced an automatic skin cancer diagnosis system for detection and segmentation. As a result of uneasy visual characteristics of skin lesion that include inhomogeneous features and fuzzy boundaries. To overcome the challenges, Adegun and Viriri [148] proposed a deep learning-based automatic melanoma lesion detection and segmentation algorithm. They evaluated their approach in terms of Dice coefficient and accuracy 92% and 95% on ISIC 2017 dataset and accuracy and Dice coefficient of 95% and 93% on PH2 datasets.

Another deadly cancer with high morbidity is liver cancer. There are no widely recommended methods for early detection of liver cancer. For patients at higher risk, an imaging test such as CT, MRI, ultrasound and angiography can be used to test for liver cancer. If the physician believes in the need, a biopsy may be used to confirm the diagnosis. Hence, deep learning methods have been proposed in assisting physicians in the diagnosis of liver cancers, including hepatocellular carcinoma (HCC), liver metastasis, cysts, hemangioma and other masses [149]. A custom CNN for classifying HCC in liver cancer from MRI images, which achieved 92% sensitivity (Sn), 98% specificity (Sp) and 92% accuracy was proposed in [150]. In [151], VGGNet was used to develop a CAD system that identifies four types of liver cancers, cysts, hemangiomas, HCC and metastatic liver cancer from ultrasound images. The developed CAD system achieved an average accuracy of 88%. A hybridized fully convolutional neural network (HFCNN) was applied in the detection of liver cancer from abdominal CT images in [64]. HFCNN accurately segments 94.7% of the tumor volume.

Stomach (gastric) cancer is also another common cancer with the fourth-highest incidence rate and the third-highest mortality rate in the world [112]. The most common screening methods for stomach cancer are UGI series, serum pepsinogen (PG) testing, Hpylori serology and endoscopy [152]. Endoscopy is the most accurate of these methods, but it is highly invasive [152]. Some popular deep learning architectures, the inception, ResNet and VGGNet that were pre-trained on ImageNet were applied using transfer learning methods has been applied to identify benign ulcer and cancer from gastrointestinal endoscopic color images in [153]. The ResNet model achieved the highest performance with normal versus abnormal accuracies of 90% and ulcer versus cancer accuracy of 77%. A pre-trained Inception-Resnet-v2 model was trained and compared with endoscopists in classifying classification of gastric neoplasms in [154]. The Inception-Resnet-v2 model performance was lower in five-class (advanced gastric cancer, early gastric cancer, high-grade dysplasia, low-grade dysplasia and no neoplasm) classification, i.e., 76.4% vs. 87.6%. The Inception-Resnet-v2 model performance is comparable with endoscopist in the differentiation of gastric cancer and neoplasm (accuracy 76.0% vs. 82.0%).

4. Conclusions

The paper review indicates that deep learning methods have achieved state-of-the-art breast cancer, cervical cancer, brain tumor. colon cancer and lung cancer detection, feature extraction, classification and segmentation. In this article, a good number of deep learning-based methods for breast cancer, cervical cancer, brain tumor and colon cancer image analysis are studied. The developed and implemented methods employed a CNN approach combined with other techniques to mitigate the existing challenge arising from a large dataset demand for such systems to learn. Problems related to noise and corrupted images have been properly addressed in some of the works as they suggest utilizing normal images and limited dataset size in modes that encompass a combination of two or more architectures to discern breast, cervical, brain and colon abnormalities.

The use of enhanced activation functions have also been recommended to improve the overall performance of deep learning-based systems in medical image analysis. Moreover, many researchers have added multiple layers in the CNN architecture to increase the performance of the system. Some researchers worked on designing unique architectures for specific task properties instead of using CNN as it is. Subsequently, most of the methods are proved to produce a successful performance in terms of specificity, sensitivity and Dice score when tested on renowned datasets and BRATS challenges. The lack of sufficient datasets can be considered a challenge for many of the deep learning-based researches. All of the reviewed papers have not used different medical images other than MRI for brain and in most cases mammograms for breast.

Author Contributions: Conceptualization, T.G.D. and S.R.K.; Methodology, T.G.D., S.R.K. and F.S.; Validation, F.S., and T.G.D.; Writing—original draft preparation, T.G.D., S.R.K. and Z.M.S.; Writing—review and editing, S.R.K., Z.M.S.and T.G.D. All authors have read and agreed to the published version of the manuscript.

References

1. Afework, Y.K.; Debelee, T.G. Detection of Bacterial Wilt on Enset Crop Using Deep Learning Approach. *Int. J. Eng. Res. Afr.* **2020**, *51*, 1–17.
2. Shen, L.; Margolies, L.R.; Rothstein, J.H.; Fluder, E.; McBride, R.; Sieh, W. Deep Learning to Improve Breast Cancer Detection on Screening Mammography. *Sci. Rep.* **2019**, *9*. [CrossRef] [PubMed]
3. Suzuki, K. Survey of Deep Learning Applications to Medical Image Analysis. *Med. Imaging Technol.* **2017**, *35*, 212–226.
4. Litjens, G.; Kooi, T.; Bejnordi, B.E.; Setio, A.A.A.; Ciompi, F.; Ghafoorian, M.; van der Laak, J.A.W.M.; van Ginneken, B.; Sánchez, C.I. A survey on deep learning in medical image analysis. *Med. Image Anal.* **2017**, *42*, 60–88. [CrossRef] [PubMed]
5. Shen, D.; Wu, G.; Suk, H.I. Deep Learning in Medical Image Analysis. *Annu. Rev. Biomed. Eng.* **2017**, *19*, 221–248. [CrossRef] [PubMed]
6. Suzuki, K. Overview of deep learning in medical imaging. *Radiol. Phys. Technol.* **2017**, *10*, 257–273. [CrossRef] [PubMed]
7. Lee, J.; Jun, S.; Cho, Y.; Lee, H.; Kim, G.B.; Seo, J.B.; Kim, N. Deep Learning in Medical Imaging: General Overview. *Korean J. Radiol.* **2017**, *18*, 570–584. [CrossRef]
8. Debelee, T.G.; Schwenker1, F.; Rahimeto, S.; Yohannes, D. Evaluation of modified adaptive k-means segmentation algorithm. *Comput. Vis. Media* **2019**. [CrossRef]

9. Kebede, S.R.; Debelee, T.G.; Schwenker, F.; Yohannes, D. Classifier Based Breast Cancer Segmentation. *J. Biomim. Biomater. Biomed. Eng.* **2020**, *47*, 1–21.
10. Rahimeto, S.; Debelee, T.; Yohannes, D.; Schwenker, F. Automatic pectoral muscle removal in mammograms. *Evol. Syst.* **2019**. [CrossRef]
11. Debelee, T.G.; Schwenker, F.; Ibenthal, A.; Yohannes, D. Survey of deep learning in breast cancer image analysis. *Evol. Syst.* **2019**. [CrossRef]
12. Debelee, T.G.; Gebreselasie, A.; Schwenker, F.; Amirian, M.; Yohannes, D. Classification of Mammograms Using Texture and CNN Based Extracted Features. *J. Biomim. Biomater. Biomed. Eng.* **2019**, *42*, 79–97. [CrossRef]
13. Debelee, T.G.; Amirian, M.; Ibenthal, A.; Palm, G.; Schwenker, F. Classification of Mammograms Using Convolutional Neural Network Based Feature Extraction. *LNICST* **2018**, *244*, 89–98.
14. Suckling, J.; Parker, J.; Dance, D.; Astley, S.; Hutt, I.; Boggis, C.; Ricketts, I. *Mammographic Image Analysis Society (MIAS) Database v1.21 [Dataset]*; Dataset; Digital Mammogram Database Exerpta Medica: Dordrecht, The Netherland, 2015.
15. Scuccimarra, E.A. *DDSM Mammography [Dataset]*; Dataset; Digital Mammogram Database Exerpta Medica: Dordrecht, The Netherland, 2018.
16. Moreira, I.C.; Amaral, I.; Domingues, I.; Cardoso, A.; Cardoso, M.J.; Cardoso, J.S. INbreast. *Acad. Radiol.* **2012**, *19*, 236–248. [CrossRef]
17. Dua, D.; Graff, C. *UCI Machine Learning Repository*; University of California, Irvine, School of Information and Computer Sciences: Newport Beach, CA, USA, 2017.
18. Bukun. *Breast Cancer Histopathological Database (BreakHis)*; Dataset; P and D Laboratory—Pathological Anatomy and Cytopathology: Parana, Brazil, 2019.
19. Aresta, G.; Araújo, T.; Kwok, S.; Chennamsetty, S.S.; Safwan, M.; Alex, V.; Marami, B.; Prastawa, M.; Chan, M.; Donovan, M.; et al. BACH: Grand challenge on breast cancer histology images. *Med. Image Anal.* **2019**, *56*, 122–139. [CrossRef]
20. Wu, N.; Phang, J.; Park, J.; Shen, Y.; Huang, Z.; Zorin, M.; Jastrzebski, S.; Fevry, T.; Katsnelson, J.; Kim, E.; et al. Deep Neural Networks Improve Radiologists' Performance in Breast Cancer Screening. *IEEE Trans. Med. Imaging* **2020**, *39*, 1184–1194. [CrossRef]
21. Alzubaidi, L.; Al-Shamma, O.; Fadhel, M.A.; Farhan, L.; Zhang, J.; Duan, Y. Optimizing the Performance of Breast Cancer Classification by Employing the Same Domain Transfer Learning from Hybrid Deep Convolutional Neural Network Model. *Electronics* **2020**, *9*, 445. [CrossRef]
22. Zhu, Z.; Harowicz, M.; Zhang, J.; Saha, A.; Grimm, L.J.; Hwang, E.S.; Mazurowski, M.A. Deep learning analysis of breast MRIs for prediction of occult invasive disease in ductal carcinoma in situ. *Comput. Biol. Med.* **2019**, *115*, 103498. [CrossRef]
23. Li, X.; Qin, G.; He, Q.; Sun, L.; Zeng, H.; He, Z.; Chen, W.; Zhen, X.; Zhou, L. Digital breast tomosynthesis versus digital mammography: Integration of image modalities enhances deep learning-based breast mass classification. *Eur. Radiol.* **2019**, *30*, 778–788. [CrossRef]
24. Zeiser, F.A.; da Costa, C.A.; Zonta, T.; Marques, N.M.C.; Roehe, A.V.; Moreno, M.; da Rosa Righi, R. Segmentation of Masses on Mammograms Using Data Augmentation and Deep Learning. *J. Digit. Imaging* **2020**. [CrossRef]
25. Zhang, Y.; Chen, J.H.; Chang, K.T.; Park, V.Y.; Kim, M.J.; Chan, S.; Chang, P.; Chow, D.; Luk, A.; Kwong, T.; et al. Automatic Breast and Fibroglandular Tissue Segmentation in Breast MRI Using Deep Learning by a Fully-Convolutional Residual Neural Network U-Net. *Acad. Radiol.* **2019**, *26*, 1526–1535. [CrossRef]
26. Zhou, J.; Luo, L.Y.; Dou, Q.; Chen, H.; Chen, C.; Li, G.J.; Jiang, Z.F.; Heng, P.A. Weakly supervised 3D deep learning for breast cancer classification and localization of the lesions in MR images. *J. Magn. Reson. Imaging* **2019**, *50*, 1144–1151. [CrossRef]
27. Huang, G.; Liu, Z.; Maaten, L.V.D.; Weinberger, K.Q. Densely Connected Convolutional Networks. In Proceedings of the 2017 IEEE Conference on Computer Vision and Pattern Recognition (CVPR), Honolulu, HI, USA, 21–26 July 2017. [CrossRef]
28. Zhang, J.; Saha, A.; Soher, B.J.; Mazurowski, M.A. Automatic deep learning-based normalization of breast dynamic contrast-enhanced magnetic resonance images. *arXiv* **2018**, arXiv:1807.02152v1.

29. Sheikh, T.S.; Lee, Y.; Cho, M. Histopathological Classification of Breast Cancer Images Using a Multi-Scale Input and Multi-Feature Network. *Cancers* **2020**, *12*, 2031. [CrossRef] [PubMed]
30. Li, X.; Shen, X.; Zhou, Y.; Wang, X.; Li, T.Q. Classification of breast cancer histopathological images using interleaved DenseNet with SENet (IDSNet). *PLoS ONE* **2020**, *15*, e0232127. [CrossRef]
31. Yan, R.; Ren, F.; Wang, Z.; Wang, L.; Zhang, T.; Liu, Y.; Rao, X.; Zheng, C.; Zhang, F. Breast cancer histopathological image classification using a hybrid deep neural network. *Methods* **2020**, *173*, 52–60. [CrossRef]
32. Sharma, S.; Mehra, R. Conventional Machine Learning and Deep Learning Approach for Multi-Classification of Breast Cancer Histopathology Images—a Comparative Insight. *J. Digit. Imaging* **2020**, *33*, 632–654. [CrossRef]
33. Vang, Y.S.; Chen, Z.; Xie, X. Deep Learning Framework for Multi-class Breast Cancer Histology Image Classification. In *Lecture Notes in Computer Science*; Springer International Publishing: Berlin/Heidelberg, Germany, 2018; pp. 914–922. [CrossRef]
34. Dembrower, K.; Liu, Y.; Azizpour, H.; Eklund, M.; Smith, K.; Lindholm, P.; Strand, F. Comparison of a Deep Learning Risk Score and Standard Mammographic Density Score for Breast Cancer Risk Prediction. *Radiology* **2020**, *294*, 265–272. [CrossRef]
35. Hagos, Y.B.; Merida, A.G.; Teuwen, J. Improving Breast Cancer Detection using Symmetry Information with Deep Learning. *arXiv* **2018**, arXiv:1808.08273v1.
36. Ferlay, J.; Shin, H.R.; Bray, F.; Forman, D.; Mathers, C.; Parkin, D.M. Estimates of worldwide burden of cancer in 2008: GLOBOCAN 2008. *Int. J. Cancer* **2010**, *127*, 2893–2917. [CrossRef]
37. Wingo, P.A.; Cardinez, C.J.; Landis, S.H.; Greenlee, R.T.; Ries, L.A.G.; Anderson, R.N.; Thun, M.J. Long-term trends in cancer mortality in the United States, 1930–1998. *Cancer* **2003**, *97*, 3133–3275. [CrossRef] [PubMed]
38. Schiffman, M.; Doorbar, J.; Wentzensen, N.; De Sanjosé, S.; Fakhry, C.; Monk, B.J.; Stanley, M.A.; Franceschi, S. Carcinogenic human papillomavirus infection. *Nat. Rev. Dis. Prim.* **2016**, *2*, 1–20. [CrossRef]
39. Patten, J. (Ed.) *Comprehensive Cervical Cancer Control: A Guide to Essential Practice*; World Health Organization: Geneva, Switzerland, 2014.
40. GençTav, A.; Aksoy, S.; ÖNder, S. Unsupervised segmentation andclassification of cervical cell images. *Pattern Recognit.* **2012**, *45*, 4151–4168. [CrossRef]
41. Tang, G.Y.; Parekh, J. Methods of Screening for Cervical Cancer. *JAMA* **2018**, *320*, 1938. [CrossRef]
42. Liang, Y.; Tang, Z.; Yan, M.; Chen, J.; Liu, Q.; Xiang, Y. Comparison-Based Convolutional Neural Networks for Cervical Cell/ClumpsDetection in the Limited Data Scenario. *arXiv* **2019**, arXiv:1810.05952.
43. Jantzen, J.; Norup, J.; Dounias, G.; Bjerregaard, B. Pap-smear benchmark data for pattern classification. In Proceedings of the Nature Inspired Smart Information Systems (NiSIS 2005), Albufeira, Portugal, 3–5 October 2005.
44. Hussain, E. Liquid based cytology pap smear images for multi-class diagnosis of cervical cancer. *Data Brief* **2019**. [CrossRef]
45. Rezende, M.T.; Tobias, A.H.G.; Silva, R.; Oliveira, P.; Medeiros, F.S.D.; Ushizima, D.; Carneiro, C.M.; Bianchi, A.G.C. CRIC Cervix Cell Classification. 2020. Available online: https://figshare.com/collections/CRIC_Cervix_Cell_Classification/4960286 (accessed on 11 August 2020). [CrossRef]
46. Franco, R.A.S.; Carvalho, M.A.G.; Coelho, G.P.; Martins, P.; Enciso, J.L. Dataset of Cervical Cell Images for the Study of Changes Associated with Malignancy in Conventional Pap Test. *ZENODO* **2018**. [CrossRef]
47. Group, A. Human Papillomavirus Testing for Triage of Women With Cytologic Evidence of Low-Grade Squamous Intraepithelial Lesions: Baseline Data From a Randomized Trial. *J. Natl. Cancer Inst.* **2000**, *92*, 397–402. [CrossRef] [PubMed]
48. MobileODT. Intel & Mobile ODT Cervical Cancer Screening. 2017. Available online: https://www.kaggle.com/c/intel-mobileodt-cervical-cancer-screening (accessed on 14 August 2020).
49. Song, Y.; Cheng, J.Z.; Ni, D.; Chen, S.; Lei, B.; Wang, T. Segmenting overlapping cervical cell in Pap smear images. In Proceedings of the 2016 IEEE 13th International Symposium on Biomedical Imaging (ISBI), Prague, Czech Republic, 13–16 April 2016. [CrossRef]
50. Zhao, J.; Dai, L.; Zhang, M.; Yu, F.; Li, M.; Li, H.; Wang, W.; Zhang, L. PGU-net+: Progressive Growing of U-net+ for Automated Cervical Nuclei Segmentation. In *Multiscale Multimodal Medical Imaging*; Springer International Publishing: Berlin/Heidelberg, Germany, 2019; pp. 51–58. [CrossRef]

51. Ronneberger, O.; Fischer, P.; Brox, T. U-Net: Convolutional Networks for Biomedical Image Segmentation. In *Lecture Notes in Computer Science*; Springer International Publishing: Berlin/Heidelberg, Germany, 2015; pp. 234–241. [CrossRef]
52. Sompawong, N.; Mopan, J.; Pooprasert, P.; Himakhun, W.; Suwannarurk, K.; Ngamvirojcharoen, J.; Vachiramon, T.; Tantibundhit, C. Automated Pap Smear Cervical Cancer Screening Using Deep Learning. In Proceedings of the 2019 41st Annual International Conference of the IEEE Engineering in Medicine and Biology Society (EMBC), Berlin, Germany, 23–27 July 2019. [CrossRef]
53. Liu, Y.; Zhang, P.; Song, Q.; Li, A.; Zhang, P.; Gui, Z. Automatic Segmentation of Cervical Nuclei Based on Deep Learning and a Conditional Random Field. *IEEE Access* **2018**, *6*, 53709–53721. [CrossRef]
54. Kurnianingsih, A.K.H.S.; Nugroho, L.E.; Widyawan; Lazuardi, L.; Prabuwono, A.S.; Mantoro, T. Segmentation and Classification of Cervical Cells Using Deep Learning. *IEEE Access* **2019**, *7*, 116925–116941. [CrossRef]
55. Zhang, L.; Lu, L.; Nogues, I.; Summers, R.M.; Liu, S.; Yao, J. DeepPap: Deep Convolutional Networks for Cervical Cell Classification. *IEEE J. Biomed. Health Inform.* **2017**, *21*, 1633–1643. [CrossRef]
56. Hyeon, J.; Choi, H.J.; Lee, K.N.; Lee, B.D. Automating Papanicolaou Test Using Deep Convolutional Activation Feature. In Proceedings of the 2017 18th IEEE International Conference on Mobile Data Management (MDM), Daejeon, Korea, 29 May–1 June 2017. [CrossRef]
57. Lin, H.; Hu, Y.; Chen, S.; Yao, J.; Zhang, L. Fine-Grained Classification of Cervical Cells Using Morphological and Appearance Based Convolutional Neural Networks. *IEEE Access* **2019**, *7*, 71541–71549. [CrossRef]
58. Deng, J.; Dong, W.; Socher, R.; Li, L.J.; Li, K.; Fei-Fei, L. Imagenet: A large-scale hierarchical image database. In Proceedings of the 2009 IEEE Conference on Computer Vision and Pattern Recognition, Miami, FL, USA, 20–25 June 2009; pp. 248–255.
59. Nayar, R.; Wilbur, D.C. The Pap test and Bethesda 2014. *Cancer Cytopathol.* **2015**, *123*, 271–281. [CrossRef]
60. Chen, T.; Ma, X.; Ying, X.; Wang, W.; Yuan, C.; Lu, W.; Chen, D.Z.; Wu, J. Multi-Modal Fusion Learning For Cervical Dysplasia Diagnosis. In Proceedings of the 2019 IEEE 16th International Symposium on Biomedical Imaging (ISBI 2019), Venice, Italy, 8–11 April 2019. [CrossRef]
61. Promworn, Y.; Pattanasak, S.; Pintavirooj, C.; Piyawattanametha, W. Comparisons of PAP-Smear Classification with Deep Learning Models. In Proceedings of the 14th annual IEEE International Conference on Nano/Micro Engineering and Molecular Systems, Bangkok, Thailand, 11–14 April 2019.
62. Ma, Y.; Xu, T.; Huang, X.; Wang, X.; Li, C.; Jerwick, J.; Ning, Y.; Zeng, X.; Wang, B.; Wang, Y.; et al. Computer-Aided Diagnosis of Label-Free 3-D Optical Coherence Microscopy Images of Human Cervical Tissue. *IEEE Trans. Biomed. Eng.* **2019**, *66*, 2447–2456. [CrossRef] [PubMed]
63. Ghoneim, A.; Muhammad, G.; Hossain, M.S. Cervical cancer classification using convolutional neural networks and extreme learning machines. *Future Gener. Comput. Syst.* **2020**, *102*, 643–649. [CrossRef]
64. Dong, N.; Zhao, L.; Wu, C.; Chang, J. Inception v3 based cervical cell classification combined with artificially extracted features. *Appl. Soft Comput.* **2020**, *93*, 106311. [CrossRef]
65. Martínez-Más, J.; Bueno-Crespo, A.; Martínez-España, R.; Remezal-Solano, M.; Ortiz-González, A.; Ortiz-Reina, S.; Martínez-Cendán, J.P. Classifying Papanicolaou cervical smears through a cell merger approach by deep learning technique. *Expert Syst. Appl.* **2020**, *160*, 113707. [CrossRef]
66. Xiang, Y.; Sun, W.; Pan, C.; Yan, M.; Yin, Z.; Liang, Y. A novel automation-assisted cervical cancer reading method based on convolutional neural network. *Biocybern. Biomed. Eng.* **2020**, *40*, 611–623. [CrossRef]
67. Garcia-Arteaga, J.; Kybic, J.; Li, W. Automatic colposcopyvideo tissue classification using higher order entropy-basedimage registration. *Comput. Biol. Med.* **2011**, *41*, 960–970. [CrossRef]
68. Wimpy, B.; Suyanto, S. Classification of Cervical and Type Image and Using and Capsule Networks. In Proceedings of the 2019 International Seminar on Research of Information Technology and Intelligent Systems (ISRITI), Yogyakarta, Indonesia, 5–6 December 2019.
69. Gorantla, R.; Singh, R.K.; Pandey, R.; Jain, M. Cervical Cancer Diagnosis using CervixNet—A Deep Learning Approach. In Proceedings of the 2019 IEEE 19th International Conference on Bioinformatics and Bioengineering (BIBE), Athens, Greece, 28–30 October 2019. [CrossRef]
70. Arora, M.; Dhawan, S.; Singh, K. Deep Neural Network for Transformation Zone Classification. In Proceedings of the 2018 First International Conference on Secure Cyber Computing and Communication (ICSCCC), Jalandhar, India, 15–17 December 2018.

71. Tang, J. *Intelligent Mobile Projects with TensorFlow: Build 10+ Artificial Intelligence Apps Using TensorFlow Mobile and Lite for iOS, Android, and Raspberry Pi*; Packt Publishing: Birmingham, UK, 2018.
72. Guo, P.; Xue, Z.; Long, L.R.; Antani, S. Cross-Dataset Evaluation of Deep Learning Networks for Uterine Cervix Segmentation. *Diagnostics* **2020**, *10*, 44. [CrossRef]
73. Guo, P.; Singh, S.; Xue, Z.; Long, R.; Antani, S. Deep Learning for Assessing Image Focus for Automated Cervical Cancer Screening. In Proceedings of the 2019 IEEE EMBS International Conference on Biomedical & Health Informatics (BHI), Chicago, IL, USA, 19–22 May 2019. [CrossRef]
74. Guo, P.; Xue, Z.; Mtema, Z.; Yeates, K.; Ginsburg, O.; Demarco, M.; Long, L.R.; Schiffman, M.; Antani, S. Ensemble Deep Learning for Cervix Image Selection toward Improving Reliability in Automated Cervical Precancer Screening. *Diagnostics* **2020**, *10*, 451. [CrossRef]
75. Sharma, M.; Mukharjee, S. Brain Tumor Segmentation Using Genetic Algorithm and Artificial Neural Network Fuzzy Inference System (ANFIS). In *Advances in Computing and Information Technology*; Springer: Berlin/Heidelberg, Germany, 2013; pp. 329–339. [CrossRef]
76. Hanif, F.; Muzaffar, K.; Perveen, K.; Malhi, S.M.; Simjee, S.U. Glioblastoma Multiforme: A Review of its Epidemiology and Pathogenesis through Clinical Presentation and Treatment. *Asian Pac. J. Cancer Prev. APJCP* **2017**, *18*, 3–9. [CrossRef]
77. Rees, J.H. Diagnosis and treatment in neuro-oncology: An oncological perspective. *Br. J. Radiol.* **2011**, *84*, S82–S89. [CrossRef]
78. Rasmussen, B.K.; Hansen, S.; Laursen, R.J.; Kosteljanetz, M.; Schultz, H.; Nørgård, B.M.; Guldberg, R.; Gradel, K.O. Epidemiology of glioma: Clinical characteristics, symptoms, and predictors of glioma patients grade I–IV in the the Danish Neuro-Oncology Registry. *J. Neuro Oncol.* **2017**, *135*, 571–579. [CrossRef]
79. Kalpathy-Cramer, J.; Gerstner, E.R.; Emblem, K.E.; Andronesi, O.; Rosen, B. Advanced magnetic resonance imaging of the physical processes in human glioblastoma. *Cancer Res.* **2014**, *74*, 4622–4637. [CrossRef] [PubMed]
80. Mohsen, H.; El-Dahshan, E.S.A.; El-Horbaty, E.S.M.; Salem, A.B.M. Classification using deep learning neural networks for brain tumors. *Future Comput. Inform. J.* **2018**, *3*, 68–71. [CrossRef]
81. Bahadure, N.B.; Ray, A.K.; Thethi, H.P. Image Analysis for MRI Based Brain Tumor Detection and Feature Extraction Using Biologically Inspired BWT and SVM. *Int. J. Biomed. Imaging* **2017**, *2017*, 1–12. [CrossRef] [PubMed]
82. Srinivas, B.; Rao, G.S. Segmentation of Multi-Modal MRI Brain Tumor Sub-Regions Using Deep Learning. *J. Electr. Eng. Technol.* **2020**, *15*, 1899–1909. [CrossRef]
83. Nadeem, M.W.; Ghamdi, M.A.A.; Hussain, M.; Khan, M.A.; Khan, K.M.; Almotiri, S.H.; Butt, S.A. Brain Tumor Analysis Empowered with Deep Learning: A Review, Taxonomy, and Future Challenges. *Brain Sci.* **2020**, *10*, 118. [CrossRef] [PubMed]
84. Akkus, Z.; Galimzianova, A.; Hoogi, A.; Rubin, D.L.; Erickson, B.J. Deep Learning for Brain MRI Segmentation: State of the Art and Future Directions. *J. Digit. Imaging* **2017**, *30*, 449–459. [CrossRef]
85. Shattuck, D.W.; Prasad, G.; Mirza, M.; Narr, K.L.; Toga, A.W. Online resource for validation of brain segmentation methods. *NeuroImage* **2009**, *45*, 431–439. [CrossRef] [PubMed]
86. Menze, B.H.; Jakab, A.; Bauer, S.; Kalpathy-Cramer, J.; Farahani, K.; Kirby, J.; Burren, Y.; Porz, N.; Slotboom, J.; Wiest, R.; et al. The Multimodal Brain Tumor Image Segmentation Benchmark (BRATS). *IEEE Trans. Med. Imaging* **2015**, *34*, 1993–2024. [CrossRef]
87. Barboriak, D. Data From RIDER_NEURO_MRI. 2015. Available online: https://wiki.cancerimagingarchive.net/display/Public/RIDER+NEURO+MRI (accessed on 15 August 2020). [CrossRef]
88. Fabelo, H.; Ortega, S.; Szolna, A.; Bulters, D.; Pineiro, J.F.; Kabwama, S.; J-O'Shanahan, A.; Bulstrode, H.; Bisshopp, S.; Kiran, B.R.; et al. In-Vivo Hyperspectral Human Brain Image Database for Brain Cancer Detection. *IEEE Access* **2019**, *7*, 39098–39116. [CrossRef]
89. Cheng, J.; Huang, W.; Cao, S.; Yang, R.; Yang, W.; Yun, Z.; Wang, Z.; Feng, Q. Enhanced Performance of Brain Tumor Classification via Tumor Region Augmentation and Partition. *PLoS ONE* **2015**, *10*, e0140381. [CrossRef]
90. Cheng, J. Brain Tumor Dataset. 2017. Available online: https://doi.org/10.6084/m9.figshare.1512427.v5 (accessed on 26 October 2020).

91. Alkassar, S.; Abdullah, M.A.M.; Jebur, B.A. Automatic Brain Tumour Segmentation using fully Convolution Network and Transfer Learning. In Proceedings of the 2019 2nd International Conference on Electrical, Communication, Computer, Power and Control Engineering (ICECCPCE), Mosul, Iraq, 13–14 February 2019. [CrossRef]
92. Amiri, S.; Rekik, I.; Mahjoub, M.A. Deep random forest-based learning transfer to SVM for brain tumor segmentation. In Proceedings of the 2016 2nd International Conference on Advanced Technologies for Signal and Image Processing (ATSIP), Monastir, Tunisia, 21–23 March 2016. [CrossRef]
93. Chahal, E.S.; Haritosh, A.; Gupta, A.; Gupta, K.; Sinha, A. Deep Learning Model for Brain Tumor Segmentation & Analysis. In Proceedings of the 2019 3rd International Conference on Recent Developments in Control, Automation & Power Engineering (RDCAPE), Noida, India, 10–11 October 2019. [CrossRef]
94. Ding, Y.; Li, C.; Yang, Q.; Qin, Z.; Qin, Z. How to Improve the Deep Residual Network to Segment Multi-Modal Brain Tumor Images. *IEEE Access* **2019**, *7*, 152821–152831. [CrossRef]
95. Mallick, P.K.; Ryu, S.H.; Satapathy, S.K.; Mishra, S.; Nguyen, G.N.; Tiwari, P. Brain MRI Image Classification for Cancer Detection Using Deep Wavelet Autoencoder-Based Deep Neural Network. *IEEE Access* **2019**, *7*, 46278–46287. [CrossRef]
96. Ramirez, I.; Martin, A.; Schiavi, E. Optimization of a variational model using deep learning: An application to brain tumor segmentation. In Proceedings of the 2018 IEEE 15th International Symposium on Biomedical Imaging (ISBI 2018), Washington, DC, USA, 4–7 April 2018. [CrossRef]
97. Sajid, S.; Hussain, S.; Sarwar, A. Brain Tumor Detection and Segmentation in MR Images Using Deep Learning. *Arab. J. Sci. Eng.* **2019**, *44*, 9249–9261. [CrossRef]
98. Wang, Y.; Li, C.; Zhu, T.; Yu, C. A Deep Learning Algorithm for Fully Automatic Brain Tumor Segmentation. In Proceedings of the 2019 International Joint Conference on Neural Networks (IJCNN), Budapest, Hungary, 14–19 July 2019. [CrossRef]
99. Zhao, X.; Wu, Y.; Song, G.; Li, Z.; Zhang, Y.; Fan, Y. A deep learning model integrating FCNNs and CRFs for brain tumor segmentation. *Med. Image Anal.* **2018**, *43*, 98–111. [CrossRef] [PubMed]
100. Kuzina, A.; Egorov, E.; Burnaev, E. Bayesian Generative Models for Knowledge Transfer in MRI Semantic Segmentation Problems. *Front. Neurosci.* **2019**, *13*. [CrossRef] [PubMed]
101. Zeineldin, R.A.; Karar, M.E.; Coburger, J.; Wirtz, C.R.; Burgert, O. DeepSeg: Deep neural network framework for automatic brain tumor segmentation using magnetic resonance FLAIR images. *Int. J. Comput. Assist. Radiol. Surg.* **2020**, *15*, 909–920. [CrossRef]
102. Fabelo, H.; Halicek, M.; Ortega, S.; Shahedi, M.; Szolna, A.; Piñeiro, J.; Sosa, C.; O'Shanahan, A.; Bisshopp, S.; Espino, C.; et al. Deep Learning-Based Framework for In Vivo Identification of Glioblastoma Tumor using Hyperspectral Images of Human Brain. *Sensors* **2019**, *19*, 920. [CrossRef]
103. Shree, N.V.; Kumar, T.N.R. Identification and classification of brain tumor MRI images with feature extraction using DWT and probabilistic neural network. *Brain Inform.* **2018**, *5*, 23–30. [CrossRef]
104. Tandel, G.S.; Biswas, M.; Kakde, O.G.; Tiwari, A.; Suri, H.S.; Turk, M.; Laird, J.; Asare, C.; Ankrah, A.A.; Khanna, N.N.; et al. A Review on a Deep Learning Perspective in Brain Cancer Classification. *Cancers* **2019**, *11*, 111. [CrossRef] [PubMed]
105. Alqudah, A.M. Brain Tumor Classification Using Deep Learning Technique—A Comparison between Cropped, Uncropped, and Segmented Lesion Images with Different Sizes. *Int. J. Adv. Trends Comput. Sci. Eng.* **2019**, *8*, 3684–3691. [CrossRef]
106. Ucuzal, H.; Yasar, S.; Colak, C. Classification of brain tumor types by deep learning with convolutional neural network on magnetic resonance images using a developed web-based interface. In Proceedings of the 2019 3rd International Symposium on Multidisciplinary Studies and Innovative Technologies (ISMSIT), Ankara Turkey, 11–13 October 2019. [CrossRef]
107. Bazin, P. Example MP2RAGEME Data Set. 2019. Available online: https://uvaauas.figshare.com/articles/Example_MP2RAGEME_data_set/7938326 (accessed on 15 August 2020). [CrossRef]
108. Tetik, B.; Ucuzal, H.; Yasar, S.; Colak, C. Brain Tumor Classification Software[Web-Based Software]. Available online: http://biostatapps.inonu.edu.tr/BTSY (accessed on 17 August 2020)
109. Selvy, P.T.; Dharani, V.P.; Indhuja, A. Brain Tumour Detection Using Deep Learning Techniques. *Int. J. Sci. Res. Comput. Sci. Eng. Inf. Technol.* **2019**, 169–175. [CrossRef]
110. Sultan, H.H.; Salem, N.M.; Al-Atabany, W. Multi-Classification of Brain Tumor Images Using Deep Neural Network. *IEEE Access* **2019**, *7*, 69215–69225. [CrossRef]

111. Badža, M.M.; Barjaktarović, M.Č. Classification of Brain Tumors from MRI Images Using a Convolutional Neural Network. *Appl. Sci.* **2020**, *10*, 1999. [CrossRef]
112. WHO. Global Cancer Observatory (GCO). 2018. Available online: https://gco.iarc.fr/ (accessed on 1 July 2020).
113. Graham, S.; Chen, H.; Gamper, J.; Dou, Q.; Heng, P.A.; Snead, D.; Tsang, Y.W.; Rajpoot, N. MILD-Net: Minimal Information Loss Dilated Network for Gland Instance Segmentation in Colon Histology Images. *Med. Image Anal.* **2018**. [CrossRef]
114. Benson, V.S.; Patnick, J.; Davies, A.K.; Nadel, M.R.; Smith, R.A.; Atkin, W.S. Colorectal cancer screening: A comparison of 35 initiatives in 17 countries. *Int. J. Cancer* **2007**, *122*, 1357–1367. [CrossRef] [PubMed]
115. Rony, J.; Belharbi, S.; Dolz, J.; Ayed, I.B.; McCaffrey, L.; Granger, E. Deep weakly-supervised learning methods for classification and localization in histology images: A survey. *arXiv* **2019**, arXiv:1909.03354v3.
116. Vázquez, D.; Bernal, J.; Sánchez, F.J.; Fernández-Esparrach, G.; López, A.M.; Romero, A.; Drozdzal, M.; Courville, A. A Benchmark for Endoluminal Scene Segmentation of Colonoscopy Images. *J. Healthc. Eng.* **2017**, *2017*, 1–9. [CrossRef] [PubMed]
117. Bernal, J.; Sánchez, J.; Vilariño, F. Towards automatic polyp detection with a polyp appearance model. *Pattern Recognit.* **2012**, *45*, 3166–3182. [CrossRef]
118. Bernal, J.; Sánchez, F.J.; Fernández-Esparrach, G.; Gil, D.; Rodríguez, C.; Vilariño, F. WM-DOVA maps for accurate polyp highlighting in colonoscopy: Validation vs. saliency maps from physicians. *Comput. Med. Imaging Graph.* **2015**, *43*, 99–111. [CrossRef]
119. Kather, J.N.; Weis, C.A.; Bianconi, F.; Melchers, S.M.; Schad, L.R.; Gaiser, T.; Marx, A.; Zöllner, F.G. Multi-class texture analysis in colorectal cancer histology. *Sci. Rep.* **2016**, *6*. [CrossRef]
120. Kainz, P.; Pfeiffer, M.; Urschler, M. Segmentation and classification of colon glands with deep convolutional neural networks and total variation regularization. *PeerJ* **2017**, *5*, e3874. [CrossRef]
121. Sirinukunwattana, K.; Ahmed Raza, S.E.; Tsang, Y.W.; Snead, D.R.J.; Cree, I.A.; Rajpoot, N.M. Locality Sensitive Deep Learning for Detection and Classification of Nuclei in Routine Colon Cancer Histology Images. *IEEE Trans. Med. Imaging* **2016**, *35*, 1196–1206. [CrossRef]
122. Chamanzar, A.; Nie, Y. Weakly Supervised Multi-Task Learning for Cell Detection and Segmentation. In Proceedings of the 2020 IEEE 17th International Symposium on Biomedical Imaging (ISBI), Iowa City, IA, USA, 4 April 2020. [CrossRef]
123. Sari, C.T.; Gunduz-Demir, C. Unsupervised Feature Extraction via Deep Learning for Histopathological Classification of Colon Tissue Images. *IEEE Trans. Med. Imaging* **2019**, *38*, 1139–1149. [CrossRef] [PubMed]
124. Ozdemir, E.; Gunduz-Demir, C. A Hybrid Classification Model for Digital Pathology Using Structural and Statistical Pattern Recognition. *IEEE Trans. Med. Imaging* **2013**, *32*, 474–483. [CrossRef]
125. Shapcott, M.; Hewitt, K.J.; Rajpoot, N. Deep Learning With Sampling in Colon Cancer Histology. *Front. Bioeng. Biotechnol.* **2019**, *7*, 52. [CrossRef]
126. Tang, J.; Li, J.; Xu, X. Segnet-based gland segmentation from colon cancer histology images. In Proceedings of the 2018 33rd Youth Academic Annual Conference of Chinese Association of Automation (YAC), Nanjing, China, 18 May 2018. [CrossRef]
127. Vuong, T.L.T.; Lee, D.; Kwak, J.T.; Kim, K. Multi-task Deep Learning for Colon Cancer Grading. In Proceedings of the 2020 International Conference on Electronics, Information, and Communication (ICEIC), Fukuoka, Kapan, 5–7 September 2020. [CrossRef]
128. Sabol, P.; Sinčák, P.; Hartono, P.; Kočan, P.; Benetinová, Z.; Blichárová, A.; Verbóová, L'.; Štammová, E.; Sabolová-Fabianová, A.; Jašková, A. Explainable classifier for improving the accountability in decision-making for colorectal cancer diagnosis from histopathological images. *J. Biomed. Inform.* **2020**, *109*, 103523. [CrossRef]
129. Suzuki, K.; Yoshida, H.; Näppi, J.; Dachman, A.H. Massive-training artificial neural network (MTANN) for reduction of false positives in computer-aided detection of polyps: Suppression of rectal tubes. *Med. Phys.* **2006**, *33*, 3814–3824. [CrossRef] [PubMed]
130. Bardhi, O.; Sierra-Sosa, D.; Garcia-Zapirain, B.; Elmaghraby, A. Automatic colon polyp detection using Convolutional encoder-decoder model. In Proceedings of the 2017 IEEE International Symposium on Signal Processing and Information Technology (ISSPIT), Bilbao, Spain, 18–20 December 2017. [CrossRef]

131. Bour, A.; Castillo-Olea, C.; Garcia-Zapirain, B.; Zahia, S. Automatic colon polyp classification using Convolutional Neural Network: A Case Study at Basque Country. In Proceedings of the 2019 IEEE International Symposium on Signal Processing and Information Technology (ISSPIT), Ajman, UAE, 10–12 December 2019. [CrossRef]
132. Liu, X.; Li, Y.; Yao, J.; Chen, B.; Song, J.; Yang, X. Classification of Polyps and Adenomas Using Deep Learning Model in Screening Colonoscopy. In Proceedings of the 2019 8th International Symposium on Next Generation Electronics (ISNE), Zhengzhou, China, 9–10 October 2019. [CrossRef]
133. Ozawa, T.; Ishihara, S.; Fujishiro, M.; Kumagai, Y.; Shichijo, S.; Tada, T. Automated endoscopic detection and classification of colorectal polyps using convolutional neural networks. *Ther. Adv. Gastroenterol.* **2020**, *13*, 1756284820910659. [CrossRef]
134. Nadimi, E.S.; Buijs, M.M.; Herp, J.; Kroijer, R.; Kobaek-Larsen, M.; Nielsen, E.; Pedersen, C.D.; Blanes-Vidal, V.; Baatrup, G. Application of deep learning for autonomous detection and localization of colorectal polyps in wireless colon capsule endoscopy. *Comput. Electr. Eng.* **2020**, *81*, 106531. [CrossRef]
135. Zeiler, M.D.; Fergus, R. Visualizing and Understanding Convolutional Networks. In *Computer Vision—ECCV 2014*; Springer International Publishing: Berlin/Heidelberg, Germany, 2014; pp. 818–833. [CrossRef]
136. Lung Cancer Screening (PDQ®): Patient Version. 2020. Available online: https://www.cancer.gov/types/lung/hp/lung-screening-pdq (accessed on 11 October 2020).
137. Hong, Z.Q.; Yang, J.Y. Optimal discriminant plane for a small number of samples and design method of classifier on the plane. *Pattern Recognit.* **1991**, *24*, 317–324. [CrossRef]
138. Armato, S.G., III; Hadjiiski, L.; Tourassi, G.D.; Drukker, K.; Giger, M.L.; Li, F.; Redmond, G.; Farahani, K.; Kirby, J.S.; Clarke, L.P. SPIE-AAPM-NCI Lung Nodule Classification Challenge Dataset. *Cancer Imaging Arch.* **2015**. [CrossRef]
139. Mader, S. Lung Nodule Malignancy. Data available at Kaggle. 2017. Available online: https://www.kaggle.com/kmader/lungnodemalignancy (accessed on 14 August 2020).
140. Suzuki, K.; Armato, S.G.; Li, F.; Sone, S.; Doi, K. Massive training artificial neural network (MTANN) for reduction of false positives in computerized detection of lung nodules in low-dose computed tomography. *Med. Phys.* **2003**, *30*, 1602–1617. [CrossRef]
141. Suzuki, K.; Li, F.; Sone, S.; Doi, K. Computer-aided diagnostic scheme for distinction between benign and malignant nodules in thoracic low-dose CT by use of massive training artificial neural network. *IEEE Trans. Med. Imaging* **2005**, *24*, 1138–1150. [CrossRef]
142. Tajbakhsh, N.; Suzuki, K. Comparing two classes of end-to-end machine-learning models in lung nodule detection and classification: MTANNs vs. CNNs. *Pattern Recognit.* **2017**, *63*, 476–486. [CrossRef]
143. Gu, Y.; Lu, X.; Yang, L.; Zhang, B.; Yu, D.; Zhao, Y.; Gao, L.; Wu, L.; Zhou, T. Automatic lung nodule detection using a 3D deep convolutional neural network combined with a multi-scale prediction strategy in chest CTs. *Comput. Biol. Med.* **2018**, *103*, 220–231. [CrossRef]
144. Sahu, P.; Yu, D.; Dasari, M.; Hou, F.; Qin, H. A Lightweight Multi-Section CNN for Lung Nodule Classification and Malignancy Estimation. *IEEE J. Biomed. Health Inform.* **2019**, *23*, 960–968. [CrossRef] [PubMed]
145. Ozdemir, O.; Russell, R.L.; Berlin, A.A. A 3D Probabilistic Deep Learning System for Detection and Diagnosis of Lung Cancer Using Low-Dose CT Scans. *IEEE Trans. Med. Imaging* **2020**, *39*, 1419–1429. [CrossRef] [PubMed]
146. Hamilton, B.A. Data Science Bowl 2017. Data Available at Kaggle. 2017. Available online: https://www.kaggle.com/c/data-science-bowl-2017 (accessed on 1 August 2020).
147. Bansal, G.; Chamola, V.; Narang, P.; Kumar, S.; Raman, S. Deep3DSCan: Deep residual network and morphological descriptor based framework for lung cancer classification and 3D segmentation. *IET Image Process.* **2020**, *14*, 1240–1247. [CrossRef]
148. Adegun, A.A.; Viriri, S. Deep Learning-Based System for Automatic Melanoma Detection. *IEEE Access* **2020**, *8*, 7160–7172. [CrossRef]
149. Azer, S.A. Challenges Facing the Detection of Colonic Polyps: What Can Deep Learning Do? *Medicina* **2019**, *55*, 473. [CrossRef]
150. Hamm, C.A.; Wang, C.J.; Savic, L.J.; Ferrante, M.; Schobert, I.; Schlachter, T.; Lin, M.; Duncan, J.S.; Weinreb, J.C.; Chapiro, J.; et al. Deep learning for liver tumor diagnosis part I: Development of a convolutional neural network classifier for multi-phasic MRI. *Eur. Radiol.* **2019**, *29*, 3338–3347. [CrossRef]

151. Yamakawa, M.; Shiina, T.; Nishida, N.; Kudo, M. Computer aided diagnosis system developed for ultrasound diagnosis of liver lesions using deep learning. In Proceedings of the 2019 IEEE International Ultrasonics Symposium (IUS), Glasgow, UK, 6–9 October 2019; pp. 2330–2333.
152. Kim, G.H.; Liang, P.S.; Bang, S.J.; Hwang, J.H. Screening and surveillance for gastric cancer in the United States: Is it needed? *Gastrointest. Endosc.* **2016**, *84*, 18–28. [CrossRef]
153. Lee, J.H.; Kim, Y.J.; Kim, Y.W.; Park, S.; Choi, Y.I.; Kim, Y.J.; Park, D.K.; Kim, K.G.; Chung, J.W. Spotting malignancies from gastric endoscopic images using deep learning. *Surg. Endosc.* **2019**, *33*, 3790–3797. [CrossRef]
154. Cho, B.J.; Bang, C.S.; Park, S.W.; Yang, Y.J.; Seo, S.I.; Lim, H.; Shin, W.G.; Hong, J.T.; Yoo, Y.T.; Hong, S.H.; et al. Automated classification of gastric neoplasms in endoscopic images using a convolutional neural network. *Endoscopy* **2019**, *51*, 1121–1129. [CrossRef] [PubMed]

Permissions

All chapters in this book were first published by MDPI; hereby published with permission under the Creative Commons Attribution License or equivalent. Every chapter published in this book has been scrutinized by our experts. Their significance has been extensively debated. The topics covered herein carry significant findings which will fuel the growth of the discipline. They may even be implemented as practical applications or may be referred to as a beginning point for another development.

The contributors of this book come from diverse backgrounds, making this book a truly international effort. This book will bring forth new frontiers with its revolutionizing research information and detailed analysis of the nascent developments around the world.

We would like to thank all the contributing authors for lending their expertise to make the book truly unique. They have played a crucial role in the development of this book. Without their invaluable contributions this book wouldn't have been possible. They have made vital efforts to compile up to date information on the varied aspects of this subject to make this book a valuable addition to the collection of many professionals and students.

This book was conceptualized with the vision of imparting up-to-date information and advanced data in this field. To ensure the same, a matchless editorial board was set up. Every individual on the board went through rigorous rounds of assessment to prove their worth. After which they invested a large part of their time researching and compiling the most relevant data for our readers.

The editorial board has been involved in producing this book since its inception. They have spent rigorous hours researching and exploring the diverse topics which have resulted in the successful publishing of this book. They have passed on their knowledge of decades through this book. To expedite this challenging task, the publisher supported the team at every step. A small team of assistant editors was also appointed to further simplify the editing procedure and attain best results for the readers.

Apart from the editorial board, the designing team has also invested a significant amount of their time in understanding the subject and creating the most relevant covers. They scrutinized every image to scout for the most suitable representation of the subject and create an appropriate cover for the book.

The publishing team has been an ardent support to the editorial, designing and production team. Their endless efforts to recruit the best for this project, has resulted in the accomplishment of this book. They are a veteran in the field of academics and their pool of knowledge is as vast as their experience in printing. Their expertise and guidance has proved useful at every step. Their uncompromising quality standards have made this book an exceptional effort. Their encouragement from time to time has been an inspiration for everyone.

The publisher and the editorial board hope that this book will prove to be a valuable piece of knowledge for researchers, students, practitioners and scholars across the globe.

List of Contributors

Xueping Chen, Jiangguo Lin, Yanru Ji, Ying Fang and Jianhua Wu
Institute of Biomechanics, School of Bioscience and Bioengineering, South China University of Technology, Guangzhou 510006, China

Yi Fu
Collaborative Innovation Center for Biomedicines & School of Medical Instruments, Shanghai University of Medicine & Health Sciences, Shanghai 200237, China

Parasuraman Padmanabhan and Satya P. Singh
Lee Kong Chian School of Medicine, Nanyang Technological University, Singapore 608232, Singapore
Cognitive Neuroimaging Centre, Nanyang Technological University, Singapore 636921, Singapore

Lipo Wang
School of Electrical and Electronic Engineering, Nanyang Technological University, Singapore 639798, Singapore

Sukrit Gupta and Haveesh Goli
School of Computer Science and Engineering, Nanyang Technological University, Singapore 639798, Singapore

Balázs Gulyás
Lee Kong Chian School of Medicine, Nanyang Technological University, Singapore 608232, Singapore
Cognitive Neuroimaging Centre, Nanyang Technological University, Singapore 636921, Singapore
Department of Clinical Neuroscience, Karolinska Institute, 17176 Stockholm, Sweden

Muhammad Waqas Nadeem
Faculty of Information and Communication Technology (FICT), Universiti Tunku Abdul Rahman (UTAR), Kampar 31900, Perak, Malaysia
Department of Computer Science, Lahore Garrison University, Lahore 54000, Pakistan

Hock Guan Goh and Vasaki a/p Ponnusamy
Faculty of Information and Communication Technology (FICT), Universiti Tunku Abdul Rahman (UTAR), Kampar 31900, Perak, Malaysia

Abid Ali and Muhammad Adnan Khan
Department of Computer Science, Lahore Garrison University, Lahore 54000, Pakistan

Muzammil Hussain
Department of Computer Science, School of Systems and Technology, University of Management and Technology, Lahore 54000, Pakistan

Ibrahem Kandel and Mauro Castelli
Nova Information Management School (NOVA IMS), Universidade Nova de Lisboa, Campus de Campolide, 1070-312 Lisboa, Portugal

Aleš Popovič
Nova Information Management School (NOVA IMS), Universidade Nova de Lisboa, Campus de Campolide, 1070-312 Lisboa, Portugal
School of Economics and Business, University of Ljubljana, Kardeljeva Ploščad 17, 1000 Ljubljana, Slovenia

Michelle Tang
Science, Math, and Computer Science Magnet Program, Montgomery Blair High School, Silver Spring, MD 20901, USA

Pulkit Kumar, Hao Chen and Abhinav Shrivastava
Institute for Advanced Computer Studies, University of Maryland College Park, College Park, MD 20742, USA

Yasuyo Urase, Yoshiko Ueno, Atsushi K. Kono, Keitaro Sofue, Tomonori Kanda, Takaki Maeda, Munenobu Nogami, Masatoshi Hori and Takamichi Murakami
Department of Radiology, Kobe University Graduate School of Medicine, 7-5-2 Kusunoki-cho, Chuo-ku, Kobe 650-0017, Japan

Mizuho Nishio
Department of Radiology, Kobe University Graduate School of Medicine, 7-5-2 Kusunoki-cho, Chuo-ku, Kobe 650-0017, Japan
Department of Diagnostic Imaging and Nuclear Medicine, Kyoto University Graduate School of Medicine, 54 Kawahara-cho, Shogoin, Sakyo-ku, Kyoto 606-8507, Japan

David La Barbera, Kevin Roitero and Vincenzo Della Mea
Department of Mathematics, Computer Science and Physics, University of Udine, 33100 Udine, Italy

António Polónia
Department of Pathology, Ipatimup Diagnostics, Institute of Molecular Pathology and Immunology, University of Porto, 4169-007 Porto, Portugal
i3S—Instituto de Investigação e Inovação em Saúde, Universidade do Porto, 4169-007 Porto, Portugal

Eduardo Conde-Sousa
i3S—Instituto de Investigação e Inovação em Saúde, Universidade do Porto, 4169-007 Porto, Portugal
INEB—Instituto de Engenharia Biomédica, Universidade do Porto, 4169-007 Porto, Portugal

Kehinde Aruleba, George Obaido and Blessing Ogbuokiri
School of Computer Science and Applied Mathematics, University of the Witwatersrand, Johannesburg 2001, South Africa

Adewale Oluwaseun Fadaka and Ashwil Klein
Department of Biotechnology, Faculty of Natural Sciences, University of the Western Cape, Private Bag X17, Bellville, Cape Town 7535, South Africa

Tayo Alex Adekiya
Department of Pharmacy and Pharmacology, School of Therapeutic Science, Faculty of Health Sciences, University of the Witwatersrand, Johannesburg, 7 York Road, Parktown 2193, South Africa

Raphael Taiwo Aruleba
Department of Molecular and Cell Biology, Faculty of Science, University of Cape Town, Cape Town 7701, South Africa

Albert Comelli
Ri.MED Foundation, 90133 Palermo, Italy

Francesco Martino, Gennaro Ilardi, Stefania Staibano and Daniela Russo
Department of Advanced Biomedical Sciences, University of Naples Federico II, 80131 Napoli, Italy

Domenico D. Bloisi
Department of Mathematics, Computer Science, and Economics, University of Basilicata, 85100 Potenza, Italy

Andrea Pennisi
Allianz Benelux, 1000 Brussels, Belgium

Mulham Fawakherji and Daniele Nardi
Department of Computer Science, Control, and Management Engineering, Sapienza University of Rome, 00185 Rome, Italy

Francesco Merolla
Department of Medicine and Health Sciences "V. Tiberio", University of Molise, 86100 Campobasso, Italy

Marcos A. M. Almeida
Departamento de Eletrônica e Sistemas, Centro de Tecnologia, Universidade Federal de Pernambuco, Recife-PE 50670-901, Brazil

Iury A. X. Santos
Departamento de Física, Universidade Federal Rural de Pernambuco, Recife-PE 52171-900, Brazil

Zemene Matewos Shewarega
Artificial Intelligence Center, 40782 Addis Ababa, Ethiopia

Taye Girma Debelee
Artificial Intelligence Center, 40782 Addis Ababa, Ethiopia
College of Electrical and Mechanical Engineering, Addis Ababa Science and Technology University, 120611 Addis Ababa, Ethiopia

Samuel Rahimeto Kebede
Artificial Intelligence Center, 40782 Addis Ababa, Ethiopia
Department of Electrical and Computer Engineering, Debreberhan University, 445 Debre Berhan, Ethiopia

Friedhelm Schwenker
Institute of Neural Information Processing, University of Ulm, 89081 Ulm, Germany

Index

www.ingramcontent.com/pod-product-compliance
Lightning Source LLC
Chambersburg PA
CBHW081545280726
48904CB00005B/323